Somatic Movement Dance Therapy

Somatic Movement Dance Therapy

The Healing Art of Self-regulation and Co-regulation

Amanda Williamson

intellect
Bristol, UK / Chicago, USA

First published in the UK in 2023 by
Intellect, The Mill, Parnall Road, Fishponds, Bristol, BS16 3JG, UK

First published in the USA in 2023 by
Intellect, The University of Chicago Press, 1427 E. 60th Street,
Chicago, IL 60637, USA

A catalogue record for this book is available from
the British Library.

Copy editor: MPS Limited
Cover designer: Tanya Montefusco
Cover image: Ella West and Jessica Cotton,
photographer Amanda Williamson
Production manager: Laura Christopher
Typesetter: MPS Limited

Print ISBN 978-1-78938-690-5
ePDF ISBN 978-1-78938-691-2
ePUB ISBN 978-1-78938-692-9

This is a peer-reviewed publication.

Dedicated to my undergraduate and postgraduate lecturers: Jayne Stevens, Jo Breslin, Michael Huxley, Ramsay Burt, Sarah Whatley, Mike Collier, Martha Eddy and Daniel Leven.

Thank you to my family and friends, Scott Closson, Tala Closson, Toby Closson, Lauren Closson, Rafferty Stewart, Emma Green and Karin Rugman. A special thank you to Laura Christopher and the typesetters at Intellect who kindly helped to organise this practice-based research book, and who have worked so hard bringing this book into being. A very special thanks to Natalie Austin, Natasha Martin, Celine Parsons, Sylvia Gregory, Heather-Larkin Jones, Vanessa Tucker, Miranda Henderson, Sara Pintch, Ella West, Jessica Cotton, Rebecca Sillence, Emma Thompson, Lizzy Le Quesne and Melanie Brierley.

Contents

Foreword: Transatlantic reflections

Sarah Whatley, Daniel Deslauriers, Celeste Snowber and Karin Rugman

Professor Sarah Whatley: Director: Centre for Dance Research (C-DaRE)

It is such a pleasure to read a book that is replete with the author's deep and unswerving commitment to researching an area with so much bodily and intellectual wisdom. What this expansive book manages to do is to provide insights to the depth and breadth of somatic movement, imbued with the author's earlier career as a gifted dance artist and since as someone who is now a leading authority in somatic movement practice and theory. The book provides a window into the author's decades of research, carried out through somatic investigations on her own body and importantly in partnership with many other movement practitioners. Her teachings have developed a pedagogy that is not only informed by a deep exploration of anatomical structures and functions but has revealed new insights to some of the more mysterious or less understood aspects of human movement.

Grounded in a deep commitment to ethical practice, the book is both complex and compelling. Whilst emanating from the author's movement research it is rooted in an extensive theoretical framework so even the more ineffable aspects of somatic movement, elucidated through references to spirit and soul, are amply substantiated through a detailed reading of the relationship between theory and experience. The book also references the work of many other somatic movement practitioners who have contributed so much to the growing discourse and understanding of somatic movement.

There are passages of quite complex theoretical explorations that are both lightened and deepened through passages of poetic writing and anatomical illustrations. The poetics are then illuminated further through descriptions of movement tasks and sequences, accompanied by movement images. What is so clearly expressed is a knowledge accumulated over many years of focused research and a curiosity that has enabled her to reach out to, and integrate, a wide range of philosophical and pedagogical perspectives. These are expertly woven through the chapters to argue for a theory of somatic movement that will contribute to fields as diverse as health, theology, philosophy whilst contributing a persuasive reminder of the healing potential of the body–mind connection. But the author goes further to acknowledge that many will experience something more than body (and) mind, which she describes as bodymind, or body-mind-spirit-soul. As the author unfolds, this is not to privilege some kind of mysticism but rather to give space for recognizing the experience of moving that exceeds physiological explanation, precisely because it lies in the individual's experience in a sensorial world of moving, breathing and stillness.

A core aspect of the author's thesis is that of self-regulation. Self-regulation is set out as an underpinning principle and serves the detailed explorations of perception, feeling, touch, movement improvisation and much more. Each chapter takes the reader through a focus on different aspects of self-regulation in relation to the body, including the nervous system and skeletal system, connective tissue and the 'fluid body', and in particular provides a new reading of the mechanics and function of fascia as a 'deeply intelligent integrative part of your being' (in Chapter 7). Each chapter concludes with 'key offerings and learnings' that beautifully summarize the main points, building one upon the other to provide the reader with a clear reference point for movement investigations. Taken as a whole, these insightful explorations show how a rigorous somatic movement practice sheds new light on anatomical and physiological systems of the body.

Professor Celeste Snowber: Simon Fraser University, Canada

This is a book that truly invites the reader into 'listening to the living tissues', which Williamson not only says, but models in a myriad of ways. *Somatic Movement Dance Therapy: The Healing Art of Self-regulation and Co-regulation* is a comprehensive text that provides a pathway for the reader to comprehend not only somatic movement practice and physiology, but integrates embodied knowledge within the soil of wisdom. Williamson is a master teacher and opens up a deeply pedagogical space for understanding on multiple levels, with the sensitivity of an open heart and a poetic eye. This book will companion me for many years and in the act of reading alone, my sensory nerve endings are awakened.

What is unique about this book is the beautiful way the practitioner, scholar, dancer, educator are woven in so seamlessly between the words, calling the reader into an intimate relationship with somatic knowing. I marvel at the breadth and depth in which this is written; also allowing for the legacy of those who have gone before and bringing the reader into so much more. This more is characterized by a portal to awe; an undertone of reverence of and for the body, fostering a deep humanness and humility. Nothing less than brilliant is found within these pages, which can serve as a mentor for so many fields. I can see how chiropractors, dancers, somatic therapists, doctors, philosophers, educators, body workers, musicians, therapists and all those who want to nurture the body, mind and soul will find this a magnificent resource.

I enter the fluidity of writing which brings me into the connectivity to my bones but also to all the facets which allow for health and consciousness in the cells. Anatomic complexity is present within, but there is also the sense of wonder of being created as whole human beings, where health can be recovered within sensing, feeling and experiencing the subtle fascia. I see this book as the connective tissue which gives the tools to repattern our bodies to wholeness. The expertise of Dr Williamson as an astute somatics scholar, working within a practice-based framework, opens us to heart-centred somatic work.

Amanda brings compassion to this journey of being bodily beings and shifts our relationship with both gravity and levity. In reading her words I am invited to slow down and sense the inner workings of my body and am inspired to continue on a journey of integrating mind, body and soul. She invites us into what she calls the sensory-moving-imaginal, leaving nothing left out, so everything available to us as humans is called upon to bring integration and wholeness. This book is not only informative but also revelatory and a sacred space to revel in the body. I am reminded that the word for sacrum is derived from sacred, meaning 'sacred bone'. This book welcomes somatic practices as the spine of who we are as humans, yet intricately connected to a sense of awe. Just as the vagus nerve runs throughout the body, this book is truly a companion to open up the miraculous bodies we are.

Professor Daniel Deslauriers: California Institute of Integral Studies: Transformative Studies

In trying to locate the sources of delight when reading Amanda's work, I first go to the pleasure of stimulation, in the right dosage. The large new scientific information about the dynamic of trauma and release, and their relationship to the nature, properties and functions of the fascia for example is a joy to discover. I am grateful for Amanda's masterful integration of knowledge, sharing her long personal somatic research in the nature of the self-regulation and co-regulation of our nervous system. This book is a compilation of her life's work as a somatic and movement practitioner and teacher. Having followed her work in print and in videos, here I am further invited to enter a dance between objective, scientific, anatomical knowledge and the subjective, lived, messy world of first-person [re]-embodiment and healing.

The second source of pleasure is in finding readily application of the concepts she shares. Seeing my partner stressed, I am in a better place to engage in a practice of co-regulation with them, seeing the immediate and contagious effect. Her work is generous and shared with care, tenderness and sensitivity. Movement scores and step-by-step protocols are accompanied by photos. Enter the gentleness of a refined phenomenology of enteroception.

The third source is in learning new materials, dwelling in new territory and delicious terms such as *thixotropy*, describing the ability of the fascia to fluctuate between its viscous and fluid states. Amanda recasts the very nature of the healing movement in scientific terms that opens the door for the enteroception of our watery and viscous body. It is not easy to translate the healing potential of movements into words, yet Amanda's prose invites us deeper into new realms of perception.

Another source of enjoyment is more intersubjective. In Amanda's world, in a parasympathetic state of softening, it is easier to genuinely connect to others. The primary aim of the book may be for self-study, yet it provides somatic practitioners deep insights on how to be with those who come to see them. Touch is recast, revealing its core aspects: attunement, receptivity, openness and support. Amanda illustrates this in detail. Once grounded in stronger interconnectivity, imagination, sensuality, social engagement is potentiated.

Amanda warns us that some chapters are not for the faint-hearted, because she pays close attention to the minutiae that underlie somatic movement. Our reward is a wider understanding of useful common practices such as work with gravity, releasing the pelvis and cranium through floor work, or unwinding and liquifying tissues. As a Contact Improvisation practitioner, I find her reference to that form enlivening. I like Contact Improvisation because it is 'stressful', it is challenging physically, emotionally, socially and creatively. It is on the 'good' side of stress, in the hormetic range. Sympathetic challenges can be overwhelming but in that beneficial range of hormesis, it can be rejuvenating. Amanda emphasizes parasympathetic release as the core practice, in our overstimulated and trauma-inducing world. This has helped me see the larger dynamics at play in the autonomic nervous system, and I leave with a far better understanding of Contact Improvisation through her work. That is a gift!

Karin Rugman: Bath Spa University, Chair of The Association for Somatic Movement Dance Therapies, United Kingdom and The Republic of Ireland

The field of somatic movement practice/therapy has grown immensely over the years, each new practice highlighting different components that emphasize the complex nature of what it means to be human. Learning how to listen to ourselves and attune to each other, to attend to our movement patterning, to notice and actively engage with our responses may seem obvious things but are skills that are keenly swallowed up by the fast and furious pace of life today. Being out of touch with ourselves is a sure sign of disease, which can be a fast-track ticket toward ill health. Amanda's work takes us back to the basics of self-regulation and co-regulation, one of the defining features of her work. The wisdom of the fundamental nature of the body that has the inbuilt mechanisms to keep us healthy and well are the focus of this book.

This book brings together the many layers of somatic practice in one beautifully crafted text. Amanda's vast experience as a somatic educator and facilitator, researcher and writer, illuminates the pages, bringing clarity and understanding to the forefront. As she excavates the different aspects of working somatically and uncovers and explains the knowledge of both the underlying science and somatic processes, Amanda draws on the innate wisdom of this practice and substantiates its significance in our world today.

Amanda's research interweaves and knits together different areas of information that together reveal a vast body of knowledge and understanding of the somatic process. Her writing explains the science behind the work, offering a systematic approach that validates the movement processes being described, whilst also acknowledging and highlighting the emotional, spiritual and social nature of being in touch with our body in this way. The care and attention to detail in this text enable the reader to gain a clear insight into the somatic processes being discussed, making it accessible and doable. The text moves from scientific understanding, to practical description, to personal narratives of practice, revealing the in-depth nature of what can be seen as a simple movement practice. Amanda uncovers this depth by reflecting on some of the key practices that have been established over the years, as well as sharing insights into her own pioneering practice, each playing their part in unfolding the multi-layered aspects of somatic inquiry, whilst examining the wonderful intelligence of the body.

The extensive nature of this book in its ability to draw vital elements of the practice of somatic movement therapy/education together in a detailed and comprehensive way provides an important and fundamental text for anyone working in this field, not only for academics in higher education or in the private domain but also for those who might be interested in understanding the incredible capabilities of our own body to self-regulate and manage pain and stress.

Introduction: The Seabed, Waves and Ripples in this Book

The focus of this book rests on my approach to practice, and key influences from the broader paradigm of applied somatics to dance and movement. I call my practice, somatic movement dance therapy, an approach that is largely improvisational, expressive, underpinned by somatic awareness, and rooted in self-regulation and co-regulation. The scholarship in this book will be of specific interest to those who are working as somatic movement educators and therapists, those who are thinking of training in this field, or students who have already embarked on this profession. Much of this book attends to the unique and subtle embodied skills that somatic movement dance therapists apply and empirically investigate in their tissues to enhance the efficiency of their artistic and therapeutic practice. Additionally, the book attends to processes and approaches that are emblematic of much international practice, such as the keen focus on soft-tissue-rolling in gravity for long periods of time, breath awareness, presence and non-duality. Within this book, I share my approach to therapeutic practice, which has grown through extensive studio-based research working with the public and training students to work in this profession. The research in this book reveals the importance of gravity, self-regulation, co-regulation, parasympathetic states of consciousness, the health of the vagus nerve, social engagement, the motility of the cranial-bones, soft-tissue-rolling in gravity, and somatic touch and myofascial unwinding. These elements are the seabed of, and waves of embodied knowing flowing throughout the book.

While the keen focus of this book is on the practice of somatic movement dance therapy, the research in this book will be of relevance to those working in somatic movement within performance contexts in higher education, and in the independent dance sector. Somatic movement education and therapy shares many intersecting herstories and histories with the enormous growth of dance underpinned by somatic awareness in higher education and performance contexts. There has always been an exchange between training programmes that qualify people to practice, and how dance is taught within university contexts, when underpinned by somatic awareness. Equally, there has always been a rich dialogue between therapeutic somatic movement modalities and performance underpinned by somatic awareness. Martha Eddy's book, *Mindful Movement: The Evolution of the Somatic Arts and Conscious Action* (2017) traces many of these intersecting histories, demonstrating a fine relationship and cross-pollination between dance and somatics in academia and the growth of applied somatics to dance in the independent sector. This fine exchange and creative dialogue can be witnessed with rigor and verve in the *Journal of Dance and Somatic Practices* (2009–present). Thus, a performer, choreographer or release-based dancer reading this text will easily resonate with the embodied training skills and somatic movement dance processes I offer. For example, in this book, I attend to myofascial unwinding and relational touch, soft-tissue-rolling in gravity, movement integration, presence and altered states of embodied consciousness. All these elements can be witnessed in the world of applied somatics to dance studies in higher education in manifold ways.

In saying this, I note early, the scope of this book does not explicitly extend its inquiry to the rich landscape of somatic awareness and dance techniques, or somatic awareness applied to choreography and performance. The scholarship in this text is firmly focused on somatic movement dance therapy, a moving-bodywork modality that intersects with many other progressive bodywork modalities in the current milieu, such as craniosacral therapy, cranio-osteopathy and massage therapies. I further note, I have extended the reach of this text to readers who know very little about this field. When outsiders witness somatic movement dance therapy in the studio, they often find it extremely hard to situate what they are seeing within their more familiar frame of reference – the mechanistic paradigm. Misunderstandings and assumptions abound largely because somatic movement/dance practitioners offer work that looks so very different to masculinist mechanistic approaches to health and movement. As such, much of this text unpicks and unearths why somatic movement dance therapists offer so much work in gravity, why they attend to tiny anatomical details, and why their work looks so very different.

I also note, this is not a book full of fancy high flying philosophical or socio-cultural theory. Much of my previous research has offered extensive research into spirituality, phenomenology and socio-cultural theory (2009, 2010, 2014a, 2014b, 2014d, 2015a, 2015b, 2018, 2020e, 2020f). We have plenty of academics and Ph.D. students taking such interesting paths, offering exquisite theoretical and philosophical adventures in the field. In many ways, this book goes right back to basics, to the art of therapeutic practice in the studio. What is it really like to be in the studio and offer somatic movement dance therapy sessions? What does this therapy look like? Why does it look so completely different to mechanistic movement? What anatomical and physiological theories underpin practice? What do we experientially sense and empirically investigate in the studio? What skills do we need to support another person's healing process? What skills do we need to support our own healing? What do I mean by healing in the first place? How do we deal with pain and sensory-motor amnesia? How long do sessions last? Why is the work different from talking therapies? What is unique to our field? How are spirituality and physiology intertwined in practice? This book attends to all these questions, supported by photographic images that demonstrate the application of theory into practice and offer the reader who is more familiar with mechanistic movement the novel opportunity to observe students self-regulating their own health through autogentic self-regulatory improvisation, while soft-tissue-rolling their fascia in gravity, or exploring their vagus nerve, for example.

I propose that applied somatics to dance and movement is one of the most difficult areas to facilitate, lecture and research in. It is a challenging and often painful field to work in. Difficulties and challenges exist in university contexts and in the independent sector. The challenges and struggles are manifold, but it is particularly the tenacity of the mechanistic paradigm that makes it extremely hard for practitioners to share the integrity of their work, its effectiveness in helping people to feel better and its importance in history, culture and society. Western culture continues to propagate disembodied work-out regimes, based on sympathetically aroused cardiovascular fitness, such as pumping-it-up at the gym, or sweating-it-out through aerobics or hot yoga. Our globalized westernized world repeatedly offers the general populous physical health programmes that treat the body as a machine that needs to be mastered, dominated and controlled by mind.

All types of approaches to health and fitness have value. I, for example, love long distance running. My point above is not to discard mechanistic fitness, but rather to be open-minded enough to witness and accept there are other approaches to health and movement circulating among the general populous and within academic contexts that approach the body differently – one being, somatic movement dance therapy. Somatic movement practitioners, whether working in performance, higher education, or in the independent sector, often face the overwhelming difficult task of explaining their work within the condescension of the mechanistic paradigm. When they do, they are often met with responses such as, 'I just don't get it' – 'that's too far out for me' – or 'that's a bit, well you know, hippie or spiritual'. Somatic movement dance practitioners face the very real situation that the body has been, and is still, overwhelmingly perceived as a machine – or a mere container, vessel, or carrier of spirit. An additional problem is evident to me, which is the inter-related pervasiveness of the positivist paradigm. I often hear the following types of comments: 'That work just looks too weird and out-there', and 'sorry I don't believe in anything spiritual; I am a scientist.' Even after decades of exquisite, elegant and superb somatic movement scholarship, I note, somatic movement dance practitioners are still up against it. Something heavy hangs over us, especially when working in patriarchal institutions, that is hard, angular, armoured, sympathetically charged, and often arrogant.

Confusion and condescension occur most obviously because somatic movement is not based on angles, levers, lines, exterior-shape, sympathetically aroused cardio, weight-baring, flexibility and strengthening. In truth, somatic movement practice does attend to all these elements of health, but they are approached very differently. The work looks so markedly different from all other physical fitness programmes, and I add even yoga, it can be extremely upfronting for people who are used to sympathetically aroused activity, using their body as a pully and lever system, and dominating their body with a positive mind-set. Most obviously to me, but certainly not the only reason, somatic movement dance augments movement that is spirilloid, curvaceous, calm, gentle, non-linear and non-directional. In fact, the spiral and water are emblematic of the somatic movement paradigm, if not the most noticeable *moving symbols* (Williamson 2015a, 2020). More than this, we invite participants to attune to their sensory-motor feedback loop. In short, our work is about sensing, feeling, perceiving and moving consciously, after years, sometimes decades, of dissociation from heart, breath and the sensate. Because breath awareness underpins all somatic movement/dance practices, the healing power of presence also underpins practice. The experiential study of presence is central to somatic movement and dance. This is an alleviating state of consciousness, where the worries from the past can no longer hold you in shame or anger, and where the future cannot riddle your tissues with anxiety and fear – perhaps momentarily – or longer if an experienced somatic movement/dance meditator.

I cannot speak to all the difficulties and problems academics and students face, but I can speak to a few. Many of these difficulties have inspired and shaped this book. The hegemony of the mechanistic paradigm is extremely painful. Don Hanlon Johnson's life's work is extremely focal about this issue and hence his work often supports students and staff in voicing the value of somatic movement and its emergence within shifting socio-cultural values. The relentless one-dimensional world-view proliferated by the mechanistic paradigm is one of the most difficult issues facilitators and academics face when they try to explain their work to the public, or with academics from other disciplines, particularly those disciplines rooted in positivism and mechanistic health. In my experience, somatic movement dance is often misunderstood, sometimes perceived as weird, and at worst, referred to as a soft science.

When I survey the field with my travelled body and keen eye, I would posit that somatic movement dance is rooted in parasympathetic release, ease, fluency, movement integration and non-duality. This lies in stark contrast to perfunctory movement focused on robotic angular movement, cardio-vascular fitness, sympathetic arousal, muscular strength and body–mind dualism. Rather than instruct someone to follow a set of prescriptive exercises, we often use improvisation underpinned by somatic awareness to invite the participant into a state of health.

In such processes, the participant is not following robotic exercises but rather is attuned to their sensory-perceptual movement awareness, self-regulatory intelligence, and I add, often their embodied imaginal awareness. For outsiders, it must look odd to witness participants lying in gravity, with eyes shut for over 30 minutes, listening to afferent sensations, resting their awareness in breath, slowing down, inhibiting their habitual motor response, and consciously choosing efferent pathways of ease and release. It must look strange to witness people releasing their jaws, softening in their face, sounding and toning, and following improvisational tails of instinct or transcendence.

Anything that looks different from mainstream dominant cultural values is often met with mockery, sheer rudeness, fear, arrogance and ignorance. Such rudeness often upsets students studying somatic movement and dance because they feel their work is under-valued and will never be taken seriously. Nonetheless, the effectiveness and exquisite holistic nature of their work usually keep them going, against extremely hard odds. Anyone studying somatic movement/dance or holding the presence of this subject in a university context are extremely courageous, often facing the difficulties and challenges described above.

The field of the somatic movement grew in response to mainstream cultural values that treat the body like a machine. In the somatic movement dance paradigm, the body is not treated like an object that needs to be pumped-up, measured, armoured, strengthened, admired through feats of flexibility, agility and strength, and shaped to look great and sexually desirable. Worth writing, but it is likely most readers are extremely familiar with this type of statement, the field of somatic movement dance does not view the body as an object, or a hard-wired machine that needs to be mastered and conquered by a positive mind-set. In contrast, we approach the body very reverently, sensitively, with gentleness and care, knowing that the body, along with the wider biosphere has taken millions of years to evolve; that our living tissues possess an intelligence that transcends, or is far vaster, than mechanical descriptions of the human body found in western anatomy. Our life and the many aspects of our being are seeded, grown, animated and maintained by living breathing tissues. In short, body and mind are one, inextricably linked. However, through the tenacious, and I would add, divisive, socio-cultural enculturation of 'mind' as superior to body, mind and body have been instrumentally divided – these two aspects of our being are often alone, lonely and estranged. Mind and body often feel qualitatively different from one another, like two entities somehow related, but in the most maladaptive, antagonistic, dissociative relationship. In contrast, somatic movement and dance invites mind to rest, soften its gaze within, and rest in gentle waves of breath. The paradigm as a whole seeks to heal body–mind dualism, and its painful dissociative outcome.

It is such a huge celebration that you can now study somatic movement and dance to MA and Ph.D. level within universities. We also have a wonderful array of highly acclaimed and beautifully researched books that are used world-wide, both in university dance departments, and by independent practitioners. The list would be too long to share them all. Below, I share several books that are frequently used in university contexts, bringing inspiration and indeed solace to academics facilitating such sensitive work, which at times, can be lonely and isolating. In terms of experiential anatomy, I always think of Bonnie Bainbridge Cohen's book, *Sensing, Feeling, and Action: The Experiential Anatomy of Body–Mind Centering* (1993), because her work lucidly explains sensing-perceptual movement awareness and embodied action. I further think of Andrea Olsen and Caryn Mchose's extremely detailed books, *Body and Earth: An Experiential Guide* (Olsen 2002), *Bodystories: A Guide to Experiential Anatomy* (Olsen and McHose 1998), and *How Life Moves: Explorations in Meaning and Body Awareness* (McHose and Frank 2006). Books by early pioneers such as Thomas Hanna, *Somatics: Reawakening the Mind's Control of Movement, Flexibility, and Health* (1980), *The Body of Life: Creating New Pathways for Sensory Awareness and Fluid Movement* (1979), and Frederick Matthias Alexander's, *The Use of the Self* (1942), continue to inspire and support academics and students. I note, I was extremely struck in my career by Peggy Hackney's comprehensive and carefully detailed book, *Making Connections: Total Body Integration through Bartenieff Fundamentals* (2002), as well as Linda Hartley's book, *Wisdom of the Body Moving: An Introduction to Body–Mind Centering* (1995). In terms of philosophy and cultural theory, Don Hanlon Johnson's books have provided a bedrock of academic activism for practitioners to progress their work academically. *Bone, Breath and Gesture: Practices of Embodiment Volume 1* (1995), *Groundworks: Narratives of Embodiment: Narratives of Embodiment Volume II* (1997), and *Body: Recovering Our Sensual Wisdom* (1992), have most certainly progressed the field of somatic movement and dance in university contexts. More recently I think of a number of extremely useful books such as, *Attending to Movement: Somatic Perspectives on Living in this World* (Whatley et al. 2015), *Dance, Somatics and Spiritualities* (Williamson et al. 2014), *Mindful Movement: The Evolution* of *the Somatic Arts and Conscious Action* (Eddy 2017), *Moving Consciously: Somatic Transformations through Dance, Yoga, and Touch* (Fraleigh et al. 2015), *Back to the Dance Itself: Phenomenologies of the Body in Performance* (2018), and *Body and Mind in Motion: Dance and Neuroscience in Conversation* (Batson 2014). Some of these later books bring many pioneers together in one volume, offering multiple perspectives on the field, and how it has been applied or grown through the exquisite and breath-full skills of dancer-academics.

There has also been a significant growth of somatic movement/dance training programmes world-wide, approved by *The International Somatic Movement*

Education and Therapy Association (ISMETA). The listing of programmes below is rather too long, but I share most of them below because they tell us something about the nature of this expanding paradigm. The programmes are: Alexander Technique Center at Cambridge, Bergin Learning Arts School of Expressive Arts, Center for BodyMindMovement, Dynamic Embodiment Eastwest Somatics Institute, Embodied Flow, EMOVE Institute, Esprit en Mouvement, Essential Somatics, EUROLAB Certificate Programs in Laban/Bartenieff Movement Studies, Institute for Integrative Bodywork and Movement Therapy, Integrated Movement Studies, Laban Bartenieff Institute of Movement Studies (LIMS®), Laban/ Bartenieff & Somatic Studies International™, Leven Institute for Expressive Movement, LLC, Mind in Motion, MA Dance & Somatic Well-Being: Connections to the Living Body, Movement Intelligence, Moving Within LLC, Rolf Movement® Training Program, Somatic Body Training, Somatic Movement Arts, Somatic Wisdom, Somatische Akademie Berlin, Sonder Movement Project, Spatial Dynamics Institute, Inc., Spiral Praxis, Tamalpa Institute, The Brook Institute: Engaged Somatics, and The School of the Topf Technique, Voice Movement Integration (VMI) Somatic Practice. (www.ISMETA.org.)

ISMETA have nurtured the field over decades and approve a large number of brilliant and artful training programmes. In 2021, I founded The Association for Somatic Movement & Dance Therapies, United Kingdom & The Republic of Ireland. The association recognizes there are many somatic movement/dance educators and therapists offering one-on-one sessions, and group work, increasingly lensed and taught through the innovative egis of free movement and dance, underpinned by somatic and imaginal awareness. This is a growing area of creative practice, and the tables 1.1 and 1.2 below, outline the association's scope and categories of practice.

We have a fantastic range of training programmes world-wide and a selection of elegant and erudite books that are found on module descriptors in dance departments across the UK, Europe, the United States, New Zealand, Australia and in many other countries. Additionally, in nearly every dance department you may find a module on somatic movement/dance, or an academic who specializes in somatic movement research, and increasingly MA and Ph.D. programmes that enable students to study this field to the highest level. Keeping this mind, the hegemony of mechanistic movement and the obstinacy of positivism still make it very difficult for researchers and students to 'come out' and say, this is what I do, this is what I want to research, and this is why it is important.

There have been many times in my career when people have laughed or mocked studio practice, especially after witnessing participants soft-tissue-rolling across the floor in fluent, smooth, curvaceous and spirilloid ways. This work certainly looks unusual to the outsider. Further, because participants are rolling across the floor in a relaxed parasympathetic state of consciousness, especially after

TABLE I.1: Scope and categories of practice: somatic movement and dance therapies, United Kingdom and The Republic of Ireland.

Sensory-perceptual motor expression	Resting, releasing, easing and softening	Hands-on, touch and bodywork
• Facilitate awareness of the sensory-motor feedback loop (through sensing, feeling, perceiving and moving consciously). • Support the development of sensory-perceptual movement awareness. • Explore interoception, proprioception, gravi-ception and kinaesthetic intelligence. • Explore interoceptive awareness, reducing exteroceptive overwhelm, in order to ease the nervous system. • Explore experiential anatomy and physiology, uniquely blending objective knowledge with subjective experience (first-person sensory-perceptual experience of the living body). • Facilitate a balance between resting (afferent sensing) and action (efferent motor expression).	• Release and ease the myofascial tissues; supporting the reduction of sympathetic arousal, inviting parasympathetic release, softening tissue tonus and releasing emotional holding. • Creatively explore the fluid nature of the human organism, supporting the free flow of fluids through tissues. • Support breath awareness and cardio-ception (heart-sensing), inviting the vagus nerve into a state of health. • Release restrictions, tension and stress in living tissues, via inviting free-flowing movement patterns, as well as applied touch and bodywork. • Support the fascia into a state of health, exploring bio-tensegrity. • Use gravity as a fulcrum to reorganise myofascial pain.	• Teach anatomy and physiology through subjective experience and objective knowledge. • Reconnect participants to their sensory-motor feedback loop. • Enhance afferent sensing and conscious efferent motor expression. • Bring awareness to living tissues and body systems that are often beneath consciousness. • Support skeletal-muscular alignment. • Balance asymmetries, releasing stress and strain, and supporting easeful posture. • Support anatomical differentiation and movement integration. • Support fascial release. • Release habituated patterns of neuromuscular holding and support movement fluidity. • Enhance moment-by-moment breath awareness and cardio-ception, reducing sympathetic arousal, and integrating mind and body. • Calm and balance the nervous system (reduce sympathetic arousal and support parasympathetic ease). • Connect with Self, others, and the community group through the nonverbal language of touch, dance and movement. • Support expressivity, creativity and the imagination-in-movement. • Support imaginative sensory-perceptual movement pathways, inviting the embodied imagination to arise.

TABLE I.2: Scope and categories of practice: somatic movement and dance therapies, United Kingdom and The Republic of Ireland.

Movement and the imagination	**Movement fundamentals and development**	**Body-mind-spirit and soul and nature**
• Explore the relationship between sensation, emotion, image, symbol, impressions and the embodied imagination. • Explore the imagination-in-movement as the bridge to the soul: a unique process where unconscious contents can be integrated into symbolic form through imaginal expression. • Work in a dyad, exploring the witness/mover container. • Explore the transpersonal as a vital source of knowledge and connection. • Offer a non-judgemental environment and heart-centred co-regularly space.	• Explore ontogenetic and phylogenetic developmental movement patterns. • Explore somatic movement fundamentals such as: gravity, weight, mass, space, time, breath. • Explore different rhythms, qualities, directions, energies, forces and planes of action. • Explore the differentiation and integration of body parts. • Explore free-improvisation, supporting fascial fluidity, skeletal-muscular dexterity, spatial awareness and movement range. • Explore movement polarities: parasympathetic/sympathetic, inspiration/expiration, up/down, high/low, left/right, direct/non-directional, inhalation and exhalation etc. • Movement observation and analysis.	• Are rooted in self-regulation, co-regulation and transpersonal awareness. • Explore the experiential study of presence (being in the present moment). • Explore the integration of mind, body, spirit and through breath awareness and the imagination. • Explore the joy of movement and kinaesthetic intelligence. • Explore the intelligence of the living body, sensing source energy. • Explore consciousness, developed through sensory-perceptual movement awareness, breath awareness and subjectively and experientially investigating the body–mind relationship. • Explore somatic movement/dance meditations. • Explore body as nature, and our connection to a wider ecosystem. • Offer processes of reflection and integration after moving.

contacting breath and the craniosacral division, the work often looks trance-like – studio practice may look spiritual and sensuous to the outsider. There are in fact physiological reasons why somatic movement dance work looks trance-like and sensual. I address these reasons in Chapters 2, 3, 4 and 5. As an early pointer, when we innervate the caudal–cranial axis (head–tail) and deepen our relationship to breath we innervate some rather pleasurable parasympathetic nerves in the cranium and sacrum. Innervating the craniosacral division of the autonomic nervous system invites participants to shift from a sympathetically aroused state into a parasympathetic relaxed state (an experience of ease, restitution and deep peace). Such relaxed sensuous movement can easily be misconstrued as sexual or spiritual.

Somatic movement dance is deeply sensuous and, as I put forward in this book, such sensual movement is often augmented by a parasympathetic deeply relaxed state of consciousness. On a physiological level, sensuality authentically arises via the gentle nature of the parasympathetic nerves. Some parasympathetic nerves emerge from the sacral region at S2, S3 and S4. Sensing and perceiving the sacrum is often very relaxing and peaceful, especially when combined with initiating movement from the cranial bones – and playing consciously with the head–tail connection. There is an incredible opening to life-energy sense–perceived in the sacrum and pelvis, moving all the way to the cranium. A very deep contact with the life-force from the sacrum and pelvis is arising, both through the parasympathetic nerves, as well as through the craniosacral system (the free flow of cerebrospinal fluid within the dural tube that surrounds the brain and spinal cord). You will notice many photographic images in this book that capture this sensuous state. You might observe how these images and this type of movement could easily be misunderstood.

Sensuality in the field refers to all our senses – attuning to the sensation of breath, heart, interoception, proprioception, cardio-ception, gravi-ception, the somatosensory system and kinaesthesia (the sheer pleasure of moving consciously within gravity, through space and time, emersed in sense–perception and the imagination). For centuries, the body has been associated with sex and base activities, whereas mind and spirit have been elevated beyond impure activities. We can thank our socio-religious institutions for relegating the body and the sensate to the impure. The pleasure of being a body and exploring the remarkable ability we have to sense our living bodies is not something western culture and society has valued or cultivated. Pleasure in our culture is relegated to things we do after dark, or after work, or for entertainment. In contrast, feeling pleasure, ease and deep relaxation innervated by the parasympathetic lies at the heart of this book, and it is absolutely central to healing.

A parasympathetic state of consciousness is the big through-line of this book; I share the importance of parasympathetic release in nearly every chapter. This state is soft-hearted, easeful, pleasurable, relaxed, meditative, open and receptive. It is extremely interesting to note early that scientists have measured sympathetic and parasympathetic states and now know that deep relaxation does indeed create altered states of consciousness. Parasympathetic states created by deep relaxation techniques (and somatic movement is a deep relaxation technique), cause the brainwaves to slow from beta to alpha to theta. Thus, the parasympathetic has been measured and it appears deep relaxation techniques slow the brainwaves to alpha (8–13 cycles/s) and theta (4–8 cycles/s) (Dispenza 2012). Altered states of consciousness are a gift we possess but are often relegated to the esoteric, new age or simply considered wacked-out. I propose in this book that there is nothing more wonderful and kinder than sharing with people how to shift from a sympathetic stressed-out state to parasympathetic ease-and-release, where they can balance their nervous system, breathe, rest, let go, dream, reflect, feel pleasure and take solace from the harsh landscapes of the exterior world. A large part of the healing process in somatic movement/dance is altering one's embodied state of consciousness and enjoying the realms of alpha (a relaxed but alert state of being), or lucid dreaming in the imaginal landscapes of theta. Such processes release participants from the mundane and expand one's awareness beyond the ego and persona, and I add, beyond the socio-economic world that constricts our sensuality and confines us to a one-dimensional barren consciousness.

The soil and landscapes that grew me

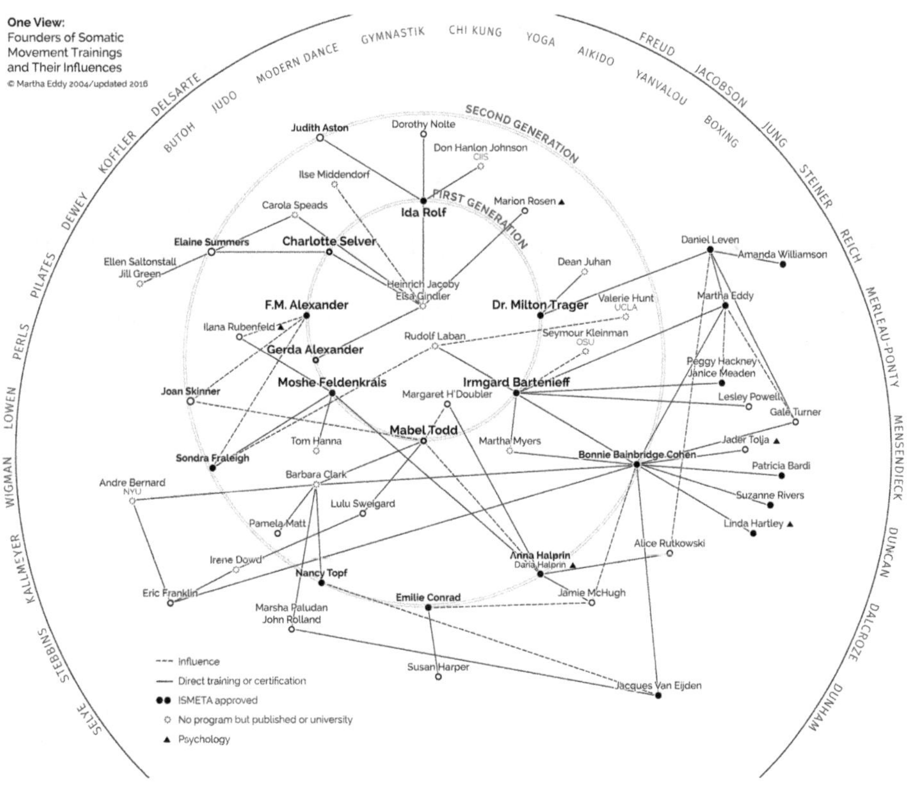

MAP 1: Map found in Eddy, M. (2017), *Mindful Movement: The Evolution* of *the Somatic Arts and Conscious Action*, Intellect: Bristol. Reprintable only with the permission of Dr Martha Eddy.

In Map 1, published by Martha Eddy in the first edition of *The Journal and Dance & Somatic Practices* in 2009, and again with slight modifications in her book, *Mindful Movement: The Evolution* of *the Somatic Arts and Conscious Action* in 2017, I am positioned as a third-generation pioneer in somatic movement education and therapy. From my standpoint, this means I have been heavily influenced by all my predecessors. In an age of fast, and not always accurate internet information, one of the issues I face as a Ph.D. supervisor is making sure younger generations of researchers fully appreciate the ground early pioneers ploughed, tilled, seeded and grew; and the emotional strength it took to offer a different world-view within the condescension of machine-like movement and positivist research. My own work is thus unthinkable without the decades of progressive scholarship established before me. My practice has been inspired by many pioneers. The first is Bonnie Bainbridge Cohen, who developed *Body–Mind Centering*. The impact of Cohen's work cannot be overstated or underestimated. Her highly specialized work in touch, the fluid systems and indeed explaining sensing, feeling and action influenced not just me, but a whole generation of dancer-academics. Equally, the progressive influence of Anna Halpin's and Daria Halprin's work cannot be overstated or underestimated. Their work developed the imaginal aspects of practice internationally, and particularly the link between emotion, sensation, feeling, the imagination and movement. These pioneers changed the landscape of somatic movement and dance, especially through the application of expressive free improvisation and multi-modal arts. Martha Eddy has deeply influenced my work, primarily through her numerous articles, that articulate the history of somatics, as well as some of the defining features of practice. Martha's work created an integral bridge between higher education contexts and independent contexts, and without her passion and concern for this field, this book would not exist.

Thomas Hanna has instrumentally inspired my work, not necessarily through the practices he developed, but rather through his books, *Somatics: Reawakening the Mind's Control of Movement, Flexibility, and Health* (1980), and *The Body of Life: Creating New Pathways for Sensory Awareness and Fluid Movement* (1979). Of all the people presented in Map 1, Don Hanlon Johnson's books gave me the most courage. His most common books are *Bone, Breath and Gesture: Practices of Embodiment Volume 1* (1995), and *Groundworks: Narratives of Embodiment: Narratives of Embodiment Volume II* (1997); and there are others that are incredibly special and healing to read such as, *The Body in Psychotherapy: Inquiries in Somatic Psychology* (1998), *Body Spirit & Democracy* (1994), *Everyday Hopes, Utopian Dreams: Reflections on American Ideals* (2006), *Diverse Bodies, Diverse Practices: Toward an Inclusive Somatics* (2018), and *The Meaning of Life in the 21st Century: Tensions Among Science, Religion, and Experience* (2008).

Johnson's first book, now out of print, *The Protean Body* (1977), is well worth reading. In terms of situating the progressive nature of somatic movement within the pervasiveness of the mechanistic paradigm, it is lucid.

I had the pleasure of being taught by Sarah Whatley, Jayne Stevens, Jo Breslin, Ramsay Burt and Mike Huxley during my undergraduate studies. This means I have been influenced by the paradigm of somatics as it grew not only in the United States, but in the United Kingdom. Eddy and Johnson's books tend to present a history of how somatic movement grew in the United States. While there has always been transatlantic exchange, the history and growth of somatic movement/dance in the UK has been rich, dexterous and creative too. I was lucky enough to study at both Coventry University and De Montford University in the early 1990s. Both universities have been instrumental movers in the growth and development of somatic movement in the United Kingdom – and with international reach. My undergraduate studies at De Montford university focused on the application of the Alexander Technique to dance and performance; thus, early in my career, I was introduced to F. M. Alexander's work and its application to dance studies. As a young person enculturated into thinking dance was about how you looked and if you could achieve the splits in the air, the application of the Alexander Technique was at first alien to me. Nonetheless, our training in depth experiential anatomy, *less is more, and releasing the head* and trusting *the labyrinth righten reflex* radically changed my perception of dance. Our bodies were stripped bare of any extra emotional expressivity, and in many ways, a phenomenological reduction was taking place. Assumptions and bias about dance were challenged and shed. We were taught to inhibit our habitual motor response and consciously direct our movement. At Coventry University, I was introduced to release-based techniques with an emphasis on softening and integrating the synovial, cartilaginous and fibrous joints, releasing over sympathetically charged tissues, and tipping, falling and spiralling into the healing power of gravity. At Coventry University, there was a lovely emphasis on softness, calmness and breath awareness.

At De Montford University we were taught in-depth anatomy, both objectively and subjectively. I am grateful for this in-depth training in applied experiential anatomy. This is perhaps my strongest influence.

Additionally, in my thirties, I undertook Daniel Leven's training programme in Massachusetts. It was during this period that my life began to radically change. I began to heal from decades of dissociation from my body, and many traumatic events in my life. I chose his programme because I was especially interested in the meditative aspects of somatic movement dance practice, and how they intersect with various forms of Buddhism. Daniel's work with meditation and heart-math particularly interested me and it was during his programme I began to understand how sense–perceiving your heart can radically alter your life. I also chose his programme because of his refined work in the application of Gestalt, the imaginal and multi-modal arts. Like many directors, his work was full of heart, breath, presence, slow-time and non-duality.

Throughout my twenties and thirties, I was leading BA (Hons) and MA programmes in Dance in the United Kingdom and latterly in the United States. Daniel Leven deeply inspired me and in my thirties I developed a university programme in somatic movement education and therapy in association with ISMETA, called MA Dance and Somatic Wellbeing: Connections to the Living Body, offered in England at UClan, and in New York at MBR.

While all the pioneers presented in the map above share common approaches, philosophical values and principles, their work looks quite different. Each pioneer developed a unique approach, specific processes and a particular language all of their own. The research presented in this book grows out of all the inspirations shared above, reaching right back to my undergraduate studies, especially the depth experiential anatomy I was lucky to learn at De Montford University. Over the years, I slowly developed a modality simply called *Somatic Dance Movement Therapy*. Much of this book explores what is shared and common across the field, but I also introduce some key areas that define my research and somatic movement dance modality. Before I differentiate what is shared and common, and what is unique to my work, let us note together that all somatic movement education and therapy programmes share the following broad scope of practice,

- focus on the body both as an objective physical process and as a subjective process of lived consciousness;
- refine perceptual, kinesthetic, proprioceptive and interoceptive sensitivity that supports homeostasis, co-regulation and neuroplasticity;
- recognize habitual patterns of perceptual, postural and movement interaction with the environment;
- improve movement coordination that supports structural, functional and expressive integration;
- experience an embodied sense of vitality and create both meaning for and enjoyment of life;
- somatic movement education and therapy are applied to both pedestrian and specialized activities for people in all stages of health and development. The work can be communicated either on an individual basis or with groups.

(www.ISMETA.org)

While all ISMETA programmes share the above scope of practice, each modality has a unique orientation; these programmes are not uniform in their approach. Further, some of these programmes use dance and expressive movement underpinned by somatic awareness, while others do not. The field is thus not a monolith. For example, a Feldenkrais session looks markedly different from Anna Halpin's modality, *Life-Art Process.* Bonnie Bainbridge Cohen's modality, *Body-Mind-Centering*, looks strikingly different from Emilie Conrad's modality, *Continuum.* Authentic Movement sessions look vastly different from Alexander Technique sessions. My key point being, there is a vast range of approaches to somatic movement and dance. While different programmes have a particular orientation, language and research trajectory, they usually enact the following elements:

- First-person perception of the living body.
- Attunement to the sensory-motor feedback loop.
- Breath awareness.
- The exploration of gravity and the biological imperative to be vertical.
- Connection to body, Other and community.
- Re-connecting the body with nature: understanding the body is nature.
- Ease, rest, fluency and release.
- Spirals, curves and non-linear movement.
- Sense–perception of motility (the free flow of fluid within the body).
- Movement re-patterning.
- Somatic touch.
- Experiential anatomy.

These elements also lie at the heart of my practice and research (for it would be very difficult to facilitate somatic movement without them). Because my background is in Dance Studies, like many second- and third-generation pioneers, improvisational dance underpinned by somatic awareness plays a large role in my work, which is evident in the forthcoming chapters. Thus, in 2009, I started to publish the extended term 'Somatic Movement Dance Education and Therapy' to acknowledge dance improvisation, and how the embodied knowledge of dancers was instrumentally shaping the field (2009). In this book, I use terms such as somatic movement dance practice, or somatic movement dance therapy – for improvisation and expressive dance underpinned by somatic awareness is a tour de force across many training programmes. Somatic movement pioneers that are dancers have expanded the field beyond the functional, notably developing *the-imagination-in-movement* as a catalyst for healing, where unconscious contents are integrated into consciousness through symbolic moving play. This approach, rooted in the healing power of expressive dance, the imagination, and improvisation, integrates body, mind, spirit and soul, inviting participants into the transpersonal, numinous and spiritual elements of practice. Dividing the human up into the aforementioned categories only causes more fragmentation. Of early note, I use words such as spirit and soul, in this book, to point to experiences and expressions of our humanness, that tend to be suppressed within the dominance of our secular technocratic globalized culture. Below I share some key elements that define my research, and programme called *somatic movement dance therapy*. These elements developed out of practice-as-research, especially working with the public, with groups, and in one-on-one sessions. These areas are explored and exampled in-depth across this book.

Self-regulatory movement: the ability to attune to your sensory-motor loop, and follow ease-full improvisational motor pathways, tracking sensation, with breath awareness. Following improvisational pathways of ease and release, resting and sense–dwelling in afferent sensation.

Co-regulation: the importance of being witnessed by a heart-centered embodied witness who has regulated their heart field.

Autogenic self-regulatory movement: the ability of the participant to shift their autonomic nervous system from sympathetic arousal to parasympathetic release.

Experiential anatomy and physiology: sense–perceiving and moving with awareness of tiny tissues and micro anatomical and physiological knowledge.

Fulcrum support and soft tissue reorganization: using gravity and the floor as a fulcrum to pivot, push, tip, roll, yield, release, soften, melt, enliven and change the viscosity of living fascial tissues.

The vagus nerve: understanding the physiological pathway, importance and role of the vagus nerve in practice, objectivity and subjectively.

Spirituality and the parasympathetic: exploring the roll the parasympathetic nervous system plays in self-regulation, co-regulation and transpersonal states of awareness.

Moment-by-moment breath awareness: exploring the healing power of presence.

The moving imaginal: trusting in the imagination as a teleological guide and preparing the receptive ground for the imagination to emerge.

Co-regulatory touch and somatic unwinding: the electricity of touch and the heart field.

The healing power of gravity: gravity is explored and offered as the very best fulcrum we have to reorganize our living tissues throughout this book and within my practice.

The healing power of gravity is a central theme in this book and can be observed in every chapter. Outsiders or people new to practice (before they experience the modality) often ask, 'why do you spend so much time lying and moving in gravity?' I propose gravity is the most powerful healer and the best fulcrum we have to reorganize our living tissues into a state of health. Among the many other details and processes I share in the forthcoming chapters, gravity is key to health because:

- When we lie and move in gravity the cardio-vascular system does not have to work so hard, and thus your heart rate and breathing regulates. Thus, gravitational play supports participants to move into parasympathetic ease because reducing the heart rate and regulating breathing is a key process that innervates the parasympathetic division of the autonomic nervous system.
- Gravitational play releases the weight of head (the heaviest part of the body) and thus reduces the load placed on the cervical, thoracic, lumbar and sacral spine.
- Lying and moving in gravity reduces the load placed on every synovial, cartilaginous and fibrous joint in the human body. Thus, gravitational play supports joint health.
- Gravitational sensing invites the inter-vertebral disks to rest and replenish. During the day these disks lose water, but when we lie down and rest for long periods of time, these disks may replenish.
- Through gravitational play, we can change the viscosity of fascia, releasing pain, resolving trigger points and healing adhesions in the fascial matrix.

In this book, I share the above aspects of my practice in detail, with a particular focus on autogenic self-regulatory movement and the importance of parasympathetic release. These distinctive areas are opened out into dialogue through theory and practice in the forthcoming chapters. Therefore, within this book, you will notice what is common and shared, but also processes distinctive to my work. Here we find a good example of how practitioners always build their work on the embodied knowledge of those who have gone before them. Additionally, I have been highly influenced by cranio-osteopathy and craniosacral therapy, building on Bonnie Bainbridge Cohen (1993), Ida Rolf (1977) and Don Halon Johnson's (1977) practice-based research trails into the common ground we share with other vitalistic therapies. You will notice this influence throughout this book.

The word healing appears frequently in this book. By healing, I do not mean esoteric healing through the hands, or the miraculous recovery from disease or that therapists can heal illness. By the word healing, I mean small shifts in one's psyche that happen during and/or after moving and sensing, however incremental. Incremental changes in one's sense of Self that help people to feel better, or support people to feel a little more whole are healing. Just connecting with breath can feel healing, or suddenly feeling the presence of the heart. Understanding how the scapulae move, or how the diaphragm invites breath can support healing. Specifically, in relation to the word healing, I mean, developing conscious awareness of something previously unknown or unfelt, for example, bringing sensory awareness to the synovial joints, connecting the scapulae, sternum and clavicles. When people sense, feel and perceive parts of their being, previously unknown, healing can take place – people begin to feel more whole.

The books in our field are so superb that I have not re-visited areas such ontogenetic or phylogenetic movement. Bonnie Bainbridge Cohen (1993) and Linda Hartley's (1995) books are superb in terms of developmental movement patterning. Nor have I delved into the application of Laban's movement principles; Peggy Hackney's work is absolutely superb in this regard (Hackey 2002). I have focused on some key areas that have not been thoroughly discussed in the field, such as the parasympathetic, social engagement, self-regulation, co-regulation and physiological states that underpin transpersonal awareness. These areas are highly relevant to anyone working in the field, but to date, have not received much visibility in publication. Additionally, I attend to tiny details that are often overlooked or not tracked in our main texts, such as the importance of co-regulation and the anatomy and physiology that underpins soft-tissue-rolling in gravity, for example. This book adds to the superb collection of books we already have, offering some new details, however small, that may enhance existing knowledge and therapeutic practice.

What type of research is in this book?

This book marks a departure from my previous research that was rooted in socio-cultural theory, phenomenology, eco-feminism and spiritual feminism (2009, 2010, 2014a, 2014b, 2015, 2018, 2020e). Over the past few years, I have turned my focus to practice-based therapeutic research, sharing the anatomical underpinnings of pedagogy (2020a, 2020b, 2020c, 2020g). This book holds and weaves all my previous research with a particular focus on asking, 'what are the practice-based elements that support effective therapeutic practice?' – 'why is somatic movement dance education and therapy so unique' – and 'why is the work often misunderstood?' These questions underpin the research in this book and, in many ways, guided me to write and present this text.

While my career has weaved between higher education (working with dance students on degree programmes) and working independently with the general public (usually non-dancers), in the past four years, I have been working almost full time as a somatic movement dance therapist, usually with non-dancers. I have also been training students to work professionally in this field. Therefore, this research has grown out of working with adults who are completely new to practice, have not moved much, other than functionally, or the odd yoga class, for years – often for decades. Working with non-dancers and in the independent sector is quite different from facilitating this work with dancers in a university context. Dancers generally have a deeper connection to their structure, fluidity, expressivity, imagination and their vast articular potential. In contrast, the general populous suffer terribly, sometimes hardly able to feel their bodies, unless in pain. Working with the general public brings you to the coal face, so to speak. It is at the coal face you hear the soulful heart-felt stories of others – their suffering, paradoxes and existential pain. As a therapist you suffer with Other, but notably always invite the transpersonal to hold the process. You observe in Self and Other just how divisive and socio-culturally inter-structured body–mind dualism is in our living tissues, and additionally, just how dissociated people are from their living body – and the incredible pain, loneliness and despair such separation causes. This book grows out of working creatively with suffering, empirically investigating processes that relieve pain, anxiety, fear and dissociation.

Somatic movement dance education has always been rooted in practice-led research, advanced by practitioners empirically investigating their own living tissues, with others, interlaced with objective knowledge about the body found in eastern and western traditions (Williamson 2010; Eddy 2017). This book grows out of this tradition. All the research presented in this book grew out of studio practice, empirically investigating my own living body, inviting theory to emerge from living experience, or applying pre-existing theory to practice. In Arts Therapy research, first-hand experimentation is valued and understood as essential to the advancement of professional practice (McNiff 2000). Thus, in kinship with arts-based therapeutic research, I am an insider, taking an emic position in understanding the materials and processes inherent in this therapeutic form (McNiff 1998, 2000, 2015). As Reed shares 'this insider view and familiarity allows for a particularly rich engagement with the material' (2020: 482). Hence, this book is seeded in, and animated by, an embodied engagement with the materials and practice-based elements of somatic movement dance therapy/practice. I pay particularly close attention to small details, and some of the unspoken elements of practice.

The structure of this book

This book is underpinned by experiential anatomy and physiology, like many other modalities in the somatic movement field. Most of the texts in the field are progressive texts, where western ideas about anatomy are reorganized into relational frameworks, and where first-person perception of the living body is balanced with objective knowledge. My work is not so different, and in this book, you will witness a great deal of applied western anatomy and physiology, underpinned by breath awareness and first-person sensory-perceptual movement awareness. I have, however, paid a great deal of attention to western anatomy and physiology in this book, in order to unpack and unearth some key elements of practice, such as the vagus nerve, the parasympathetic division of the autonomic nervous system, the craniosacral system, relational touch and myofascial unwinding. These areas are so important to health

I have attended to their physiological and anatomical underpinnings in-depth. Our bodies are often riddled with stress, tension and fear – an in-depth understanding of these areas feels particularly important in the current milieu.

It is of course true you can facilitate somatic movement/dance without any anatomical language at all. Practices such as *Authentic Movement* and *Skinner Releasing* do not use anatomy explicitly in the way I do in this book. Poetic language and carefully chosen embodied language using symbol, image and metaphor, and beautifully crafted phrases arising out of the moving/dancing experience itself, often hold and tone processes. Notably, many somatic movement dance practitioners mix it up, using anatomy as a pathway into the senate, but sounding, toning and unfolding anatomical ideas within a poetic language that drops participants into the sensate in a less mechanistic way. The erudite practitioner will know that exploring anatomy and physiology within a progressive relational framework, that supports movement integration, structure, fluidity and the imaginal, but does not mechanize the body, marks the departure from masculinist approaches and discourses about the body. First-person perception of the living moving body always transcends the mechanical and functional descriptions of the human body found in western anatomy and physiology books. However, a keen knowledge of anatomy and physiology has always underpinned the field, but notably, this knowledge is applied experientially and explored through first-person perception of the living body.

I confess, however, that at times, this book is heavy in anatomical and physiological detail. Reading anatomy and physiology is not easy. I find it hard. I often retract within myself because the terminology feels disembodied, dismembered and objectified; and notably, it is an androcentric language – the body was dissected and classified primarily by men, prior to, during and after the renaissance. Over the past ten years, I have been working increasingly with relational anatomy and physiology. I find anatomical and physiological details incredibly important when they are invited into living sensory awareness. Such details influence the efficacy of practice, offering sensory-perceptual trails and pathways into living tissues, where subjectivity and objectivity dance, dialogue and find balance. Following Dean Juhan's Goddess trail (2002), in this book I am inviting Hygeia (the goddess of health) to meet Asclepius (the Greek God of medicine). I combine the feminine sensitivity that drives the somatic movement dance paradigm with the masculine approach of western physiology and anatomy. Of course, I am not alone in this. So much somatic work combines anatomy and physiology with the phenomenological world of lived experience, or reconfigures disembodied mechanical descriptions of the human body into a holistic relational anatomical framework (Hartley 1995; Hackney 2002; Olsen and Mchose 2002).

Throughout this book, I offer processes captured through photography. The photos are offered to support the application of theory, but also offer readers more familiar with mechanistic approaches the novel opportunity to observe how soft tissue reorganization can be explored through self-regulatory movement that does not rely on lines, right angles and linear movement. Noted earlier, curves, spirals, circles, undulating, rippling, wave-like movements are emblematic of much international practice – this is such an extraordinary and lifegiving phenomenon I purposely wanted to capture this in the book. For readers outside the field, the photos are offered to share the uniqueness of somatic movement dance modalities underpinned by sensory-perceptual improvisation and why this work looks so sensitive, gentle, attuned and parasympathetically relaxed.

This book is structured in a particular way that deepens inquiry into the parasympathetic division of the autonomic nervous system or explores different ways to soften into fluency, ease and restitution. In Chapter 1, 'Autogenic self-regulatory movement', I introduce the importance of the self-regulation. In doing so, I share some defining features of the field internationally, in relation to somatic movement modalities underpinned by experiential anatomy, the imagination and improvisation. Within this wide frame I introduce readers to the importance of the parasympathetic nervous system in supporting autogenic self-regulatory movement. This chapter deals with the complexity of the term self-regulation, and what it might mean in the field of somatic movement and dance.

Chapter 2, 'Sympathetic holding and parasympathetic release', deepens topics introduced in Chapter 1, such as parasympathetic release and autogenic self-regulatory movement. At the heart of this chapter is how to release stress, anxiety and fear in the studio. Throughout, I offer practice-based examples of how to contact and move with awareness of the vagus nerve, the craniosacral and lumbar-thoracic divisions of the autonomic nervous system, as well as the ventral branch of the vagus nerve, supporting social engagement. This chapter is rich in anatomy and physiology, but presented is such a way that readers can observe how theory is applied to practice.

Chapter 3, 'Fulcrums of support and soft tissue reorganization', continues to deepen the anatomy and physiology of the parasympathetic, taking an in-depth look into why releasing into gravity and landing in the bony structural supports of the occiput, scapulae and sacrum help participants reorganize neuromuscular holding. This chapter is the longest and most dense chapter in terms of anatomy and physiology. It is a harder read, but vitally important because it unpicks why releasing into gravity, tipping and pouring our cranial bones, and inviting the rest of the body to tenderly follow is so healing. This is especially important for the reader who is new to the field, who upon witnessing participants rolling in gravity may make assumptions about practice, not realizing just how important it is to self-regulate in gravity. Each section attends to tiny physiological details that are vital to my practice and the way I facilitate self-regulation.

Chapter 4, 'Co-regulation, cardio-ception and the transpersonal witness', introduces the importance of co-regulation, and the therapist's ability to create a heart-space. The heart has been conceptualized and perceived as an organ of consciousness and of great significance since antiquity, and in this chapter, I share the importance of *cardio-centric* (heart-centered) dyadic witnessing. Within this chapter, I share some of the scientific research undertaken by the HeartMath Institute – research that was rather beautifully inspired by asking why so many ancient mystical, religious and philosophic traditions focus on the organ of the heart?

Chapter 5, 'Co-regulatory touch and myofasical softening', elucidates why touch is so important and the type of touch I faciliate. It is a shorter chapter that sheds light on the many photographs in this book that evidence the centrality of touch in practice. Chapter 6, 'Sense–perceiving the craniosacral system', focuses on the craniosacral system and the importance of sense–perceiving the cranial bones. In western anatomy, we have been taught the cranium is solid and fused. In contrast, in progressive anatomy, the cranium is re-perceived as biotensile – there is a small degree of motility between the sutures and the bones in the cranium. Again, this chapter is rich in anatomy and physiology, with examples of studio practice throughout. Releasing the cranial bones and attuning to the craniosacral system is emblematic of much international practice, and therefore this chapter offers a glimpse into the sensitivity of what I have come to term *craniosacral somatic movement dance therapy*. Chapter 7, 'Soft-tissue-rolling and myofascial unwinding', shares the importance of fascia, experientially and objectively. I attend to how soft-tissue-rolling in gravity changes the viscosity of the fascial matrix.

This book is offered with the knowledge that this is my perspective on practice, and only one perspective out of many existing, and potential future voices, in the field. Research is always biographic – from a postpositivist feminist standpoint, researchers always write from their positionality, acculturation, passion, situatedness and limitations. So too – this book grows out of my life experiences, my suffering, my research expertise and my deep passion for the subject. It also bares my limitations. I acknowledge my knowledge is partial, and every academic book is partial and limited, growing out of the author's life-journey. The scope of this book traces some extremely important elements found of current practice, but for every detail I draw attention to, there are many more. While I present and share important knowledge, through a postpositivist frame, I acknowledge the book is unfinished, for I am always growing and changing – and every time I teach or read, I learn. The aim of this book is to open-out topics and areas that have not been shared explicitly in publication, or revisit existing ideas and practices through a different lens. My hope is, this book brings courage, insight and peace, offering support to students, lecturers and practitioners with their ongoing work, which, I know, always requires strength and methodological ingenuity.

1

Autogenic Self-regulatory Movement

Through the practice of experiential learning, personal enquiry and reflection, I am offered the space to slow down and deepen my awareness of my physical body, and the relationship between mind and body. I am then able to share this knowledge with others, through moving, talking and listening, as well as witnessing the somatic movement of others. This has been a profound and healing process for me as I learn to self-regulate my nervous system, and become aware of other's nervous systems.

(Emma Rockford)

Preliminary reflections on self-regulation

Throughout this book, I use the words self-regulation and co-regulation. I also use related terms such as self-regulatory movement and autogenic self-regulatory movement. These terms underpin most of the practices and processes offered in this book. From my standpoint, self-regulatory movement and co-regulatory support are two of the most important terms that define the uniqueness of the somatic movement dance field, particularly in relation to movement modalities rooted in free improvisation underpinned by sensory awareness. Exploring these terms is not easy. It requires both physiological and spiritual knowledge, and the latter is of course harder to quantify in academic study. When applied to practice, the term self-regulation is complicated and multidimensional. For example, in this book, I offer self-regulatory processes rooted in anatomy and physiology, and additionally, self-regulatory movement processes rooted in the imaginal, supporting the integration of different dimensions of the psyche (body, mind, spirit and soul). Therefore, somatic movement dance therapy does not reduce self-regulation to physiology alone; although, one is always invited to release the body first, to reduce sympathetic arousal and suffering held in tissues.

I note early, applying Stephen Porges's term in a new context, somatic movement dance therapy is a 'bottom-up' feeling therapy (Porges 2017). Mostly, people are used to cortico-centric approaches to healing and therapy. These are top-down therapies that prioritize language and cognition. While language and cognition play an important role in somatic movement sessions, and are interwoven in the healing process, the body and breath always come first.

The body comes first because while talking about problems and the complexities of life can offer tremendous healing, if a person's physiology has been damaged by trauma, anxiety and depression, talking alone will not necessarily bring the nervous system and living tissues back into balance. For example, if you are depressed, anxious and afraid it is likely your sympathetic nervous system is over-riding your ability to sense parasympathetic ease, peace and restitution. Somatic movement dance therapy is a bottom-up healing approach to trauma, offering processes and practices that release stress and strain held in living tissues first. Therapists invite sensory awareness of breath and breathing tissues first, followed by sensory-perceptual movement, and then, figurative, symbolic and metaphorical reflections, noticing how developing sensory awareness first and foremost invites change in the whole psyche (body/mind). All sessions are grounded in sensory-perceptual movement processes (bottom-up). This way of working invites the right hemisphere into expression, where therapists work with sensation, vibration, energy, intuition, e-motion, feeling, touch and the imagination. For example, bringing awareness to breath, releasing the jaw, relaxing in the mouth, sounding, toning and softening the muscles in the face, neck and shoulders starts to repair the ventral branch of the vagus nerve (Williamson 2020c). In addition, soft-tissue-rolling in gravity releases tension held in the fascial matrix and skeletal-muscular system and reduces sympathetic arousal (Williamson 2020a, 2020b, 2020c). This deep release of stress held in the tissues offers participants a completely different sense of Self; expansive, peaceful and socially engaged. From this place of balance and rest, other areas of life can be tilled through movement, artwork and reflection. If our original source (our living tissues) are riddled with stress and grief, it is difficult to heal trauma through talking alone, namely because anguish and strain, over time, are patterned in the nervous system, particularly the autonomic nervous system (ANS) (Porges 2017; Rosenburg 2017). Therefore, self-regulation in the somatic movement dance field necessitates softening and releasing our tissues first, in order to reduce stress, ease pain, soothe and dissolve sympathetic arousal.

In saying this, it is worth remembering, somatic movement/dance is aligned with postpositivist arts therapies and therefore does not reduce health to physiology alone. We are more than a physiological body – we are *body–minds*. Additionally, many people sense they are more than a *body–mind*. They sense transpersonal and transcendental dimensions to their being. Following this trail, we might say we are *body–mind–spirit* or *body–mind–spirit–soul*. We often read that somatic movement integrates body, mind, spirit and soul (Halprin 2002, 2014; Eddy 2017; Hayes 2007,

2014, 2013). These words are not definable things or objects that can be dissected, quantified, analyzed and known in their totality; rather these words point to experiential sensory expressions of our being that often feel fragmented or dissociated, and arise into awareness when people sense there might be more to their life than their job, persona or ego. Somatic movement dance therapy, when it opens into imaginal realms is a holistic practice that attends to materia, conceptualized as earth, body and mass; *spirit* which inspires *mater*, breathing life into and illuminating the *body*; mind, a developmental stage in the growth of our consciousness (often disassociating from our body as we develop into adults); and soul, considered the most delicate part of our being, which expresses through the imagination, bridging the spiritual centre of Self with the ego and the external world (Williamson 2018; Hayes 2007, 2014, 2013).

Our life-force is severely compromised in a world that mechanizes the body and assaults nature, culturally constructing mind as superior, and indeed humans as superior to nature. Participants often express dissociation followed by re-association to their life-energy in the studio. Further, some participants express dissociation and re-association to their soul (the deeper meaning of their life-journey or a timeless eternal sense-feeling). All these fragmented aspects of our being are given space, sense–perceived and integrated in somatic movement dance modalities that explore the imagination-in-movement as a teleological guide. Many participants attend sessions because they feel isolated, dissociated from their body, and lacking in vitality. Thus, I use the words spirit and soul in this book as pointers to existential and spiritual dimensions of our being that often feel suppressed within the dominance of the mechanistic paradigm and in a world marked by increased secularization. Spirit and soul allude clear definition and academic quantification. They are elusive slippery words for some. I use these words later in Chapter 4 to explore the transpersonal aspects of practice, largely rooted in Carl Jung's theories.

While somatic movement dance therapy is a bottom-up feeling therapy, easing the distress and suffering held in our tissues first and foremost, we must not hide the fact that participants often access a wide spectrum of consciousness during their moving experience. Carl Jung referred to this as *the material-spiritual continuum*, spiralling from infra-red (*materia*) to transcendental spirit (ultra-purple) (Jung [1969] 2003, [1933] 2002, [1972] 2003). Sensory-perceptual-moving processes are earth bound, temporal, finite, and paradoxically, non-spatial, infinite, and timeless (Hayes 2014, 2013; Kieft 2020; Hartley 2014, 2020; Williamson et al. 2014a; Halprin 2014; Stromstead 2014; Fortin 2014; Fraleigh 2014). The psyche (body/mind) is thus vast and paradoxical in nature. On the one hand, for example, we are bound by time and space, yet on the other hand, people often sense a timelessness and expansive non-spatiality to their being. We are finite, moving towards death, yet some people sense an eternal soul.

Self-regulation thus attends to the vast and paradoxical aspects of our being. For example, we might offer a process rooted explicitly in sense–perceiving the sensory-motor loop, or a process specifically oriented to moving with sensation, emotion, image and symbol. Both are valuable and contribute to participants sense–perceiving and integrating unconscious aspects of Self. Very often a process will transverse and integrate both, attending to our body tissues and the imagination. For example, we might offer a process initially rooted in sense–perceiving the skeletal–muscular system (sensing bones and soft tissues) that unfolds out into imaginative symbolic movement play, followed by reflective artwork and dialogue with the therapist. Such holistic processes offer participants the opportunity to self-regulate and integrate many aspects of their being. In this chapter, I specifically attend to the physiological aspects of self-regulation.

Self-regulation is a frequently used term. It has become a bit of a buzz word in the world of bodywork therapies (Shea 2016, 2010; Porges 2017; Rosenburg 2017). It is often assumed that the reader or listener knows what the term means, but self-regulation is a complex term and does not necessarily mean the same thing across the wonderful array of bodywork modalities circulating in the current milieu. Dean Juhan defines self-regulation as 'hedonic self-regulatory behaviours', meaning the innate bodily instinct somas have to move towards 'useful, live-preserving or life-enhancing' activities (Juhan 2002: 29, 31). In 2020, I published the following:

> Self-regulation in its broadest sense tends to mean the ability to sense imbalance within the organism and move towards balance through conscious awareness and embodied action. Furthermore, it tends to mean listening to the self-regulatory intelligence of the body and following the body's desire for easeful functioning.
>
> (Williamson 2020d: 178)

The biological imperative to be well is one element of self-regulation. However, this instinct often becomes deeply buried underneath sympathetic stress and trauma, losing its teleological drive. These types of definitions, while common in our field, do not really explain how somatic movement dance practitioners and therapists support their participants to self-regulate. Let us take a detailed look.

Breath awareness and the healing power of presence

The human body is always self-regulating beneath our conscious awareness. For example, our cerebrospinal fluid, which is produced in the ventricular system in the brain, continuously circulates and reabsorbs fluid beneath the level of our everyday awareness. As it does this, the brain and spinal cord are cleansed of toxins, and you are protected from unwanted intruders that would ultimately threaten your life. The lymph system picks up waste products and removes toxins left behind by your venous blood flow (lymph moves diligently and conscientiously below the threshold of your awareness, keeping you safe in a toxic world). The nervous system regulates your being after a period of stress or fear, restoring your body to homeostasis by innervating the parasympathetic, reducing sympathetic arousal. These are just three out of millions of self-regulatory processes that take place beneath the threshold of our awareness. The autonomic aspects of our being are intent on our survival – one could say they are a loving part of us. As Sumner and Haines so beautifully state,

> The smartest thing in the room is the intelligence expressed in our bodies. There are millions of years of evolution behind the shapes and forms and movements in the body. There are lots of coordinated self-regulating processes that respond to events and maintain an internal balance and flow. This intelligence defines the chemistry, nervous activity and alignment of the body. Health is an active principle: it is a living breathing reality.
>
> (2010: 24)

However, the term self-regulation does not just point to the extraordinary processes that autonomically take place beneath our conscious awareness. It suggests there is a 'self' that can further support your body to regulate. The term might also suggest there is a 'self' who can attune to autonomic bodily processes and thus bring unconscious aspects of our being into conscious awareness. While mind and body are of course inextricably linked, the populous have been enculturated on mass into body/mind dualism, and thus people often feel dissociated from their body. At heart, the term self-regulation is referring to the cultivation of a *body–mind* – an integrated sense of self, where chattering (often worrying) mind is invited rest, direct its awareness inwards, land softly in living tissues, and settle awareness in the diaphragm. Breath awareness is commonly positioned as the bridge between mind and body, and thus self-regulation involves the integration of body and mind, through conscious awareness of breath (Halprin 2014). In somatic movement dance practice, we invite mind to surf the waves of breath, settle awareness in the diaphragm, linger on the inhalation, follow the exhalation, and sense–perceive the motility of tissues inspiring. In short, we invite mind to settle awareness on source and life-energy. We can therefore say a key aspect of self-regulation is healing body/mind dualism. Body and mind are unified through bringing awareness to breath (life-energy or source energy) (Fortin et al. 2014). When our enculturated egoic mind is invited to turn inwards, soften and relax into its original source, our consciousness expands. We become a *body–mind*. Because breath awareness is the bridge between body and mind, as we breathe, we oxygenate. Hence, we can also say, self-regulation involves integrating body, mind and spirit (breath).

Developing and sensing–perceiving an integrated experience of body–mind–spirit is not a taken-for-granted state consciousness. It is not easy. It does not happen overnight. It requires learning to breathe, sense and perceive one's living tissues again, after years, perhaps decades of dissociation and fragmentation. It is a lifelong process of recovery and discovery. Recovering from dualism, and its outcome, dissociation from source energy, takes slow-time sensing and perceiving. When mind is invited to sense–dwell in the breath, gently land in sensory receptors and travel consciously with motor neurons, mind, body and spirit start to flow together in a state of non-duality. Self-regulation thus requires moving our central identity, often located in a disembodied *mind* (where one's sense of self floats above the intelligence of the body so to speak), to identifying 'self' with body, mind and spirit. Self-regulation is thus fully dependant on the disruption the body/mind dualism, and the expansion of consciousness. Thus, self-regulation involves non-duality, where differing aspects of 'self', usually perceived as opposites, assimilate and heal. western culture has identified and enculturated *mind* as the centre of our identity, personality, ego and the pinnacle of western civilization. Hence, most of us are enculturated into living distally, always thinking rather than sensing and feeling, separated from our source. While mind serves us very well as we develop, needing to individuate from pre-personal states, at some point in our life journey we may notice identifying with mind and ego as our centre, serves to keep us distant and disconnected from other aspects of our being, especially our living breathing tissues.

When we have no time to reflect, *to still*, to meditate, to imagine, to dream, rest in our tissues and direct awareness to our original source, we become trapped in the dualistic world of the egoic mind and persona. In short, on a collective level, mind/body dualism reflects our societal institutions that require the mass population to think and live dualistically to uphold the cultural values of mind as superior to body, of humans as superior to nature. From a somatic point of view, institutionalized dualism requires a firm physiological foundation to keep up its disembodied values and one-dimensional consciousness. Put simply, western institutions require stress-out bodies, dissociated from breath, heart, soul and the imaginal. The dominant cultural values we inhabit (or inhabit us) require us to work fast, hard and relentlessly, using and discarding our bodies to keep up the speed of production and consumption. It does not serve economies to support breath awareness, non-duality, reflection, restitution and dream-time. It serves our economies very well to enculturate people into a sympathetically charged state, to identify with mind as the centre of their personality and thus to live distally from their life-energy. Economies need disembodied minds, and bodies riven with stress. In contrast, therapeutic somatic movement dance processes support participants to experience breath awareness, deep rest, organismic ease, and precious moments of non-duality (however fleeting), often after years (perhaps a lifetime) of dissociation.

Of self-regulation Michael Shea writes the following,

> Understand that self-regulation is modulated by two pathways. One pathway is from the body and heart to the brain via sensation and feeling (bottom-up), which is slower. It is processed by the right hemisphere of the brain. The second pathway is from the brain to the body via cognitive thinking (top down). It is processed by the prefrontal lobe in the left hemisphere of the brain.
>
> (Shea 2016: 59–60)

In terms of self-regulation, somatic movement dance therapy sits easily with the first pathway described by Shea above. The first thing we do in the studio is invite people to close their eyes, contact breath flow, sense, feel, perceive and move with conscious awareness; we invite participants into slow-time sensory-perceptual movement awareness. However, self-regulation requires the mind to care for the body; it necessitates inviting our awareness to soften its directive intelligence into the rich and lush landscape of the body. In order to self-regulate, the mind, often wildly upset in emotional trauma and looping thoughts, needs to reorientate its gaze from outer to inner, and soften into its original source. Mind must slow, sense spirit-breath, land in the heart and take presence in the diaphragm. When our awareness has landed curiously in our tissues, we can sense, feel and perceive with far more acuity. Thus, while somatic movement is a bottom-up feeling therapy that values sensing, feeling and perceiving, calming and inviting one's dissociated mind to acknowledge the body is equally important. Mind is invited to focus its attention on living tissues (that are often lonely, tense and in pain). In doing so, mind is no longer dissociated, and the body is no longer alone, forgotten and abandoned. We can further say that self-regulation in the field of somatic movement is modulated by both pathways shared by Shea above.

In 1997, Eckhart Tolle published *The Power of Now: A Guide to Spiritual Enlightenment*, selling over two million copies world-wide. The main offering in this book is there is a transpersonal Self (or experiential state of consciousness) behind the egoic enculturated self. Tolle managed to articulate this message in a way that was accessible to the western world. This is the Self we feel when our roaming over excited mind is invited to land in breath and heart. This is Carl Jung's transpersonal Self (the centre of the mandala) who I propose is always available, sense–perceived in breath and heart, behind the little self – the egoic mind, the enculturated self – the mask and persona (Williamson 2015, 2020e). Of note, this expanded and integrated sense of Self, as Tolle points out, can only be reached and animated through breath and interoceptive awareness (internal sensations). It is only though moment-by-moment breath awareness and heart-sensing that egoic babbling and chattering mind can rest, take-a-break, settle and *still* in living tissues.

The other inter-related message in Tolle's work is that through breath awareness we become present. While attending to breath awareness, we are simultaneously moved into *the present*, alleviated from worries from the past, and no longer riddled with anxiety and fear about the future (perhaps momentarily, or for longer if an experienced meditator). Thus, contacting the transpersonal Self emerges through moment-by-moment breath awareness, simultaneously bringing us into *the present moment*. Somatic movement shares many things in common with eastern meditative practices, such as moment-by-moment breath awareness, heart-centeredness, presence, being, non-doing and non-duality (Eddy 2009; Williamson 2009, 2010). This is of course no great surprise given the eastern and non-western influences underpinning many pioneers work (Reed 2020; Eddy 2009; Williamson 2010, 2014a). Experiencing the healing nature of *presence*, cultivated through breath awareness is also a key aspect of self-regulation in the field.

While somatic movement dance shares many concepts and principles in common with Buddhist practices (Fraleigh 2015, 2020; Blum 2015a; Blum and Williamson 2015b; Kittikong 2015), our work is however different. For example, we do not just focus on stilling the chattering mind in sitting meditations, but rather focus our mind throughout our living tissues as we move – or listen to the life-energy in tissues and the mind of the cells as we move. Thus, somatic movement meditations invite mind to focus tenderly on the moving body, resting awareness in organs, in sensory receptors, in bones and soft tissues. We might for example rest our awareness on our clavicles, in our heart, diaphragm, thorax, sacrum or toes, inviting movement underpinned by breath awareness to emerge and express from this experience. We also may follow imaginal improvisational trails underpinned by breath awareness – hence the common term *movement meditation*. As participants move, they sense–track their movement, simultaneously surfing the waves of breath. Rather than identifying self with egoic mind, often riddled with past and future anxieties, and disassociated from the body, movers experience breath as deeply integrative, cultivating a sense of, or experience of Self, who resides peacefully in breath, heart and the present moment.

Contemporarily, the term self-regulation is often related to the health and balance of the ANS. In the extensive work of Steven Porges, Stanley Rosenburg (2017), Michael Shea (Shea 2016, 2010), and my own (Williamson 2020a, 2020b, 2020c), one of the most important aspects of self-regulation is sense–perceiving the state of the ANS. In many somatic movement practices, the ANS is invited into conscious awareness, so participants can learn to reduce sympathetic aroursal and soften myofascial tissues riddled with tension, asymmetries and stress. Slowing down in the studio, when combined with conscious awareness of breath and afferent sensing, naturally invites the parasympathetic into expression (Williamson 2020a, 2020b, 2020c). The parasympathetic is a potent and powerful part of the ANS and will usually override sympathetic arousal if the participant feels safe. Somatic movement dance therapy offers participants creative ways to deduce stress, anxiety and manage life's suffering through gentle movement processes that innervate the parasympathetic. The parasympathetic, by its nature, invites reflection and the possibility of finding ease within the organism. Attuning to the parasympathetic engages the vagus nerve and, through this experience, participants begin to sense a profound difference between a parasympathetic state and their more normal state of sympathetic arousal. Therefore, another aspect of self-regulation in the field is attuning to the ANS through sensory-perceptual movement processes underpinned by interoception – particularly breath and cardio-ception. This aspect of self-regulation forms the foundation of this book.

Additionally, with the advent of Polyvagal theory, it has been scientifically established that feeling safe is an integral element of self-regulation (Porges 2017). Put simply, when we feel safe, the ANS will naturally shift from deregulation to homeostasis. When we feel unsafe, the autonomic nervous becomes sympathetically aroused. Self-regulation, in this context, is enhanced by the co-regulatory presence of the therapist who has balanced her own nervous system, in turn supporting the client to self-regulate. Porges's work, discussed further below, and in Chapter 2, highlights that any worthy definition of self-regulation needs to include safety. We can self-regulate much more effectively when we feel safe, held in the presence of the compassionate witness, or when receiving the artful attuned touch of the therapist.

I note early in this chapter, somatic movement dance therapy, in comparison to other bodywork modalities, such as massage and craniosacral therapy, takes the term self-regulation to whole new level, because we offer processes that support participants to self-regulate by attuning to their own sensory-perceptual movement awareness, and often their sensory-perceptual-moving-imaginal; the latter rooted in the expansion of imaginal consciousness moving us far beyond the ego, into transpersonal realms. In short, we support people to attune to their own sensory-motor feedback loop, through sensing, feeling, perceiving, and moving consciously. In these processes, the participant is actively involved in the healing process through sense–dwelling and sense–tracking their own movement. They are the authority of their experience, witnessed by the compassionate co-regulatory presence of the somatic guide or therapist. The presence of the witness is vital to the efficacy of self-regulation because the ability to self-regulate depends on safety and sociality (Porges 1997). Thus, the definition of self-regulation in this book is advanced through the concept of co-regulation, shared in Chapter 4.

The heart of self-regulation: Attuning to the sensory-motor feedback loop

One of the most significant differences between the paradigm of somatic movement dance education and therapy and other forms of restorative bodywork, such as massage therapy, craniosacral therapy or yoga, for example, is the focus on how sensory-perceptual movement awareness supports self-regulation. While other bodywork modalities, such as craniosacral therapy are rooted in an extensive and rich dialogue about self-regulation and co-regulation (Shea 2010, 2016), we must note, clients attending these sessions are not *moving*. They are lying down on the bodywork couch receiving the therapist's knowledgeable touch, which helps them to self-regulate. Self-regulatory movement, imaginatively unfolding out of sensory-perceptual movement awareness is absent in other forms of restorative bodywork. In most bodywork modalities, the client is dependent on the therapist's erudite physiological and anatomical knowledge to help them feel better. Bodywork aims to bring homeostasis to deregulated nervous systems. However, somatic movement dance therapy and practice is the only bodywork modality that involves self-regulating through moving, underpinned by sensory-perceptual awareness. Sensing, feeling, perceiving and moving consciously lies at the heart of practice. Thus, while the broad paradigm of somatic movement shares some things in common with the wider field of restorative bodywork, it is also significantly different.

The greatest difference, which I believe we should celebrate, is the invitation to *move and express* with attuned sensitivity to one's sensory-motor feedback loop. We invite participants to move with awareness of afferent sensation and awareness of efferent motor pathways. These processes, while reliant on co-regulation (the heart-centered non-judgemental witness), are different from other forms of bodywork in numerous ways. Most obviously, clients are invited to be actively involved in their own health through sensing, feeling, perceiving, moving and reflecting. Thus, clients are not passive receivers, but rather sensitively attune to the unique ability humans have to sense, feel and perceive the state of their own living tissues. This is a distinctive aspect of somatic movement practices. I note early, it is perhaps one reason why somatic movement dance practices have not reached the same status or level of acceptance by the general populous, as craniosacral therapy, cranio-osteopathy, yoga or massage work, for example. Inviting participants to be actively involved in sensory-perceptual movement explorations, rather than lie on a couch, or follow specific poses, requires developing the imagination and improvisatory agency in movement. For practice to be transformative, participants are invited to be actively involved in sensing, feeling, perceiving and action (expressing and motoring out with conscious awareness). Researchers in myofascial bodywork, such as Schleip (2003a, 2003b) have put forward the idea that if a client is actively engaging with their sensory-motor feedback loop, myofascial bodywork is more effective. While this idea might be revelatory in other bodywork modalities, developing an intimately sensed, felt and perceived relationship with one's sensory-motor feedback loop lies at the beating heart of somatic movement dance practices, and is synonymous with the art of self-regulation.

Since the inception of the somatic movement, and the ground-breaking work of Thomas Hanna (1988, [1973] 1993), Frederick Matthias Alexander (1932, 1942) and Moshe Feldenkrais (1977), the field has been underpinned by self-regulatory movement that involves conscious awareness of the sensory-motor feedback loop. Very uniquely, practitioners discovered that if participants develop a sensed and perceived relationship with their own sensory-motor feedback loop, they can learn how to re-pattern their own posture and alignment, release skeletal–muscular tension and undo habitual dysfunctional neuro muscular pathways. Somatic movement invites the participant, for want of a better word, to take conscious 'responsibility' for their health. Practice invites participants to sense, feel and perceive, and then make conscious choices about to move easefully, paying attention to quality, energy, temporarily, space, alignment and posture. Conscious and creative awareness of the sensory-motor feedback loop underlies all somatic movement dance modalities. All the theorists noted above, wrote extensively about the sensory-motor feedback loop and the incredible ability people have to attune to their own body, sense disfunction and move towards healthy functioning.

Your sensory-motor feedback loop has both afferent (sensory) receptors and efferent (motor) neurons. Afferent pathways carry information away from your peripheral nervous system (PNS) (both your somatic and ANS), back to your spinal cord and brain where information can be perceived. *Afferent sensing* in the studio, supports participants to sense–perceive the state of their PNS, both their somatic and ANS. In contrast, efferent neurons carry information away from your brain and spinal cord, to your PNS (your somatic and ANS); this is called your motor response. *Efferent expression* in the studio supports participants to move with conscious awareness of their motor neurons – their expressive neuromuscular pathways. Participants are invited to dwell in afferent sensation, enabling them to sense the state of their internal visceral body (their ANS), and the state of their somatic nervous system (SNS) (their joints and muscles). Slow-time dwelling in afferent sensation, decelerates the efferent motor response, inviting participants to slow-down enough that they can inhibit their habitual motor response and make conscious choices about how to respond and express (to motor out). I call this *slow-time afferent sensing* and *consciously sensed efferent motor expression*. People are supported to make healthy movement choices about how, where and what to move, and with what quality, energy, directionality, force, spatiality and temporality. Slowing down, *afferent sensing* and consciously *sensed efferent motor expression* is another key aspect of self-regulation. Therefore inhibiting the habitual motor response also supports the art of self-regulation.

Sensory nerve endings are wonderfully sensitive and receptive; they receive sensation from both our inner world and the exterior environment. *Efferent* motor nerves are wonderfully active and directional, carrying impulses away from the central nervous system (CNS), bringing movement to all our muscles. We have trillions of nerves in our bodies (and billions of neurons). Thus, in somatic movement dance, the cerebral cortex is not celebrated as the pinnacle of western achievement and civilization, but rather the entire nervous system is highly distinguished. The CNS (the brain and spinal cord), the PNS (which encompasses both the ANS and SNS) and the enteric nervous system are all celebrated as intelligent parts of our living wholeness (Eddy 2017).

Somatic movement/dance modalities underpinned by improvisation have a unique emphasis on self-regulation in comparison to other forms of restorative bodywork; we might call this, the ability of the participant to influence change in their own system. In short, there is less intervention by the therapist trying to solve problems for the client through deduction, observation and the instruction of set exercises. Unique to somatic movement dance is the unwavering belief in the capacity people have to self-regulate and influence the state of their own living tissues. A large part of the therapist's role is supporting participants to cultivate their ability to listen to afferent information streaming into the CNS, and additionally, creative agency in terms of how to respond (to move) with conscious awareness of their efferent motor neurons and expressive pathways.

In reality, the sensory-motor feedback loop is superfast, and neuromuscular activity happens mostly beneath the threshold of everyday awareness. Because it happens so fast, our inherent ability to sense–perceive our own sensory-perceptual and motor response is easily forgotten. Thus, our motor responses become habitual, unconscious and often dysfunctional. On top of this, we live in a Euro-American (globalized) dominant culture that has placed our sensitive *feeling-full* bodies within dehumanized socio-economic systems driven by production, consumption and speed. Our sensitive tissues are deregulated by disembodied heady institutions. Patriarchal institutions are certainly not invested in supporting people to slow-down, dwell in sensation and enjoy their motor expression consciously. The sensory-perceptual and imaginal capacities of the general populous has been greatly diminished by our sympathetically charged socio-economic world and our patriarchal institutions (both religious and medical) that have positioned, and continue to position our bodies, either as a machine or transient shell. In somatic movement dance practices, the body is re-claimed from these dehumanizing societal institutions and cultural values. This is achieved through slow-time sensory-perceptual moving awareness, where people learn to sense, feel, perceive, and move consciously, attuned to the intelligence of their living body (Johnson 1995).

The sensory-motor feedback loop is an exceptionally beautiful and intelligent aspect of our being, but often falls beneath consciousness. Conscious awareness of the sensory-motor loop is certainly not something that is taught in main-stream education. When young people learn about the sensory-motor feedback loop at school, it is objectified and taught as *Other*; this is what it is, where it is and what is does. Rarely are children invited to sense–dwell in their sensation, receiving afferent information streaming into their CNS, telling them how their body is feeling. Rarely are they invited to sense–perceive their ANS (breath and heart), which provides information if they are stressed or calm. Our young people, and the general populous, are rarely shown how to soothe a sympathetically charged nervous system into a state of balance. In contrast, in somatic movement dance practices, the sensory-motor feedback loop is slowed right down. Slowing down enables participants to sense–perceive tensions, torsions and pain in their own organism, and further, make conscious choices about how to unwind in order to alleviate suffering.

To use Don Hanlon Johnson's phrase, somatic movement is marked by *slow-time* sensory-perceptual movement awareness (1992). When you slow down, and direct your awareness to breath, heart, skin or muscle, for example, you can begin to sense the living presence and intelligence of your sensory receptors (so full of feeling). In the studio, I invite participants to attune to different sensory receptors. Cutaneous receptors, for example, are sensory receptors found in the dermis or epidermis. Mechanoreceptors are found in the muscles and joints. Visceroceptors are found in the organs (in the ANS). How lovely it is to invite participants to soft-tissue-roll, sense–perceiving their cutaneous receptors, or to delicately explore their synovial joints, sensing their proprioceptors. How wonderful it is to invite participants to stretch, lengthen, compress and decompress in gravity, sensing their mechanoreceptors. How calming it is to invite participants to sense–dwell in their own heart and breath, contacting their visceroceptors.

When participants rest, settle, soften and yield in gravity, contacting their sensory-motor feedback loop, pain often arises. The arising and perception of pain offers the unique opportunity to ease-out suffering through self-regulatory movement. Sensing and acknowledging the living presence of nociceptors (pain receptors) is particularly relevant in studio practice because these intelligent receptors are communicating with you; they are telling you something is wrong, vying for your attention (nociceptors care about you). Nociceptors are located all over your body, in your muscles, skin, joints, blood vessels and organs. These intelligent receptors sense damage to your tissues and communicate this information to your spinal cord and brain, where it can be perceived. The human body is rich in pain receptors. Sometimes participants arrive in acute pain, after a recent injury. Other participants express chronic pain, which may have lasted for years, leaving their muscles tense, with limited mobility. Many participants express what might be termed neuropathic pain, where there appears some sort of damage to their nervous system. Mostly, participants express myofascial pain, sharing a tightness and soreness in their muscles, and often inflammation. Moving away from and dissociating from pain is common. However, being invited to soften into your own living tissues and listen to where and how pain is expressing and then reorganize your tissues through slow-time sensory-perceptual movement underlies self-regulation in the field. As I share later in this book, the vagus nerve plays a central role in somatic movement/dance practices, and when the vagus nerve is engaged and healthy, it supports the reduction of pain (Hinton 2020; Richards 2020).

Developing an intimate relationship with one's own sensory-motor feedback loop (sensory receptors and motor neurons) is highly effective in resolving pain and dysfunction. While a somatic movement therapist is trained to observe patterns of sympathetic holding and offer processes that help to resolve tensions and asymmetries in the tissues, we must note, the client can sense tension and pain in their own organism far more acutely than a therapist can observe or deduce. Human beings are blessed with the ability to sense–perceive and make conscious choices about how to move – to ease – to soften – to release – to compress and decompress. In short, the incredible intelligence of the sensory-motor feedback loop is a key to self-regulatory health but is not advanced as a method within popular and dominant cultural values, that still place enormous emphasis on *body as machine* that requires intervention by an authority if it breaks down (Johnson 1992, 1987). And, noted earlier, the living body is thoroughly inter-structured within dehumanized socio-economic systems that augment sensory-motor amnesia. Supporting people to resolve and ease pain, or heal sensory-motor amnesia, by attuning to their sensory-motor feedback loop is one of the unique gifts somatic movement dance practitioners bring to the world of health.

In sports therapy or physiotherapy, for example, the therapist makes observations and offers restorative movements based on their erudite deductions. In contrast, rather than diagnose and instruct someone to perform specific movements, somatic movement dance therapists facilitate self-regulation by inviting participants into sensing, feeling, moving and perceiving. The attuned participant learns how to ease-out tension, resolve trigger points, and reduce sympathetic overcharge. These processes are crafted in manifold ways and are often underpinned by exploring gravi-ception, interoception, proprioception and kinaesthesia. This is often a delicious experience, where participants can dwell in afferent sensation and sensitively motor out, creatively attuned to their own motor neurons.

We must take a pause here – and digest – if humans have the ability to sense their own pain, why is the outside observer and therapist considered a greater authority than the client in mechanistic models? A participant attuned to their own sensory-motor feedback loop can sense where they feel tension, where they are riddled with pain and if they are sympathetically charged, with far more precision and acuity than the therapist. This is a very significant difference between somatic movement dance and other forms of restorative bodywork. We offer processes that support intimacy with one's own sensory-motor feedback loop. Participants can feel pain, where it is expressing, and most importantly, learn how to ease-out pain through self-regulatory movement. This is one reason why the word agency is synonymous with the field; we invite participants to be the authority in their own healing process.

Somatic movement dance practitioners share ways to relieve pain and alleviate human suffering by inviting participants into slow-time sensory-perceptual-movement awareness and reflective dialogue with the somatic guide. We strictly do not diagnose. We do not manipulate bodies lying on the bodywork couch or prescribe functional movements to alleviate pain. Our role is to provide a peaceful safe space where the intelligence of the human organism can arise into awareness and move towards healthy functioning. Through self-regulatory movement, for example, we support participants to release trigger points in the myofascial tissues, and inevitably 'more oxygen and glucose' flows 'into the muscle tissues' (Warren 2019: 18). It is particularly soft-tissue rolling in gravity that eases myofascial pain. Because there are ten times more sensory receptors in fascia, and six times more pain receptors, than found in muscle tissue, attention to our soft fascial tissues enhances proprioceptive awareness, and the release of pain (Albini 2021). Through softening, melting, releasing, or pushing and applying different degrees of force and pressure, the sympathetic charge and the viscosity of fascia can change as fluid is pushed through the cells, detoxifying and replenishing. I often, for example offer processes that help crystallized, stiff and damaged fascia into fluency, or facilitate cerebrospinal fluid to flow freely, via inviting people into initiating movement from the head–tail connection. The work is non-diagnostic, but nonetheless, still rooted in health.

Self-regulating through water-based fluency

The work invites people to move, but not functionally, robotically or mechanically. Rather, somatic movement dance supports softening, rolling, pouring, yielding, melting, easing, releasing, flowing and tissue fluency. In osteopathy and craniosacral therapy this is referred to as *motility*, which means augmenting the autonomic flow of internal fluids within the human organism (Shea 2016, 2010). I note, the fluency of our work is challenging for people new to practice or may look strange to the outside observer. Mainstream media continues to enculturate the populous into the mechanistic paradigm, propagating disembodied work-out regimes, advertising angular mechanized movement, usually sympathetically charged by speed and cardio-vascular activity.

Believing one's health relies on being corrected by an authority or is dependent on following set exercises, or rarefied poses, set out by instructors, is common. Thus, a significant difference between somatic movement and dance practices and mechanistic health is the focus on improvisation underpinned by awareness of the fluid body. In somatic studios world-wide, you can witness free-flowing, tidal, wave-like, rippling, pooling, curving and spiralling improvisational movement underpinned by sensory-perception of internal bio-flows. Improvisational spirilloid expressivity is initiated and sense–perceived from the bio-logical reality we are water-based beings (Juhan 2003).

Our fluid systems move, circulate and transform below the threshold of our awareness, but all can be enhanced by slow-time sensory-perceptual movement awareness. For example, the flow of cerebrospinal, which is approximately 99% water, can be enhanced by moving with awareness of the caudal–cranial axis (the head–tail connection). This is because the circulation of cerebrospinal fluid retains its rhythm in relation to the movement of the cranial bones (the sphenoid and occipital bones in particular), the entire vertebral column and the sacrum. Another example of augmenting fluid movement is supporting the lymph, which is approximately 95% water, to return from the periphery of the body towards the heart. This can be supported by attuning to breathing and sensing the movement of thorax, or through gentle self-touch, guiding this clear fluid from the lymph nodes back towards the heart. Another wonderful example of enhancing bodily fluids through consciously aware movement is supporting crystallized, stiff and dried out fascia to soften into fluency via soft-tissue-rolling in gravity, breaking up adhesions and resolving trigger points. Participants are supported to rest, settle, tip, pour, yield, roll, glide and slide, or compress, decompress and release their tissues into the ground with breath awareness. This starts to change the viscosity of fascia, which is approximately 70% water.

> The earth's surface and the human body are both approximately 70% water, with 97.5% of it salt water and 2.5% fresh water. Blood and most bodily fluids are salt-water based. In humans, fresh water exists in the form of cerebrospinal fluid CSF, salt-free and as close to pure water as can be found in the body [...] We are indeed part of one bio-ecosystem that encompasses us both.
>
> (Gintis 2007: 78)

We are thus a fluid microcosm reflecting the wider bio-eco system, and attending to the movement of fluids through the tissues is an integral part of self-regulation. As Gintis shares, 'Bio-logical systems are primarily fluid-based, so that most nutrients, waste products, and other things that need to be transmitted are exchanged most freely through fluid' (2007: 92), and 'water is the single most abundant chemical found in living things and water is the medium through which we stay alive, providing the liquid environment for essential functions that keep us alive' (2007: 91–92). The fluid systems are a primordial water-based part of our *being*. Examples of such fluids are:

- *circulatory flow* (venous and arterial blood)
- cerebrospinal fluid (dural tube head-tail)
- lymph fluid (throughout the body)
- synovial fluid (fluid within the joints)
- intracellular fluid (the fluid within the cell)
- extracellular fluid (the fluid around the cell)
- interstitial fluid (the extracellular fluid living outside of the blood) and
- transcellular fluid (the fluid found within epithelial lined spaces).

All these fluids are water-based. They are a vital and integral part of our being, and their flow can be encouraged by movement.

Free-flowing, non-directional, curvaceous and spirilloid fluid-based movement can be extremely challenging for the general populous, who may be used to robotic lines, yoga poses and pumping it out at the gym. Thus, self-regulation in the field, while highly efficacious, looks extremely unusual to some because it breaks so imaginatively from the mechanistic paradigm. However, it is this fluency, this water-based nature of our being that supports self-regulation in the field of somatic movement dance education therapy. Where there is stagnation, there is dis-ease. Where there is flow, there is health. Augmenting fluid flow is thus another key aspect of self-regulation in the field.

Self-regulation and the imagination

Throughout this book, you will see images where participants are dropping their awareness deeply into their sensate (through anatomical and physiological focus points and pathways) and simultaneously engaging their imagination, as they unwind and release. This is another distinctive difference between somatic movement dance education and therapy and mechanistic health. The imagination-in-movement plays an essential role in health and healing. On a physiological level, movement underpinned by the imagination supports the discovery of novel and playful neuromuscular pathways and may open and release energy through the myofascial meridians. Imaginative movement also augments the dexterity and fluidity of the skeletal–muscular system. However, the imagination is also considered a teleological guide. Often lensed through a Jungian frame, the imagination is considered the subtle bridge between consciousness and the unconscious. When we dance with the imagination, it is believed unconscious contents are expressed in symbolic form and can then be integrated into consciousness. This starts to open participants to a path that Jung called *individuation*. Individuation is, in a sense, the holy grail – a life-long process in which the psyche (including conscious and unconscious parts) seeks integration, unification, balance and wholeness. We have many dimensions of our being that need attention, care and encouragement to self-regulate, such as our inner world of emotions, and our existentiality. The high value placed on the imagination-in-movement (as a bridge to the unconscious) expressed via free improvisation is another defining feature of the field, and plays a key role in the efficacy of self-regulation.

Touch and self-regulation

Touch is used across a variety of bodywork health professions. Just as cranio-osteopaths, chiropractors and massage therapists use touch, somatic movement and dance therapists/specialists also use touch. In fact, the skilled use of touch is one of the defining features of the field. Qualified practitioners are often trained in somatic touch and bodywork processes underpinned by experiential anatomy and physiology. Touch is offered to help participants develop sensory-perceptual movement awareness, and subjective and objective anatomical/physiological knowledge. Touch is also offered to release myofascial tension and holding, and to enhance proprioceptive and interoceptive awareness. Most notably, touch soothes the nervous system and softens the fascia, and is one of the most effective ways to support self-regulation and parasympathetic release. The production of cortisol is reduced when safe touch is applied, cascading healthy chemicals through the tissues, such as oxytocin, dopamine and serotonin. Touch is offered in one-on-one practice and in community groups. Touch is used for the following reasons, greatly enhancing a client's ability to self-regulate. For example, practitioners might use touch to:

- reconnect participants to their sensory-motor feedback loop
- enhance afferent sensing and conscious efferent motor expression
- support expressivity, creativity and the imagination-in-movement
- bring consciousness to living tissues and body systems that are often beneath consciousness
- support fascial release through soft-tissue rolling and easeful motor pathways
- support skeletal-muscular alignment
- support anatomical differentiation and movement integration
- calm and balance the nervous system (reduce sympathetic arousal and support parasympathetic ease)
- teach anatomy and physiology through subjective experience and objective knowledge
- release habituated patterns of neuromuscular holding

- support movement fluidity
- connect with Self, others, and the community group through the non-verbal language of touch, dance and movement
- enhance moment-by-moment breath awareness and cardio-ception, reducing sympathetic arousal, and integrating mind and body
- offer processes that explore presence with Self and other.

(Williamson 2021: The Association for Somatic Movement Dance Therapies, UK and The Republic of Ireland)

Moving into practice: Autogenic self-regulatory improvisatory movement

In this part of the chapter, I offer one early example of a self-regulatory movement process. It is one example out of many self-regulatory processes I offer in the studio, and in this book. It is a practice-based framework that supports participants to slow-down their sensory-motor feedback loop and attend to different parts of their nervous system. This specific framework invites participants to sense–perceive and initiate self-regulatory improvisational movement attuned to different parts of their nervous system. Within this framework, I offer that participants stay in contact with the parasympathetic division of the ANS throughout the process. I have come to term this approach *autogenic self-regulatory improvisational movement.* Autogenic self-regulatory improvisational movement broadly refers to the ability of participants to bring their own nervous system into a state of balance, via learning how to shift from sympathetic arousal into parasympathetic release. Thus, autogenic self-regulatory movement invites participants to release sympathetic arousal in their tissues and sense–dwell in the peaceful nature of the parasympathetic. Key aspects of autogenic self-regulatory improvisation are:

1. The ability to move from sympathetic arousal into parasympathetic release through attending to breath awareness and cardio-ception (interoceptive awareness).
2. The ability to release sympathetic holding in the tissues via sensing where there is tension, strain and pain, and noticing how the tissues need to ease, decompress, loosen, soften, yield, lengthen – sometimes stretch, push, press and pull – and sometimes weight bare.
3. The ability to slow-down your motor response, inhibiting habitual movement pathways and through slow-time sensory-perceptual awareness find new motor pathways of ease and release.

4. The ability to attune (direct awareness) to different parts of the nervous system, such as interoception and proprioception, as well as awareness of the somatosensory system (sensing the external world touching your skin and how your internal structures and tissues touch each other within).
5. The co-regulatory presence of the witness or somatic guide, creating a holding environment of safety, sociality and peace. (I attend to this aspect of practice in Chapter 4.)

Somatic movement dance therapists often use improvisation as a catalyst for healing. Improvisation, or free movement (following your own unique movement expression) ignites the dexterity, biotensility and playfulness and of the fascial matrix and skeletal-muscular system. Improvisation opens movers to infinite movement possibilities, each person sense–dwelling in afferent sensation and sense–tracking their distinctive movements, with a wonderful array of different qualities, spatiality, directionalities, rhythms, temporalities, forces and energies. Being invited to move freely rather than following another person's body or their instructions plays a central role in self-regulation. This is because each person's body is unique. The tensions, torsions, asymmetries and pain people feel, are specific to their psyche and life journey. Working with a one-size fits all mentality does not attend to the unique life storey of each individual, or till and unpack how the exterior world has impacted their tissues and psyche. Thus, improvisation offers the unique opportunity to attend to your own tissues – to listen, respond, follow and sense–perceive how you are feeling and how you need to move (to ease-out and soften your tissues). Therefore, improvisation in the field of somatic movement not does simply mean moving your body freely to music or expressing how you feel emotionally. The following often underpins somatically orientated improvisations (this list is not exhaustive):

- sense–dwelling in breath awareness and cardio-ception (interoceptive sensing/attuning to your autonomic nervous system), slowing-down and dwelling in afferent sensation;
- inhibiting your efferent motor response, so you no longer follow habitual neuro muscular movement pathways, but rather seek new pathways of ease and release;
- following sensation as you move (sense–tracking your sensory receptors and motor pathways);
- staying in touch with breath awareness as you move through the process, and noticing how breath underlies and supports movement;
- shutting the eyes to remove extroceptive overwhelm and support interoceptive sensing;
- being led by an embodied facilitator who leads while in a parasympathetic state, languaging the improvisation while staying in touch with their own body

experience. As they lead, they also sense, feel, perceive and move with conscious awareness of Self and others. As such, the facilitator enters the sensate with the participants, toning, sounding and languaging the process through their heart and breathing tissues.

In short, for readers new this field, somatic improvisation is not simply free dance or expressive movement, but rather is underpinned by sensitive attunement to living breathing tissues. Below, I offer a process rooted in autogenic self-regulatory improvisation, unpinned by all of the above delineations. However, before we dive into practice, let us briefly take a look at the divisions of the nervous system.

Directing awareness: Interoception, gravi-ception and proprioception

The western divisions of the nervous system are extremely useful, even though they are undoubtedly reductive because they do not work discretely. However, we can support participants to experience different aspects of their nervous system through sensing and initiating movement from specific tissues. The nervous system comprises *the* CNS, which includes the brain and spinal cord. All the nerves that extend beyond the geography of the brain and spinal cord, via the cranial nerves and the spinal nerves together form *the* PNS. The PNS system is divided into *the* SNS and *the* ANS. The ANS is further sub-divided into *the sympathetic* and *the parasympathetic* divisions, together forming the ANS. Often people are dissociated from their ANS, their SNS and their somatosensory system (sense of touch), not realizing that all these parts of the nervous system can be attuned to through sensory-perceptual movement play, in turn, healing degrees of sensory-motor amnesia, inviting integrative wholeness.

The areas of the nervous system that inform the practice-based process below are the following.

Exteroceptors

Exteroceptors receive information from the external environment, through touch, sight and smell, for example. Shutting the eyes removes the exteroceptive visual sense and reduces exteroceptive overwhelm. Shutting your eyes and attuning to interoception (the ANS) begins to invite the nervous system into homeostasis.

Interoceptors

Interoceptors receive stimuli from the ANS and tell you about your internal state (if you are stressed or if you are calm). Interoceptors are sensory neurons that bring information back to your brain, so you can perceive the internal state of your ANS. These sensory neurons are located in your organs and blood vessels. Interoceptive awareness is absolutely vital to self-regulation because sensing your breath, heart and diaphragm, in particular, invites the autonomic nervous to shift from sympathetic arousal to parasympathetic release. Interoceptive awareness involves sense–perceiving *afferent* information streaming into the central nervous from the ANS. Sense–dwelling in your heart and breath, for example, contacts sensory neurons and receptors in your organs and blood vessels.

Proprioception

Proprioception is part of the SNS. Proprioceptors receive stimuli from skeletal-muscles, tendons, joints and the inner ear. Proprioceptive awareness, especially when combined with parasympathetic release, supports ease of movement in the fiberous, cartligenous and synovial joints. Proprioceptive awareness involves sense–perceiving information streaming into the CNS from your joints, muscles and inner ear, in particular.

Gravi-ception

Gravi-ception is the ability to sense–perceive the earth's gravitational pull and explore the earth's ground reaction force; the latter is the delightful equalizing force that counter-balances your weight, force and movement. The continuous smooth surface of the studio floor plays an essential role in gravi-ception, offering a fulcrum to release your weight and reorganize painful and sympathetically charged tissues. Gravi-ceptive play, while maintaining good vagal tone (staying in contact with interoception), offers incredible release as participants tip, pour, roll, yield, and glide and slide across the floor for long periods of time.

The somatosensory system

The somatosensory system contains an extraordinary array of sensory receptors that help you feel touch on the surface on your body, and indeed how your internal tissues and structures are touching each other. The somatosensory system underlies all the other senses, and thus developing an attuned relationship with how the world is touching you, how you touch yourself within, and how you touch the world underlies self-regulation. Being touched soothes the CNS because the skin is empirically explored as the outmost layer of your CNS.

Diving into practice: Sensing interoception and visceroception

The two divisions of the ANS, the sympathetic and parasympathetic, are particularly significant in autogenic self-regulatory improvisation. These divisions are the extensive topic of Chapter 2, but for now I would like share early that innervating the parasympathetic is absolutely vital for the recovery of a stressed and sympathetically charged nervous system (Power 2020). These two divisions offer an incredibly clear framework enabling participants to shift from stress and tension, to ease and release. The sympathetic division is often referred to as *fight-or-flight* because this part of the ANS responds to danger and keeps you safe. In contrast, the parasympathetic is often referred to as the *rest-and-relax* or *rest-and-repair* response, because this part of the autonomic nervous system re-balances you after a period of stress. Sometimes the ANS is referred to as the involuntary nervous system because it is remarkably busy regulating the body beneath our conscious awareness. The ANS regulates our digestive system, breathing, heart and blood vessels, bladder, genitals, exocrine glands and adrenal glands, for example.

Our bodies are often riddled with stress. Sympathetic stress creates dysfunctional and often painful neuromuscular patterns and pathways. I call this *sympathetic holding in the tissues*. Sympathetic stress is caused by overactivity (excitement) in your sympathetic nerves. The sympathetic nerves exist on either side of your vertebrae between T1 and L2 (in your thoracic and lumbar spine). The sympathetic division neurologically extends far beyond the vertebral column, expanding out into your thorax and abdomen, arms and legs, affecting the heart, blood vessels, solar plexus and many other organs. When these nerves become over-excited, the body is preparing you to fight or flee. When you are in danger or feel unsafe, your sympathetic division does all it can to save you. In this way, your sympathetic division is a very protective part of you. When the sympathetic chain is activated your heart rate and breathing changes because your heart has to work much harder, delivering more oxygen and blood to your muscles, preparing you to run or fight (Rosenburg 2017).

Participants (including me) are often highly stressed when they arrive in the studio. Their (my) muscles are often tense, their mobility is impaired and they are disconnected from breath. This is a clear indication the body is sympathetically charged. Perhaps their job has given them little time to rest and breathe, or perhaps they are carrying childhood or institutional trauma, which has sympathetically charged their body for years, perhaps decades. All of us carry stress, which is multidimensional; usually there is more than one stressor in our lives. One of the best ways to ease sympathetic holding in the tissues is to lie down on the floor and actively release into gravity, shut your eyes, rest, settle and breathe. Moving your awareness away from your exteroceptive sense (the external public world of seeing and hearing), to your interoceptive sense (your internal private world of sensing and feeling) is the first stage of self-regulating an over-sympathetically charged nervous system. The simple act of lying down and closing your eyes stops information from the exterior environment over-whelming your nervous system. Interoceptive awareness supports people to release sympathetic over-charge (Porges 2017; Rosenburg 2017). In the studio, participants are invited to listen and sense–dwell in afferent information streaming in from the sensory neurons in their organs and blood vessels. This is most easily achieved via sensing the tissues of cardio-respiration, particularly the heart, lungs, thorax and diaphragm. Lying, softening, resting and easing your tissues in gravity with breath awareness further invites your myofascial tissues to release sympathetic arousal (Williamson 2020a, 2020b, 2020c).

Interoceptive awareness, especially sense–dwelling in breath, innervates the vagus nerve (Rosenburg 2017; Williamson 2020c). The vagus nerve is the topic of Chapter 2, but here I would like to share that the vagus nerve is the longest parasympathetic nerve, and it plays a vital role in helping you to re-balance your nervous system after a period of stress. It emanates from your brainstem, moves out of your cranium and down into nearly every organ in your body. We know scientifically that sensing breath, shutting the eyes and developing interoceptive awareness innervates the vagus nerve (Rosenburg 2017). When the vagus nerve is engaged, less oxygen needs to get to your muscles, so your heart rate slows and your breathing regulates.

Most participants that attend sessions have a degree of sympathetic arousal – a catabolic expenditure of energy has dominated their life, sometimes for decades. Often people express burnout, tiredness and lethargy. In such cases, the sympathetic branch of the autonomic nervous is in over-drive. The last thing a somatic movement practitioner should do is invite participants into catabolic movement expression – this may serve to create more sympathetic arousal in their tissues. Thus, all good practice, I suggest, should initially invite people to shift from *sympathetic holding* into *parasympathetic release*.

In the studio, the parasympathetic is invited into living awareness, so participants can learn to reduce tension, balance asymmetries and ease pain in the mysofascial tissues. Slowing down in the studio, when combined with conscious awareness of breath and afferent sensing (attuning to the sensory neurons in your viscera), invites the parasympathetic to override the sympathetic (Rosenburg 2017; Power 2020). The parasympathetic will usually override sympathetic arousal and dysfunction, especially if the therapist has also calmed her nervous system and produced a safe holding environment (Williamson 2020c).

Thus, the first stage of autogenic self-regulatory improvisation in the studio is inviting participants to sense–dwell in afferent information streaming into the

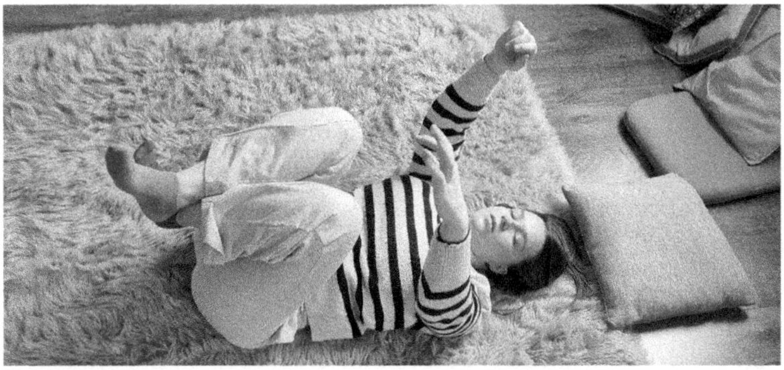

FIGURE 1.1: Natasha Martin: releasing into gravity and dropping into interoceptive awareness. Photographer: Amanda Williamson.

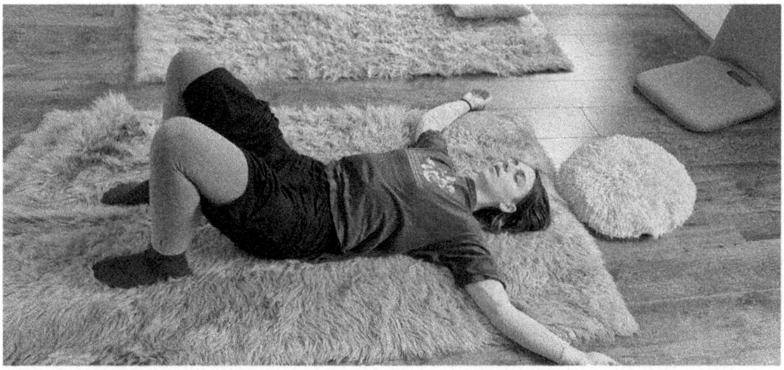

FIGURE 1.2: Jessica Cotton: releasing into gravity and dropping into interoceptive awareness. Photographer: Amanda Williamson.

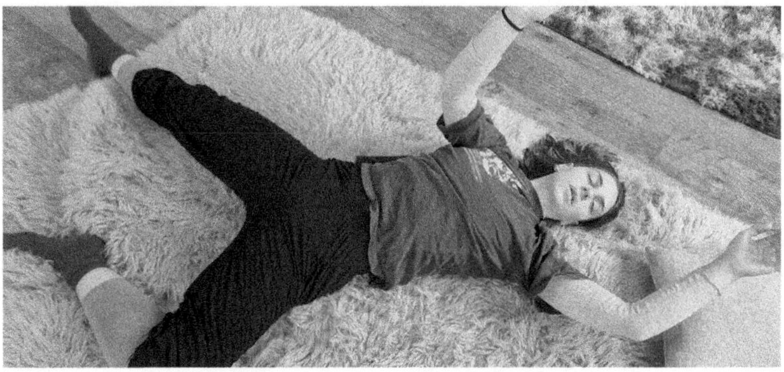

FIGURE 1.3: Jessica Cotton: sense–dwelling in interoception. Photographer: Amanda Williamson.

CNS through their viscera, particularly their heart and breath. This is referred to as interoception or sometimes visceroception. In contrast to receiving sensory information from your muscles, joints and inner ear, interoceptive awareness is the sensory-perceptual ability we have to listen to stimuli arising from within. Interoceptive awareness is extraordinary because it tells you immediately about your internal state, especially if you are stressed or calm.

In contrast to the sympathetic chain, parasympathetic nerves emanate from your brainstem. These nerves are called *the oculomotor nerve*, *facial nerve*, *glossopharyngeal nerve* and *vagus nerve*. At this point in our study, their names are not as important as their location. Note they emerge from the brainstem in your cranium. You also have parasympathetic nerves that emerge from your sacral region, specifically S 2 3, 4. Note then, the caudal–cranial (head–tail) axis is the delightful location of your parasympathetic nerves, which by their nature invite peace, restitution and calm. In order to innervate the parasympathetic at the beginning of sessions I invite participants to,

- close their eyes, removing exteroceptive overwhelm;
- rest in gravity, softening, loosening, curling and uncurling, and relaxing their tissues, easing out sympathetic arousal;
- bring awareness to their breath, particularly the movement of breath in the thorax and diaphragm;
- explore and cultivate moment-by-moment breath awareness, supporting presence;
- bring awareness to the living tissues of their heart;
- initiate movement and stimulate the parasympathetic nerves located in the caudal–cranial axis; softening and easing the cranial bones, and all along the vertebral column to the sacrum.

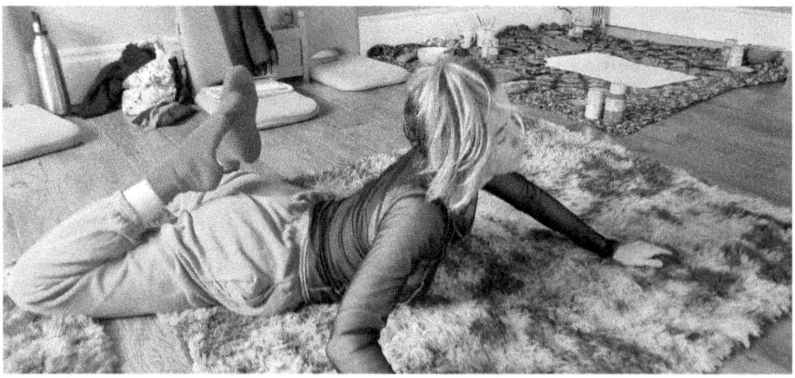

FIGURE 1.4: Sylvia Gregory: sense–perceiving the caudal-cranial. Photographer: Amanda Williamson.

Gravity the healer: Gravi-ceptive awareness

Autogenic self-regulatory improvisation always starts in gravity. Gravity and the continuous smooth surface of the studio floor offer themselves to our well-being. The studio floor is the finest fulcrum we have to reorganize our tissues. By fulcrum, I mean a pivotal place around which body tissues can be reorganized. Sometimes tissues call to be compressed so they can decompress. At other times tissues call for lengthening, reaching, expanding and stretching. Often tissues call for rest – asking for softening, loosening, melting and yielding. The floor is a continuous horizontal fulcrum which offers itself to you so completely. You can pivot, tip, pour, roll, yield, push, reach, pull, lengthen, soften, squeeze, ripple and undulate along the floor. As you sense–perceive your tissues desires you can release sympathetic holding and augment fluency. The floor is always there, inviting you to self-regulate. Self-regulatory gravitational play is extremely nutritious for all your tissues. There are multiple reasons why developing a sense–perceived relationship with gravity enhances well-being. Gravitational processes are offered throughout this book because when we release our weight into gravity and reorganize the mass of our tissues along the floor, the stress of being vertical and sympathetically charged can soften and liquify. Tension, strain and pain can be eased by softening, loosening, melting and relieving the tissues. If you sense your nociceptors (pain) calling, notice how these sensory receptors desire different qualities, pressures, tempos, energies and forces to ease and dissolve pain. Inviting participants to follow pathways of comfort, pleasure and fascial unwinding is key to self-regulation – movement that feels delicious.

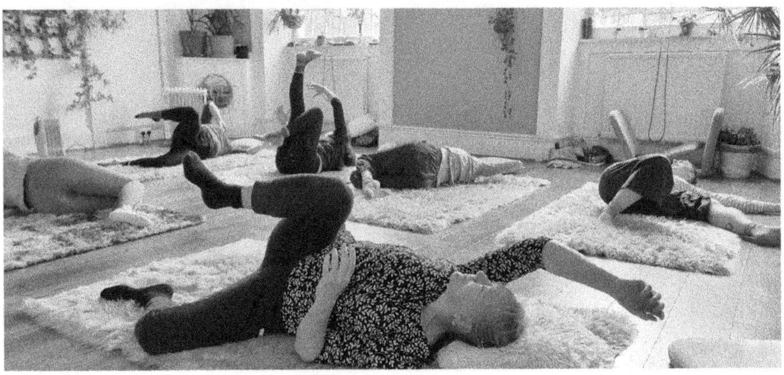

FIGURE 1.5: Karin Rugman and movingsoma students: using gravity as a fulcrum to ease-out tissues. Photographer: Amanda Williamson.

When we lie down and release our weight, we have a fantastic opportunity to release the sympathetic suffering held in our tissues. On the one hand, we can let go and sink into gravity, releasing, softening, melting, yielding and surrendering to the earth's gravitational pull. The earth calls, 'you belong to me'. On the other hand, the earth's ground reaction force, which matches your weight and force exactly, meets you – balances you – supports you. The earth says, 'go forth'. These complimentary forces have shaped us from infants to adults. They are a constant and always there. Usually beneath conscious awareness, we invite participants to sense–perceive these forces, so they can feel the earth's call (which offers release and embrace) and the support of the earth (which is integral to our biological imperative to become vertical and our movement across the earth's surface and out through space).

The uncomplicated act of lying down in the studio might appear simple, yet it is the most powerful friend we have to support self-regulatory tissue re-organization. When we lie down at night, we often go to bed with intense neuromuscular holding. The day's stress and tension, as well as accumulations of neuromuscular anxiety that may have built up over years, sometimes decades, fall into bed with us. Thus, the act of lying down in bed does not necessarily resolve the many torsions, twists and tensions accumulated in the body in vertical waking life. Mattresses are soft and often made to emulate weightless. Integrated health is dependent on yielding into and pushing away from gravity. Thus, building an active relationship with gravity is vastly different from sinking into a soft mattress.

In somatic movement modalities, such as the Alexander Technique, posture and alignment is often corrected while standing (not always). Certainly, it is effective

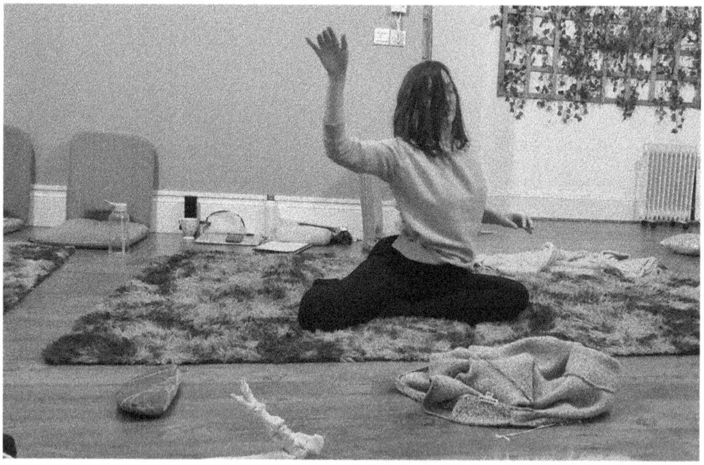

FIGURE 1.6: Louise Furmenge: sensing her proprioceptive Intelligence. Photographer: Amanda Williamson.

to use touch in a vertical plane to support realignment. In other modalities, such as my own, far greater emphasis is placed on surrendering one's weight and mass into gravity, to reorganize fascial restrictions. Curling, uncurling and extending and lengthening our tissues, as well releasing hypertonic asymmetries influences our posture and alignment in the vertical plane. In terms of our midline, the vertebral column is under the constant pull of gravity. As Thomas Hanna so beautifully notes, as we stand tall and face the world, we often hyperextend or somatically collapse (Hanna [1973] 1993). All humans have the innate desire to stand. Verticality is a mark of our humanness. However, people's extensor muscles often become riddled with tension through hyperextension. Other people somatically collapse with lack of tonus in their flexor muscles. Surrendering into gravity offers participants the opportunity to repattern 'hyperextension' or 'somatic collapse'. Hanna points out the biological imperative to become vertical is not a neutral process as we grow from infants into adults. Our standing is enculturated, often stressed, tense and thus distorted. The way we stand reflects how we feel about the world and simultaneously how the exterior world has infringed and patterned our standing – thus somatic distortions in our alignment and posture often reflect the crushing pressures and stresses we feel in our lives. In gravi-ceptive play we surrender to the earth with eyes closed specifically to let go of the exterior world, and the many ways culture and society has pathologically disturbed our alignment. Gravi-ceptive play is an invitation to repattern our antigravity reflexes (so intent on standing tall). Gravitational play invites hyperextension in the neck and back to soften, and/or lack of tonus in the flexor muscles to build, find strength and integrity.

There are many ways to bring support to the vertebral column, but I note, unwinding in gravity is a superb way to realign. Uncurling, reaching and stretching, and curling, folding and softening in gravity for example, enables participants to unwind tension in their sympathetic chain (T1–L2). Gravitational sensing offers participants the opportunity to sense and integrate their concave curves (the cervical and lumbar regions) and their convex curves (the thoracic and sacral regions). Realigning, through curling and uncurling, with attention to both the primary and secondary curves is a superb way to bring sensory awareness to the vertebral column and repattern alignment. When you invite participants to furl and unfurl, or spiral in and spiral out, the convex and concaved curves start to move as a fluid continuum. Here we are working specifically with the integration of the cervical, thoracic, lumbar and sacral regions, which are often misaligned or segmented. Through attuned curling and uncurling participants can release holding in the cervical–thoracic junction (C7–T1), the thoracic–lumbar junction (T12–L1) and the lumbar–sacral junction (L5–S1). These are junctions where weight is transferred from one area of the spine to another, but they often become junctions of stress and misalignment. Resting in gravity, the load is reduced on these junctions.

The load is also reduced on every joint in the human body (the cartilaginous, synovial and fibrous). The intervertebral disks also have the opportunity to replenish in gravity; throughout the day these disks lose water. Working in gravity for long periods of time soothes and nurtures the intervertebral disks that are under the constant pull of gravity (Williamson 2020b).

Yielding and softening in gravity in a supine and/or prone position, and then gently pushing, tipping, pouring, rolling and surrendering your body weight and mass across the floor (for long periods of time) offers participants the incredible

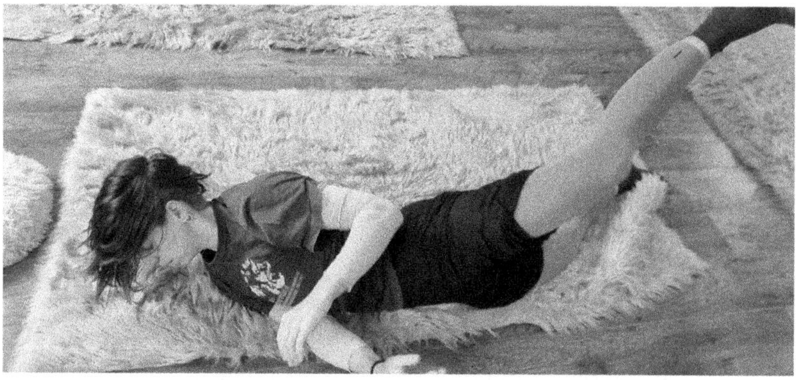

FIGURE 1.7: Jessica Cotton: curling and uncurling. Photographer: Amanda Williamson.

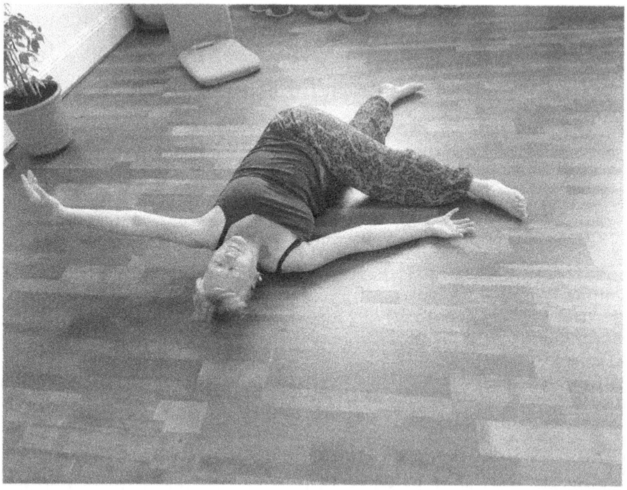

FIGURE 1.8: Karin Rugman: sensing the integrative fluency of the vertebral column. Photographer: Amanda Williamson.

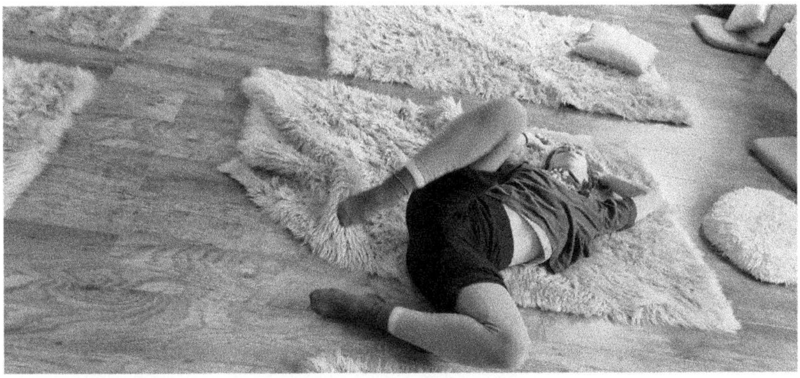

FIGURE 1.9: Jessica Cotton: sensing ease after curling and uncurling. Photographer: Amanda Williamson.

experience of sense–perceiving 'the omnipresent and omnipotent' presence of gravity. In the somatic movement/dance field gravity is generally approached with great reverence. Thomas Hanna went as far as to say,

> Gravity is, if you will, the universes nearest approximation to what theologians might call an immanent deity: namely a God that is universal, ubiquitous, law-giving, and all powerful. I think it quite impossible to conceive of the incredible nature of gravity without entertaining a quasitheological concept.
>
> (1993: 103)

Augmenting gravity's great law of swirling objects or mass via circles and spirals is something one can witness in somatic studios world-wide. Thus, we often invite participants to explore movement that spirals away from gravity and then releases back into gravity. Movers are experientially playing with the non-linear law of gravity. We also purposely invite participants to tip off balance, surrendering their weight into gravity, but then notice the power of the *labyrinthine righting reflex*. As soon as the body tips off balance the vestibular system corrects the head. Participants are being invited to play with (1) The omnipresence of gravity and (2) the biological imperative to be vertical. Participants are learning to balance two opposing forces that have shaped their organism from infanthood to adulthood, the earth's gravitational pull and the somas biological drive to stand tall.

When you invite participants into gravi-ceptive play, quite intuitively and instinctively, participants start to yield and push or reach and pull. In doing so, they are enacting and revisiting two early *ontogenetic* developmental patterns: *yield and push* and *reach and pull* (Hackey 2002). Equally when participants

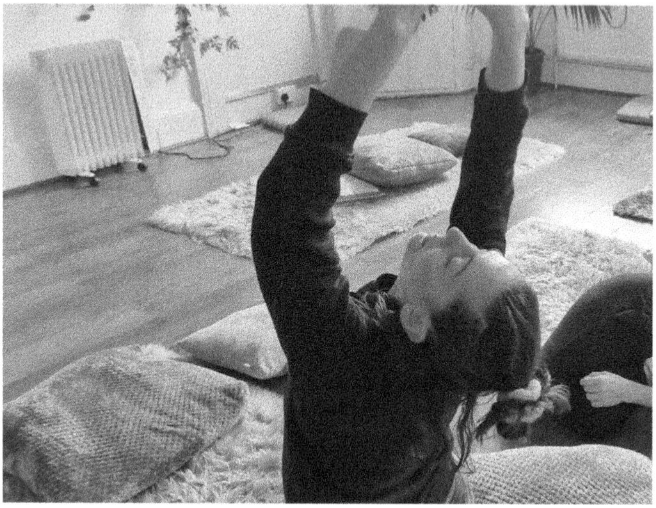

FIGURE 1.10: Louise Furmenger: sensing proprioception: Photographer: Amanda Williamson.

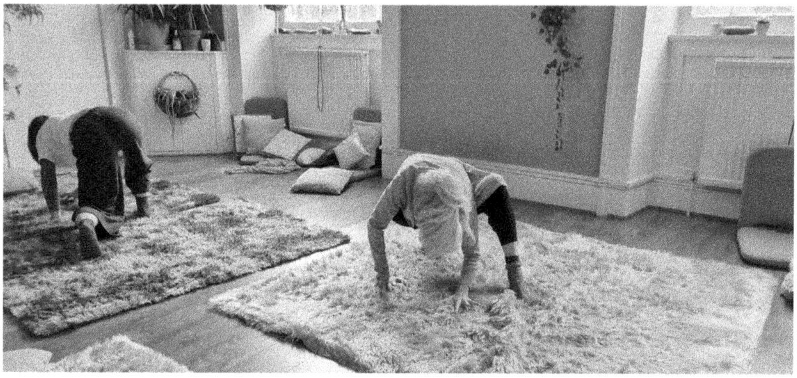

FIGURE 1.11: Movingsoma students: pushing away from and compressing into gravity. Photographer: Amanda Williamson.

are invited to sense–dwell in the fluid body (focusing on breath and the organ system), *phylogenetic* movement patterns often appear (Cohen 1993). Participants frequently start to undulate, swell, surge, squeeze, ripple and wave through their fluid body. All of these early developmental movement patterns are essential to self-regulatory health. In autogenic self-regulatory improvisation, I offer it is essential to stay in contact with the parasympathetic nervous system, attending to interoceptive awareness and breath as you yield, push, tip, pour, roll, soften, dissolve and liquefy. This keeps your tissues relaxed and offers greater release and fluency.

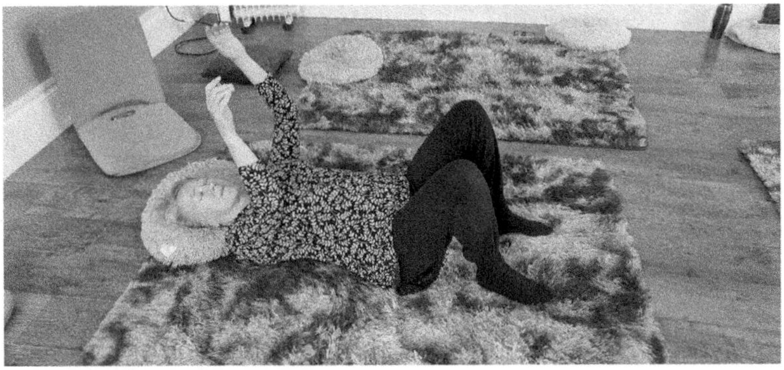

FIGURE 1.12: Karin Rugman: sensing proprioception, and floating her synovial joints. Photographer: Amanda Williamson.

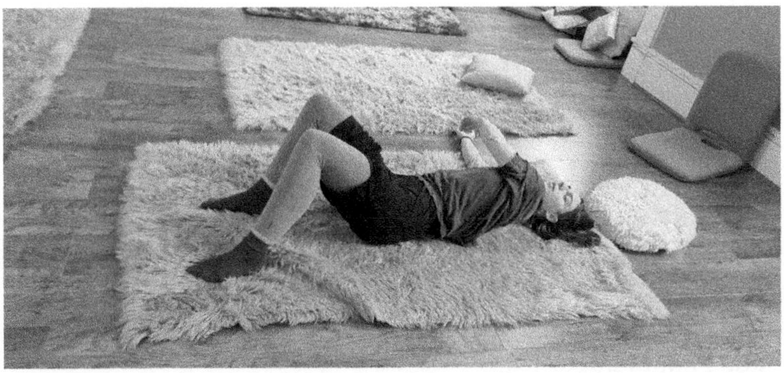

FIGURE 1.13: Jessica Cotton: soft-tissue rolling her scapulae in gravity. Photographer: Amanda Williamson.

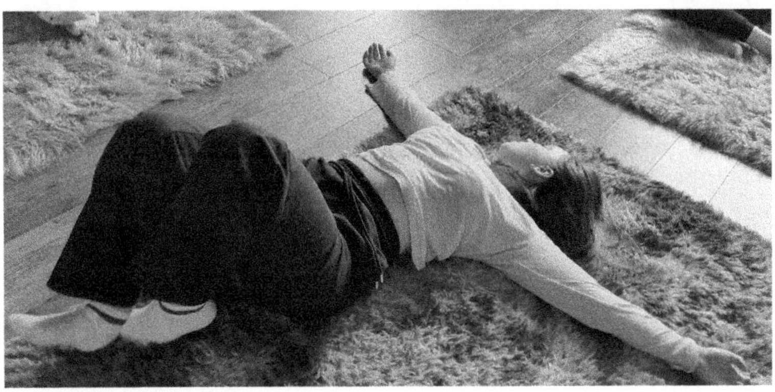

FIGURE 1.14: Movingsoma students supporting each other to surrender into gravity. Photographer: Amanda Williamson.

Gravity and the somatosensory system

Gravi-ceptive play also stimulates the *somatosensory system*. The somatosensory system contains a wonderful selection of sensory neurons and neural pathways that respond to touch on the surface of your body (your skin), and within the skeletal–muscular and organ system (how your internal structures are touching each other). This is an extensive and vast network of nerve endings, and these touch receptors enable us to sense–perceive an extraordinary range of sensations, as well as vibrations. We usually associate touch with touching others, or being touched in somatic movement work, but gravitational play also offers the experience of being continuously touched by the floor as you roll across every surface of your body. When we receive touch from the floor, we can begin to integrate the somatosensory system into our awareness.

Inviting participants to receive and enjoy the floor's touch is particularly soothing for the brain. In somatic literature, we often read, when we touch the skin, we are also touching the brain. It is incredibly important to note that the central nervous and the skin develop out of the same primitive tissues, called *the ectoderm*. In somatic literature, we note how the skin is experienced as the outmost layer of your CNS. Thus, when your skin is touched, your CNS is touched (Juhan 2003: 35). When we invite participants to soft-tissue-roll in gravity, sensing the floor touching their skin or explore how their internal structures are touching within, we are inviting them back to their first language of growth, development, enfoldment and emergence. Touch underlies all the senses and is a vital element of self-regulation (Sumner and Haines 2010: 19).

When I facilitate gravi-ceptive play, I invite participants into a combination of the following, and always with breath awareness and interoceptive sensing underlying the process. I invite participants to:

- Sense breath moment-by-moment as you move or dwell in *stillness*.
- Sense–perceive the earth's gravitational pull and ground reaction force.
- Use the floor as a fulcrum to rest, push, pivot, press, soften and yield – following delicious, nutritious pathways of ease and release.
- Play gently with different pressures, compressions and decompressions (sensing your internal structures touching), and your tissues touching the ground.
- Gently furl and unfurl, spiraling throughout the vertebral column, easing the cervical–thoracic (C7–T1), thoracic–lumbar (T12–L1) and lumbar–sacral junctions (L5–C1).
- Sense skin being touched by the floor, and on every surface of the body.
- Sense lengthening, contracting, stretching, reaching, pulling and expanding.

- Explore spirals, curves, waves, ripples and undulations throughout the vertebral column and soft fascial tissues in the organ body.
- Tip off balance, release into gravity and sense the labyrinth righting reflex.
- Integrate the atlanto-occiptial, cervical, thoracic, lumbar and sacral-tail vertebrae into fluency through curling and uncurling, with gravi-ceptive and cranial-caudial awareness (delineated in the next chapter).

Sensing proprioception

When participants have contacted interoceptive awareness, moved into parasympathetic release, loosened and softened in gravity, you can further invite a shift in sense–perception to proprioception. Proprioceptors are found throughout your body, in your inner ear, synovial joints, tendons and the muscles, for example. Proprioception tells us where we are in space, the relationship between our body parts, and indeed how we are moving through space. We have different proprioceptors, for example, *muscle spindles*, embedded in our muscle fibres, as well as *Golgi tendon organs*, found in muscles and tendons. We also have joint receptors, called *mechanoreceptors* found in our joint capsules. Therefore, proprioception invites you to sense–dwell in your joints, muscles, tendons and inner ear. Proprioception is often unconscious because sensory-perceptual processing happens so fast, and with such complexity, we barely notice these extraordinary proprioceptors supporting and guiding us through the world.

In contrast to interoception, we can bring proprioception into conscious awareness, offering sensory-perceptual improvisations unfolding and expressing with awareness of muscles and joints. Attuned sensory awareness with the central, proximal and distal joint system, is the easiest way to support proprioceptive awareness. Of note, proprioceptive awareness is best brought to consciousness when participants have dropped into *parasympathetic release* and with heightened gravi-ceptive awareness. If you try to bring proprioceptive awareness to a sympathetically charged nervous system in the vertical plane, the potential to find ease and release in the joints, and loosening, lengthening and softening in the myofascial tissues is highly compromised. Noted earlier, gravit-ceptive play reduces the load placed on every joint in the human body, as well as every muscle. Thus, contacting proprioception lying down and floating the long bones and joints, offers the opportunity to decompress all the joints and sense their fluid nature. Inviting the synovial joints to open and decompress is particularly soothing.

Proprioception is part of the somatic nervous system and thus described as under our conscious control. And it is, to a degree. However, we must

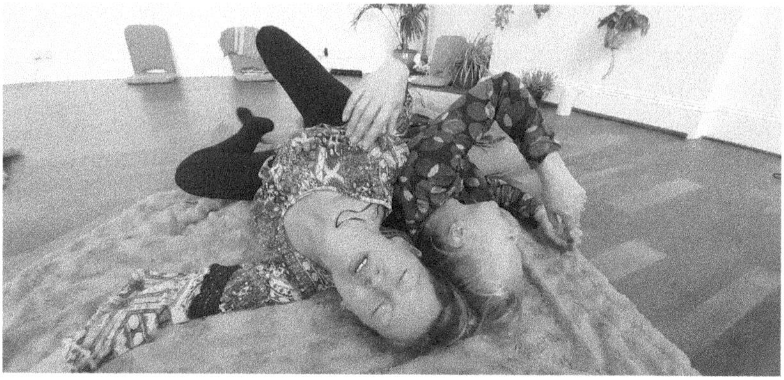

FIGURE 1.15: Amanda Williamson and Karin Rugman: sensing gravity. Photographer: Scott Closson.

note, this part of the nervous system also falls beneath conscious awareness. The somatic nervous system is riddled with habits, many dysfunctional. While we can consciously direct movement through our SNS, enculturated sensory amnesia has created a great distance from our playful, creative and dextrous somatic nervous system. Sensory-motor amnesia means we have not only lost contact with sensory receptors (our ability to be in the sensate) but also our conscious ability to be present and direct movement through our motor neurons. Proprioceptors are an extraordinary part of our being, full of both sensory receptors and motor nerves. Sensory receptors, often called afferent, give us our ability to sense, feel and perceive. Motor neurons, called efferent, give us our ability to move, to express, to direct and motor out with conscious awareness in the world. Bringing conscious awareness to proprioceptive intelligence develops an intimate and coherent relationship with one's sensory-motor feedback loop. Through proprioceptive play, we can attune to the incredible ability we have to not just sense and feel our bodies moving through space, but also our ability to make conscious choices about how, where and what to move, and with what quality, temporality, spatiality, energy and force.

Proprioception often feels delicious. Proprioceptive attunement can be electrifying, vivifying and illuminating, as well as pooling, trickling, watery and fluid. Dwelling and sense–tracking movement within your synovial joint system, tendons and muscles is a beautiful way to feel your body again, especially if you have suffered years of dissociation. However, I note, attuning to interoceptive and proprioceptive awareness simultaneously is particularly profound. Moving with ease and restitution further loosens the joints and

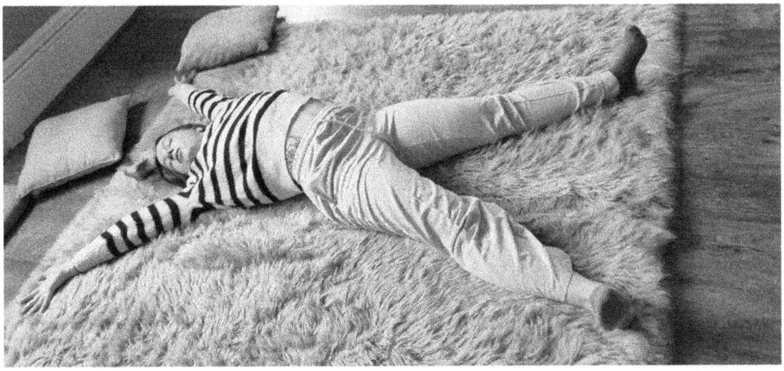

FIGURE 1.16: Natasha Martin: sensing proprioception and interoception. Photographer: Amanda Williamson.

softens the skeletal-muscular system. Thus, another stage of self-regulation is slowing down enough to sense and feel the living presence and intelligence of proprioception, with interoceptive awareness underlying the process. Proprioception is often referred to as the sixth sense (Eddy 2017). It is a profound intelligence full of illumination. When we contact our sensory receptors and motor neurons with our eyes shut, our proprioceptors become our eyes. In sessions, I invite participants to

- to move with proprioceptive awareness, but simultaneously with interoceptive sensing underlying the process (awareness of breath and heart);
- move with gravi-ceptive awareness and awareness of breath, initiating gentle movement from their distal synovial joints;
- move with gravi-ceptive awareness and awareness of breath, initiating movement from their proximal synovial joints;
- move with gravi-ceptive awareness and awareness of breath, initiating movement from their central joint system, the cartilaginous and synovial joints in the vertebral column;
- move with gravi-ceptive awareness and conscious awareness of breath, sense–perceiving their fibrous joints in the skull (the sutures). Soften the weight of cranium into gravity, gently tipping and pouring the weight of the cranium from side-to-side;
- sense–perceive and listen to the proprioceptors in the inner ear. Notice how the inner ears become the eyes when we move with eyes shut;
- initiate movement from the distal, to the proximal and to the central joints, and back out again from the central, to the proximal, to the distal joints

(integrating the central, proximal and distal joint system is vital to integrative health);

- move awareness to soft myofascial tissues, lengthening, reaching, expanding, stretching, softening and folding;
- move between eyes open and eyes shut, integration exteroception, with interoception and proprioception.

Supporting participants to sense–perceive different parts of their nervous system helps them attune to their sensory-motor feedback loop and integrates different parts of the nervous system. Maintaining awareness of heart and breath supports vagal tone and innervates the parasympathetic throughout the process, offering ease and restitution. Cultivating moment-by-moment breath awareness supports the healing power of presence. Working in gravity for long periods of time and reorganizing the tissues through autogenic self-regulatory movement releases sympathetic holding and supports realignment. This is just one example out of many self-regulatory processes offered in the studio.

Key offerings and learnings

Before we move into the next chapter that deepens the concept of self-regulation, let us remember some key aspects of self-regulation discussed so far. Below is a list of key learnings and offerings. Many elements listed below will be built on as we move through the book and revisited in more detail. Self-regulation is offered through the following processes, concepts and principles:

- Self-regulation requires integrating mind and body. Mind is invited to turn its gaze from outer to inner, settle awareness in breath and sense–perceive the life-force inspiring and expiring.
- Self-regulation is underpinned by breath awareness – breath awareness is the bridge between mind and body. Breath awareness supports participants to experience *presence*. Presence supports participants to let go of past worries and fear about the future (even if only momentarily).
- Self-regulation involves bringing conscious awareness to autonomic processes that normally function below the threshold of everyday awareness, such as breath awareness and cardio-ception.
- Self-regulation involves augmenting motility (the free-flow of fluids within the body), attuning to the water-based reality of our being.
- Self-regulation is dependent on cultivating the ability to sense, feel, perceive and move with consciousness awareness. Thus, the concept of self-regulation

is synonymous with developing a conscious relationship with the sensory-motor feedback loop.

- Self-regulation involves attuning to afferent sensation, slowing down, inhibiting the habitual motor response and consciously choosing efferent motor pathways of ease. Thus, inhibiting the habitual motor response is a key aspect self-regulation.
- Self-regulation involves listening to our living tissues, noticing where and how pain is expressing and then reorganizing our tissues into a state of ease and balance through slow-time sensory-perceptual movement awareness.
- Attuning to the ANS through breath and cardio-ception is a key aspect of self-regulation. This slows the heart rate and regulates breathing, and engages the vagus nerve.

When I first came to the studio, the doctor had diagnosed me with myelofibrosis. My life for over 3 years has deteriorated and I am frightened. The pain makes me feel weak, and I feel I have no strength in my bones and muscles. I just couldn't believe I could attend a therapy where I was allowed and invited to move while lying down in the floor, and for ages. Moving in gravity and getting the fluids in my body to move and my joints to ease is very special to me now. I feel my breath and tissues, and then invite my body to follow a pathway that feels good – sometimes really good. A pain-pleasure thing starts to arise. What a simple thing. My pain hasn't gone, but I have found a way to invite the pain to subside and I notice a reduction in pain for about three days. I sometimes just rest in breath for ages and then might make a few simple movement responses. What a simple thing. I have learned about my body, my joints and fascia and new ways to ease myself in gravity. I think my spine is so much healthier from playing in gravity and all my joints feel more fluid. After these sessions I know my lymph has moved. This also reduces the pain in my arms. It is the pressure into gravity, and decompression that helps my pain.

(Rosie Nevins)

2

Sympathetic Holding and Parasympathetic Ease-and-release

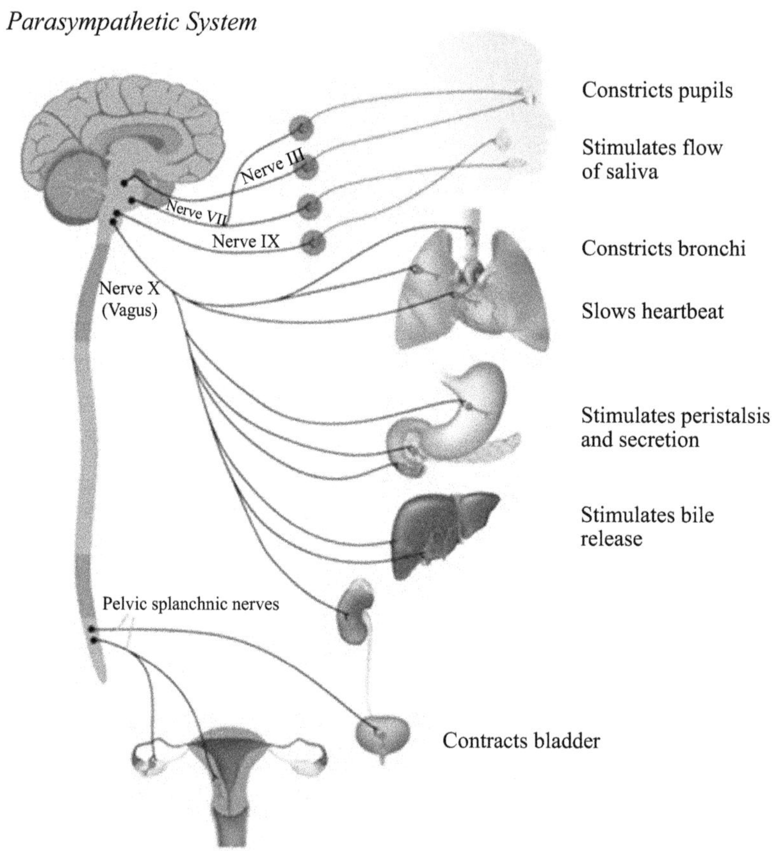

FIGURE 2.1: The vagus nerve.

Lying, settling, sensing ground
Bodies broken. Hard bones.
restrictions. tight shoulders
grounding, I sense a trickle of breath
Life Pushed Down
Suffocated
Life Sucked Out
I reflect I am drunk with tiredness, drinking stress.
Slammed Pushed Compressed
Rung-out and drinking fear
Grief fills my cells
Tears salty dry rivers

Shaking, I open my eyes.
I see you, tending to your pain
I hear your breath
You begin to breathe me

Thickly tight breath
expanding a little
two BIG breaths.
Bellow within.
Filling. Enlarging. Breathe me
I begin to make a home within
'Come home says my diaphragm,
you have been gone so long. Where have you been? I am also lonely without you'

(Eve O'Rafferty, reflective writing, after moving)

In Chapter 1, we explored the concept of self-regulation broadly, and the many unique aspects of practice that support self-regulatory health. Part of this chapter focused on autogenic self-regulatory movement and the importance of supporting participants to ease their tissues, sense peace and rest in sensory awareness. In this chapter, I take a detailed look at the parasympathetic and sympathetic divisions of the autonomic nervous system (ANS), deepening anatomical and physiological theory shared in Chapter 1. This chapter is rich in anatomy and physiology, exploring the vagus nerve, the craniosacral and thoracic–lumbar divisions of the ANS, and information about Polyvagal theory, the new vagus and social engagement. I have presented this knowledge in a stimulating and digestible way, weaving theory and practice throughout. As such, this chapter enhances and magnifies areas presented in Chapter 1. Throughout I offer detailed processes that help participants to balance their nervous system.

When I facilitate and transmit information about the ANS, with clients and students, I cover the following areas in theory and practice:

- The vagus nerve and its long journey through our living body tissues.
- The geography of the sympathetic and parasympathetic divisions of the autonomic nervous system, sometimes referred to as *the craniosacral* and *the thoracic–lumbar divisions.*
- The cranial nerves.
- Polyvagal theory.

In a world of high stress and incredible trauma, what is more important than developing somatic agency? By somatic agency, I specifically mean, intellectual knowledge and a set of embodied skills that reduce stress, support ease and bring balance to living tissues. My hope is, this chapter supports students, practitioners and lecturers to find more ease and enjoyment in their lives, as well as bring compassion to their journey, which may be fraught with long-term and daily struggles. A further aim of this chapter is to support detailed facilitation processes and provide inspiration for those working in both higher education and independent contexts.

When participants attend a session, without exception, they express stress and pressure – and usually some degree of pain. Life is pressured and people are stressed. Pressure comes from all angles, often leaving people in a state of chronic sympathetic holding, or sometimes what is referred to as *a dorsal shutdown state.* Societal and cultural values that cause dissociation, as well as institutional, familial and childhood trauma, socio-economic pressure, stress at work and the strain of parenthood all impact the body. Organisms can only take so much pressure; people start to implode, shut down, retract, fall apart and, at worst, feel crushed. There have been many times in my life where I felt overwhelmed by work pressure, cut off from my body, sympathetically stressed – and edging towards fight-or-flight. Like many people I work with, I have felt devastated by life's curve balls, broken and deeply shocked. Suffering is a very real aspect of human life.

The human organism is responsive and quick to respond to stress. Unfortunately, stress directly affects the endocrine system, which surges and cascades chemicals through the glands, upsetting the ANS. After a period of stress, ideally the ANS should return to a state of balance. However, the constant pressure that people are under tends to create fear, in turn, arousing the sympathetics. As noted in Chapter 1, this means the sympathetic branch of the ANS remains habitually over excited. Sympathetic excitation expresses in all our tissues – in our glands, fascial tissues, skeletal–muscular and vascular systems. Peter Levine refers to this as *global high activation*, pointing to how the populous on mass are enculturated into sympathetic charge (2008). Stephen Porges calls this 'faulty neuroception', emphasizing how our societal institutions are not safe, causing dysfunction in the cranial nerves and the ANS (Porges 2017). Porges iterates, through his exquisite research, the importance of feeling safe, which enables the ANS to regulate. The importance of feeling safe in the somatic studio is a key theme in this chapter.

Given the pressure people are under, I have dedicated a great deal of time empirically investigating through practice-as-research how to support people to rebalance their ANS through self-regulatory movement. The therapeutic processes I offer in the studio vary, and many are offered throughout this book. In this chapter, I specifically share vagus nerve engagement, which calms and soothes the body – and notably for anyone in pain, engaging the vagus nerve reduces inflammation (Henton 2020). Inflammation is the main cause of pain and thus the processes presented in this chapter are of paramount importance to anyone in pain. I will also attend to the sensory stimulation of the cranial nerves, many of which support the ventral branch of the vagus nerve to enliven into a state of health (Porges 2017). Additionally, I share how to innervate the craniosacral division (the parasympathetic) and release stress and strain in the thoracic–lumbar division (the sympathetic). All these areas are key to restoring balance, managing pain and reducing fear and anxiety.

The parasympathetic started to interest me when my clients started to report reduced pain and an incredible sense of well-being after class, often expressed in a surprised jubilant manner upon leaving the studio (packing up their stuff with smiles on their faces). After many years of practice, working with students in university contexts and the general public, I came to realize that the most effective somatic movement is reliant on what I have come to broadly call *parasympathetic ease-and-release*, which softens and eases sympathetic holding in the tissues, enabling participants to return to a state of balance.

Participants are often surprised that a bottom-up feeling therapy can create such change, and not just physically, but emotionally. Many participants who attend sessions are used to cortico-centric approaches to healing and therapy. These are top-down therapies that prioritize mind, language and cognition. In short, top-down therapies use talking. Noted in Chapter 1, while language and verbal dialogue play a vitally important role in somatic movement sessions, the body comes first. Talking about problems certainly offers relief, but it is important to remember that trauma, stress, anxiety and depression damage our physiology. If you are depressed, stressed, afraid and anxious, your vagus nerve is likely to lack strength and potency (Francis 2020). Additionally, the sympathetic division of your ANS is likely to be in overdrive. Thus, in order to support healing, I invite participants to sense–perceive and move with conscious awareness of their vagus nerve, and their *craniosacral* and *thoracic–lumbar divisions*.

Noted in Chapter 1, somatic movement sessions often start in gravity. I usually invite participants into gravitational processes for well over 30 minutes. With very experienced groups, I often work in gravity for an hour. Gravity is a superb healer and possibly the best fulcrum (and friend) we have to reorganize our tissues, release sympathetic holding and realign our bodies.

Gravity, breath and self-regulatory movement, together, engage the parasympathetic division of the nervous system, release sympathetic holding and improve vagal tone (Williamson 2020a, 2020b).

This chapter shares how to do this. I have divided this chapter into nine sections to share micro-physiological details that underlie and inspire somatic movement dance processes oriented to vagal health and parasympathetic release. The nine sections are the following:

1. the intelligence of the ANS
2. the traditional divisions of the ANS: the sympathetic and parasympathetic
3. the cranial nerves
4. sense–perceiving the journey of the vagus nerve
5. sense–perceiving the geography of the craniosacral and lumbar–thoracic divisions
6. releasing sympathetic holding in the vertebrae through somatic touch
7. polyvagal theory
8. immobilization without fear: a deep parasympathetic release
9. open-hearted social engagement: the ventral vagus.

The intelligence of the ANS

The ANS plays a vital role in our physiological, emotional and mental health. Our thoughts, emotions and the exterior environment directly impact the ANS. The ANS continuously responds to our experience of the exterior world, and markedly, also, our inner world of thoughts and emotions. Our thought patterns and emotionality invest themselves deeply in our neurochemical, cardiovascular and skeletal–muscular systems. Very often, our emotions and thoughts become repetitive, expressing and firing through habitual neuromuscular pathways. Does this sound familiar? Stressful thoughts, emotions and fear release chemicals that increase sympathetic holding, while peaceful thoughts and emotions release chemicals that increase parasympathetic ease (Lipton 2015). When you are stressed, the hypothalamus, pituitary and adrenal glands are all involved in a hormonal cascade that flows through your nerves and associated tissues. This is referred to as *the hypothalamic–pituitary–adrenal axis*. In short, the *hypothalamic–pituitary–adrenal axis* prepares you for fight-or-flight, or indeed gives you enough energy to carry out a physical or demanding task. When you burn out, you can be sure your *sympathetics* have been overactive; this is true for many people who have survived for years in extremely demanding, fearful and stressful situations. For our purposes in this chapter, it is important to note that the *hypothalamic–pituitary–adrenal axis* controls levels of cortisol, as well as other stress-related hormones. When it is overactive, sympathetic charge excites all the interrelated living systems in our body.

It is thus our tiny glands that create the chemical torrent that causes sympathetic arousal in our body. Of note, the endocrine system works so closely with the nervous system, the skeletal–muscular and the cardiovascular system that it is extremely hard to write about the endocrine system discreetly. The endocrine system is extremely sensitive. Many of its glands are so small that 'it is hard to imagine they do anything at all' (Wiley 2016: 19). To paraphrase Wiley, this could not be further from the truth because the glands are major energy centres, supporting homeostasis, affecting all your nerves, tissues and blood vessels. The glands of the endocrine system support our well-being below the threshold of awareness. Many are concerned with keeping you safe and thus are highly responsive to fear.

Fear and stress enter our system as soon as the limbic brain and the amygdala start signalling to the hypothalamus that the environment is dangerous or unstable. This initial signal is followed by a cascade of chemicals that surge through your glands and body tissues, moving you into fight-or-flight, or sympathetic arousal. Thus, fear and stress are embodied at the get-go and flood through our *tissues*. There are four body systems involved in sympathetic arousal: glands, nerves, muscle tissues and blood vessels. Because stress and fear are embodied, it is often hard to resolve biochemical and neuromuscular patterns through talking therapies alone. Fear is thus deeply visceral, expressed in our chemicals, hormones, tissues, blood, muscles and nerves. Bringing awareness to these tissues and learning how to ease and soothe them are the key to the art of self-regulation.

The sympathetic part of the ANS is sometimes referred to as *the sympathoadrenal response*. It fires into neuromuscular expression to keep you safe, responding to threats in the external environment. Our health is severely compromised by the external world, our responses to the external world and our emotionality. For example, when we are stressed, upset or frightened, there is increased activity in the sympathetic part of the ANS. Our muscles may become tense and tight, and our *cardiac plexus* and the *coeliac plexus* may become overactive and overstimulated. If a person is continuously upset, depressed, anxious and afraid, sympathetic expression becomes habituated, leading to chronic sympathetic holding, or sometimes what is referred to as a dorsal vagal shutdown state (Porges 2017). My point being, stress and anxiety do not manifest and express in mental thoughts alone, dissociated from the visceral body. Stress and anxiety manifest in our living tissues. The link between our response to the external world, our inner world of emotions, and the health of the ANS has been researched and documented by many scientists who have a keen socio-cultural, spiritual and political awareness (Dispenza 2012; Pert 1997; Lipton 2015).

In somatic movement dance sessions, we work sensitively and gently with living tissues, through touch, movement and sound, inviting the ANS to rebalance.

The traditional divisions of the ANS: The sympathetic and parasympathetic

> The autonomic nervous system (ANS) is one of the most significant systems in human function. It plays a vital role in maintaining life supporting organs such as the heart and lungs, as well as all the viscera. It is one of the principal networks linking the physical body with our emotions and our psyche. It is significantly involved in the majority of health disturbances. It is actively participating in every moment of our lives and is an essential factor in our ability to respond to circumstances from moment to moment in everyday life.
>
> (Attlee 2012: 365)

In Chapter 1, we noted that the ANS was traditionally divided into two parts called *the sympathetic* and *the parasympathetic*. We noted that the sympathetic is often referred to as *fight-or-flight* because this part of the ANS responds to danger and keeps us safe. In contrast, the parasympathetic is often referred to as the *rest-and-relax* or *rest-and-repair response*, because this part of the autonomic nervous rebalances us after a period of stress. Notably, the parasympathetic is deeply restful and has a spiritual quality; when the *parasympathetic is engaged*, people's muscle tonus softens, the heart rate slows and feel-good chemicals are produced that help them to feel relaxed (Attlee 2012; Rosenberg 2017; Lipton 2015). When we sense into the parasympathetic division, we often feel a peaceful life-energy regulating our being that brings us spaciousness, relaxation, peace and release.

With the advent of Polyvagal theory, the two divisions of the ANS were overturned and are now considered rather outdated and reductive. However, the two divisions of ANS are especially useful to share in the studio with students, because they provide a clear framework for participants to sense and perceive how they are moving through the world. 'Am I moving catabolically, expending a lot of energy in my life, feeling fearful, utterly exhausted and burned-out?' Or, 'am I moving through life in a soft relaxed anabolic way, feeling calm, conserving energy and feeling safe?' From a therapist's perspective, I note with compassion, that most participants (and I include myself) arrive in the studio with some degree of sympathetic arousal. Fear and anxiety can dominate people's lives, sometimes for decades. In fact, we can go a whole lifetime in a predominantly sympathetically aroused state. Many people arrive with tight muscles, tense shoulders, and sometimes their mobility is impaired. Many express burnout and myofascial pain. Because of this, it is vital to initially invite people to shift gently from a sympathetic state into parasympathetic release. And, I add, this process can be observed world-wide, when somatic movement dance practitioners invite participants into gravitational play, breath awareness and free-flowing movement that loosens the myofascial tissues. Before we dive into more anatomical detail about the parasympathetic, I offer some lucidly useful quotes below. Observe in the quotes, how the two divisions of the ANS have clear locations in the geography and landscape of your body. This geography is extremely useful to map in therapeutic practice and is integral to this chapter.

> The parasympathetic is 'primarily concerned with vegetative processes. This division is anabolic, meaning that it builds up and conserves resources'.
>
> (Attlee 2012: 365)

> The nerve fibres that innervate your parasympathetic division are located in your cranium and sacrum. Coming into sensory awareness with the parasympathetic can be initiated by softening the cranium in gravity (releasing the tissues around the sub-occipital triangle, sensing breath, and initiating slow-time movement from your caudal-cranial axis (this is referred to as the cranio-sacral division).
>
> (Williamson 2020c: 202)

> The sympathetic is 'primarily concerned with responses to the environment (including responses to stress). This division is catabolic, meaning that it uses up or expends resources'.
>
> (Attlee 2012: 365)

> The nerve fibres that innervate your sympathetic division are located between T1 and L2 in your vertebral column. In studio practice it is extremely helpful to release holding in the spinal nerves exiting your thoracic and lumbar vertebrae.

> Unwinding tension and discharging energy held in these nerves and throughout your vertebral column and limbs (neck/cranium) invites sympathetic holding to resolve.
>
> (Williamson 2020c: 202)

Attlee shares, 'in our pressurised modern society', the

> two divisions are often set against each other, creating conflict and dysfunction – for example, 'eating a rushed meal under pressure of work, or living under persistent pressure and stress, leading to exhaustion of the ANS and confusion and malfunction of both divisions'.
>
> (Attlee 2012: 372)

He further notes that sympathetic arousal and stress manifests physiologically in many other body systems, such as

- in the organs – as indigestion, ulcers, asthma, irritable bowel in the nerves – causing overstimulation, potentially affecting in and around all the body systems
- in and around the vertebral levels associated with entry and exist of the nerves – leading to facilitated segments
- in the muscles of the back surrounding the associated vertebral levels – leading to back pain
- in the central nervous system – leading to disturbed function in the psycho-emotional state – leading to agitation, anxiety, irritability and exhaustion.

(Attlee 2012: 372)

The cranial nerves

When I introduce the parasympathetic nervous system, I share the cranial nerves first. Many participants are inspired, if not a bit shocked, to learn that exploring their parasympathetic nervous system means learning about and attending to their cranial nerves through self-regulatory movement play. Note that the cranial nerves are located in your cranium and many of them (not all) start from your brainstem. Thus, releasing the weight of the cranium (and the tissues around the sub-occipital triangle) and sensing into the occipital bone and brainstem underlie engagement with the parasympathetic in my practice. You have twelve pairs of cranial nerves that are an integral part of your peripheral nervous system. These nerves are incredibly important and related to your survival (and our survival as a species). They are involved in searching for food, seeing food, smelling, tasting,

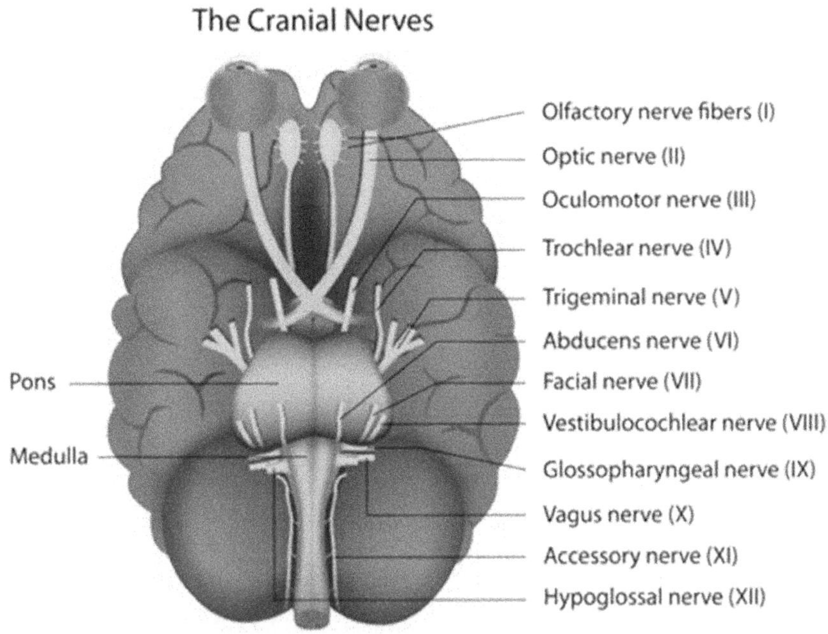

FIGURE 2.2: The cranial nerves.

chewing and hearing, as well as sociality, communication, safety and balance. For clarity, I have listed the twelve pairs of cranial nerves in detail below, sharing Rosenburg's superb work. As you read, notice how all these nerves are related to your survival.

Wandering

> The Vagus nerve is 'one of the cranial nerves' that 'wanders through the body, coursing from the brainstem into the chest and abdomen to regulate many of the visceral organs. It innervates the muscles of the throat (pharynx and larynx), and the organs of respiration (lungs), circulation (heart), digestion (stomach, liver, pancreas, duodenum, small intestine, and the ascending and transverse sections of the large intestine), and elimination (kidneys).
>
> (Rosenburg 2017: 7–8)

Smelling for food

The Olfactory nerve enables our sense of smell (CNI). 'The fibres of CNI originate in sensory organs of the nose and have a direct pathway to the forebrain'. 'In terms of evolution' the olfactory nerve 'was the first cranial nerve to develop' [...] 'The sense of smell is vital to human beings and all other mammals; it is crucial in first finding food and then discriminating whether a morsel is edible. Smells create an immediate response of attraction or repulsion – does my mouth water when I bring a morsel closer, or do I turn my head away in disgust?'

(Rosenburg 2017: 9–10)

Aiding our vision

The Optic nerve CNII, aides our vision and thus also helps us find food. This nerve originates in the forebrain, specifically the telencephalon and diencephalon. 'It transmits signals from rods and cones in the retina of the eye to a synapse, and across that synapse to the visual centres in the back of the (occipital) lobe of the cerebral cortex. The brain interprets these nerve impulses into what we see'.

(Rosenburg 2017: 10)

Finding food and moving our eyeballs

The oculomotor nerve CN III, the trochlear nerve CN IV and the abducens nerve CN VI work together and control the movement of our eyeballs. 'These allow us to roll our eyes up, down, right or left.' Note, these nerves are also involved in finding food.

(Rosenburg 2017: 10)

Expanding our field of vision with an articulate neck

The spinal accessory nerve CN X1 'controls the trapezius and sternocleidomastoid muscles. These muscles move our head so that we can look up, down, and to the sides. This allows our search for food to include bringing a morsal closer to smell it, and, if it does not smell good, to turn our head away'. As Rosenburg notes, the spinal accessory nerve helps us to find food because it 'expands our field of vision' as we extend and move our neck.

(Rosenburg 2017: 10)

Eating and mastication

The Trigeminal nerve CN V, The Facial nerve CN V11, and the Glossopharyngeal nerve CN1X, all 'innervate the salivary glands' and thus are involved in eating. For example, the trigeminal nerve innervates 'the muscles of mastication, opening and closing the jaw and grinding the food with a side-to-side movement'. The glossopharyngeal nerve moves 'our tongue to shift the food around in the mouth, and on and off the surfaces of our teeth'. The facial nerve 'relaxes and tightens the muscles of the cheeks, creating a pouch for the food and emptying it to move food back onto the grinding surfaces of the teeth'.

(Rosenburg 2017: 11)

Tasting and swallowing

'For the actual tasting of food, we use the taste buds on the tongue, which connect to branches of three cranial nerves: CN V11 (the facial nerve), CN IX (the glossopharyngeal nerve), and CN X (the vagus nerve).' We swallow food with muscles in the throat that are innervated by CN IX, the glossopharyngeal nerve, and tongue muscles innervated by CNX11, the hypoglossal nerve, as well as other muscles innervated by CN V and CN V11.

(Rosenburg 2017: 11)

Hearing and regulating the ear muscles

The Acoustic nerve (CNVIII) is obviously to do with hearing; however, as Rosenburg further notes, 'in mammals, the trigeminal nerve (CN V) and facial (CN VII) nerves also have important roles to play in listening and in understanding human speech by regulating the middle-ear muscles'.

(Rosenburg 2010: 12)

You can playfully explore the health of all these nerves, especially by bringing gorgeous and different types of food into the studio, placing the food in different locations and inviting the students to see, smell, move towards and choose what to eat – and eat. While the students are choosing, eating and sharing, communicate how the nerves above are all involved in our survival. However, the cranial nerves that are the focus in this chapter are the:

vagus
facial nerve
glossopharyngeal
trigeminal
and the spinal accessory nerve.

Some of these nerves make up the craniosacral division of the parasympathetic nervous system, such as *the facial nerve*, *the glossopharyngeal nerve*, *the vagus*, and *the oculomotor nerve*. Others together stimulate the ventral branch of the vagus nerve, such as *the vagus*, *facial*, *glossopharyngeal*, *trigeminal* and *accessory nerve*. But let us start by exploring the vagus nerve, the longest and most extraordinary nerve in the parasympathetic division of the ANS.

Sensing-perceiving the journey of the vagus nerve

> Our nervous system is made up of about 100 billion nerve cells, which releases information from the brain to the body and vice versa. The vagus nerve is one of the most critical command centers responsible for bi-directional communication between the brain and the body. A nerve probably 90% of the population have never heard of or have no clue of its location, nor how powerful this nerve is to the human body.
>
> (Henton 2020: 17)

The vagus nerve is the longest nerve in your parasympathetic nervous system. It plays a central role in regulating bodily functions, such as heart rate, breathing and mood, and reduces inflammation (the main cause of pain) (Power 2020; Richard 2020). The vagus nerve carries a range of signals back from your digestive system and other organs to your brain and vice versa. Thus, there is communication between your brain and your gastrointestinal tract through the vagus. The vagus nerve extends all the way from your brainstem down your neck, into your thorax and down into your abdomen. This wonderful winding nerve is predominantly afferent (it is a deeply feeling nerve, bringing a wealth of information back into your central nervous system). This exceptionally long nerve wanders through your tissues and touches nearly every organ in your body – and so, we find the word vagus, from Latin 'to wander'. Note that the vagus nerve is innervated by breath awareness and good diaphragmatic breathing. Thus, breath awareness underlies all the processes I offer in this chapter and throughout the book.

While the path of the vagus is extremely complex, below is a little of its journey:

> The vagus nerve originates in an older part of the brain, called the brainstem. Specifically, the vagus nerve originates in the part of the brainstem called *the medulla oblongata*. Sensing into the brainstem just behind the occipital bone is vital in studio practice, supporting participants to sense the emanating location of this nerve. I invite participants to move their attention away from their neocortex and frontal lobe into their brainstem, just behind their occipital bone.
>
> The vagus nerve weaves out of the medulla oblongata and leaves the skull through *the jugular foramina* (discussed in more detail in Chapter 3). The jugular foramina are two small holes between the occipital bone and temporal bones. Hence, bringing awareness to the occipital bone and temporal bones, as well as the brainstem supports participants to sense–perceive the early part of the vagus nerve's long journey through the body.
>
> Of note, the vagus nerve travels together with *the accessory nerve* and *the glossopharyngeal nerve* within *the carotid sheath*, along with *the internal jugular vein* and *common carotid artery*. Thus, I offer that unwinding the soft tissues in the neck

(particularly releasing *the sternocleidomastoid* and *the trapezius*) further supports participants to sense–perceive the long journey of the vagus nerve.

Wandering down into the neck on both sides, the vagus nerve also innervates most of the muscles of *the pharynx* and *the larynx*. Hence, releasing the jaw and oral cavity, softening in the mouth, and sounding/toning, helps participants to sense–perceive the journey of the vagus nerve.

Continuing, and moving into the thorax, the cardiac branches of the parasympathetic nerves supply the heart. When the vagus nerve is engaged, noted earlier, there is often a reduction in the heart rate. Therefore, in practice, sensing into the thorax and the heart further invites participants to sense–trace their vagus nerve.

Moving on, the vagus nerve penetrates the abdomen via the oesophageal hiatus. Sensing the diaphragm also brings awareness to the vagus and its amazing journey through the body - breathing with conscious awareness also stimulates this nerve.

As it moves into the belly, vagal branches regulate the abdomen, the stomach, oesophagus, and the small and large bowel. Moving into the intestines, the vagus nerve continues regulating the smooth muscles. Inviting participants to feel and breathe into their abdomen is particularly efficacious in terms of bringing the vagus nerve into sensory awareness. Soft-tissue rolling onto the belly, and breathing deeply into the organs of digestion helps us to sense the vagus nerve.

It is fascinating and enlivening to share with participants that the vagus nerve starts from the brainstem, behind the occipital bone, and travels all the way to the abdomen, touching and bringing health to nearly every organ in the body. Because this nerve is so vital to our health, I offer processes that help participants to sense–perceive the living presence of this nerve and its journey through their body. The process offered on pages 54–58 is a slow-time gravitational process, encouraging participants to sense where this nerve lives and travels through the landscape of their body. Note that the order of the process below is a guide, highlighting the path of the vagus. It can be developed and adapted, of course. I acknowledge that each somatic movement/dance practitioner is uniquely creative, and noted in the introduction, the ingenuity of each practitioner continues to develop the field. In the process below, I explore specific areas of the vagus nerve more than once. When you are facilitating, it is more effective to move down and up the vagus nerve, and any combination in between, rather than offer a linear journey from top to bottom only. For readers new to this field, note the photographic example is short; in the studio, this process would last for 30–45 minutes. This work does not offer quick-fix exercises, but rather slow-time explorative sensing, perceiving, and moving, supporting incremental shifts towards well-being, developed via daily practice.

Example of practice: Sensing-tracking the journey of the vagus nerve in gravity

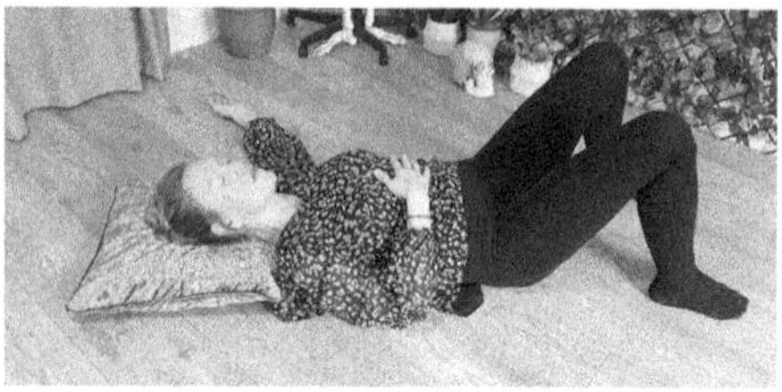

(a)

Rest your tissues and bones in gravity, releasing your weight. Settle into ground (earth) inviting your mass and tissues to spread. Invite your eyes to close. Enjoy landing, resting and settling in bones and soft tissues.

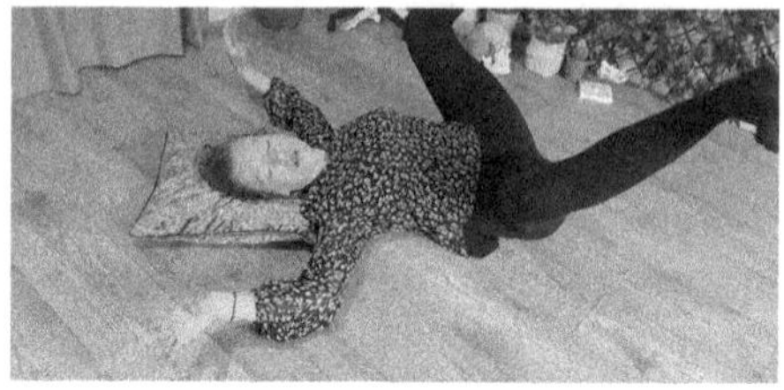

(b)

Bring awareness to your brainstem, living and breathing behind your occipital bone. This is where the vagus nerve starts its journey. Invite your cranial bones to relax. Release and soften the tissues all around the sub-occiptial triangle.

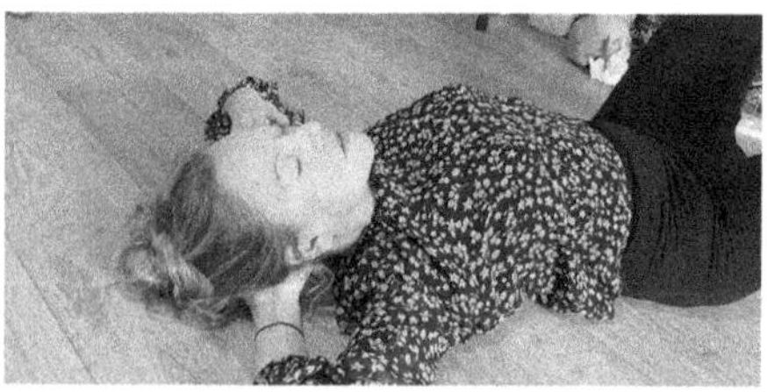

(c)

Move your attention away from the neocortex and posteriorly into your occipital bone. The brainstem lies approximately behind the base of the occiput.

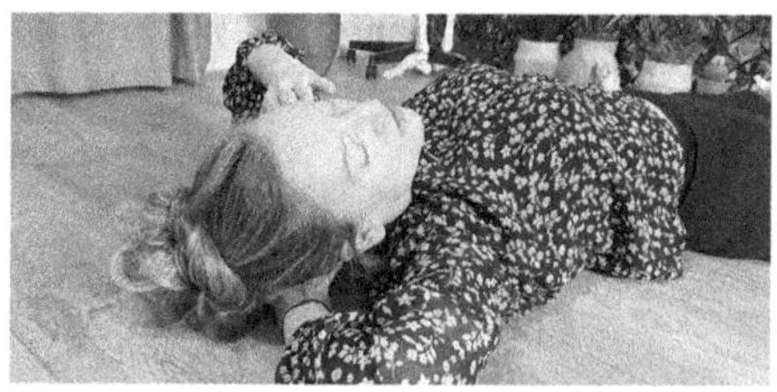

(d)

Bring awareness to breath and sense–dwell in your occipital bone. Invite participants to rest their occipital bone in the palm of one hand, and follow how the occipital bone wants ease, yeild and release.

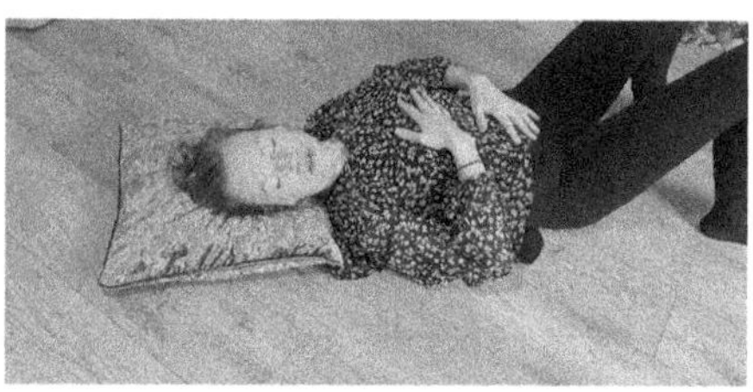

(e)

Notice how the diaphragm breathes you. Invite the diaphragm to take space, moving within you. Relax your oral cavity and throat, noticing breath passing into the pharynx and trachea.

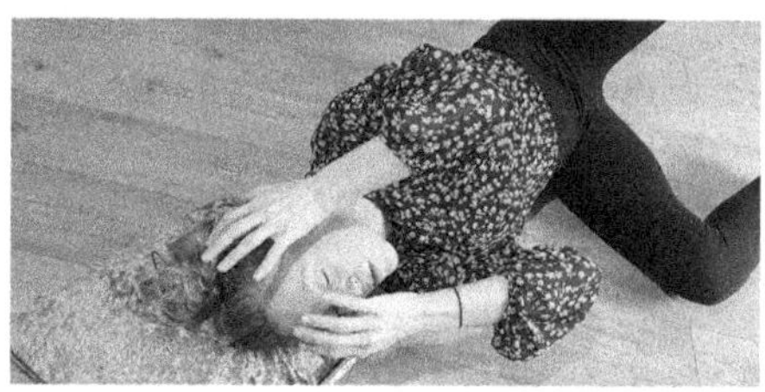

(f)

The vagus nerve also weaves down into your larynx (voice box). Invite any type of sound, tone, or sigh to emerge from sense–perceiving your oral cavity and larynx.

FIGURE 2.3A–R: Amanda Williamson. Photographer: Scott Closson.

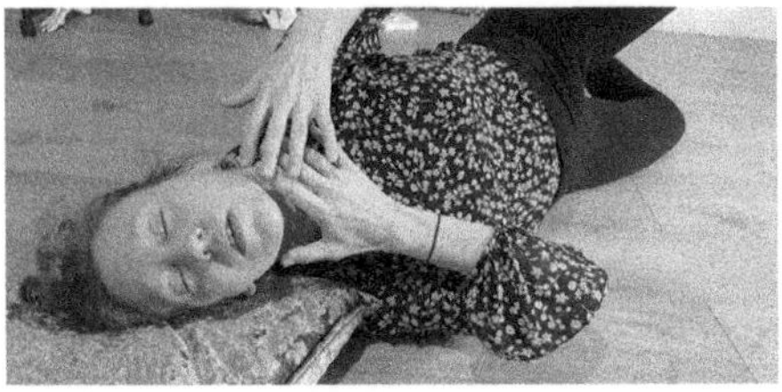

(g)

Release the weight of the cranium, gently pouring the weight of your head from side-to-side, moving off the occipital bone onto the temporal bones or parietal. Remembering the vagus moves out of the cranium through the jugular foramina (two small holes between your occipital bone and temporal bones). Invite the soft tissues of your neck to soften, melt and unwind. Soften the tissues around the suboccipital triangle. The vagus nerve makes a pathway down into the soft tissues of your neck along with the accessory nerve.

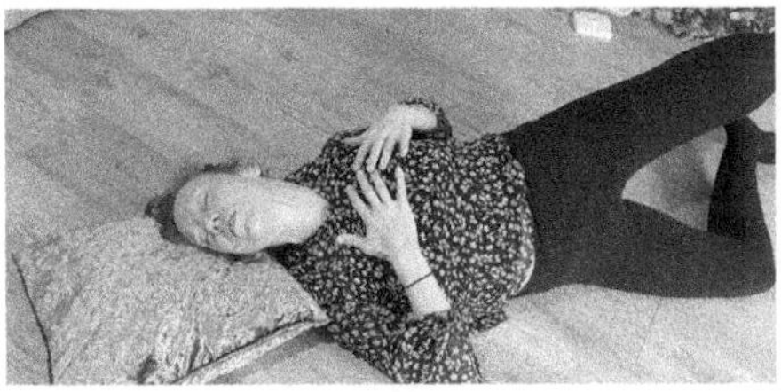

(h)

Sense–perceive your heart with breath. Place one hand on your heart space. The cardiac branches of the vagus nerve supply the heart. Sensory awareness of the heart stimulates a reduction in the heart rate.

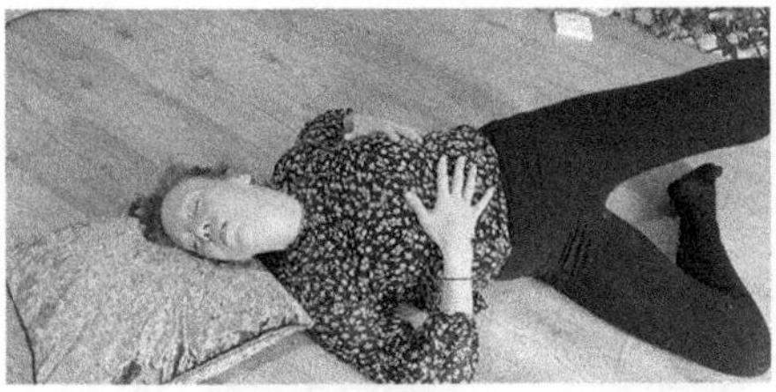

(i)

Sense–perceive the gentle flow of breath, inspiring your tissues. Bring one hand to just below your ribcage, where the diaphragm attaches. The vagus nerve penetrates the abdomen via the oesophageal hiatus. Invite the diaphragm to take space within you; notice how much space the diaphragm loves to take.

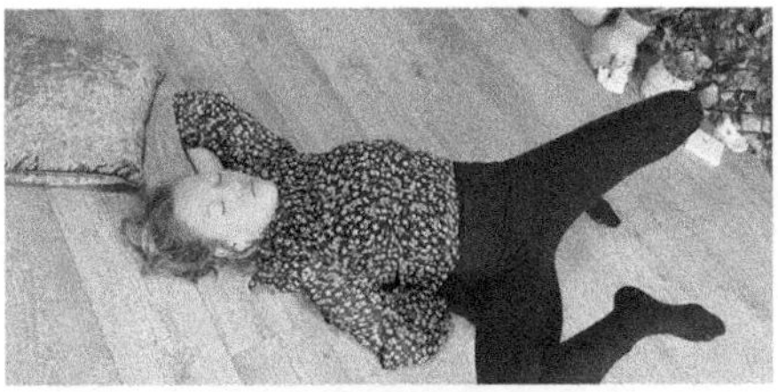

(j)

Continue to soften and release the tissues in your neck with breath awareness; invite the sternocleidomastoid and the trapezius to release and soften. Remember, the accessory and the vagus nerve travel together; they are sometimes viewed as the same nerve.

FIGURE 2.3A–R: Amanda Williamson. Photographer: Scott Closson. (*Continued*)

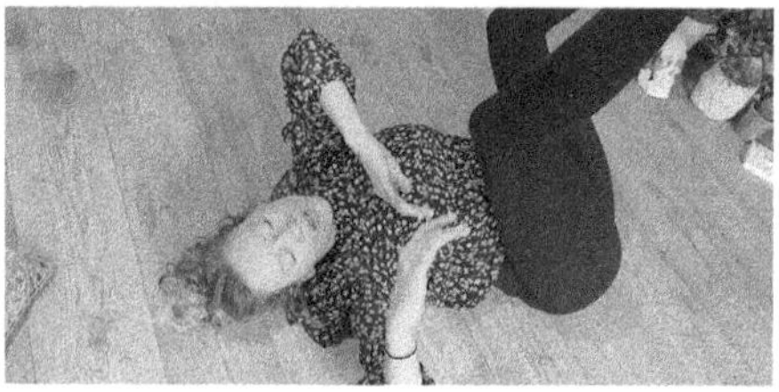

(k)

Continue to notice your breathing, inviting your hands to move around the thorax. The vagus nerve moves into your thorax, and supplies your airways and lungs.

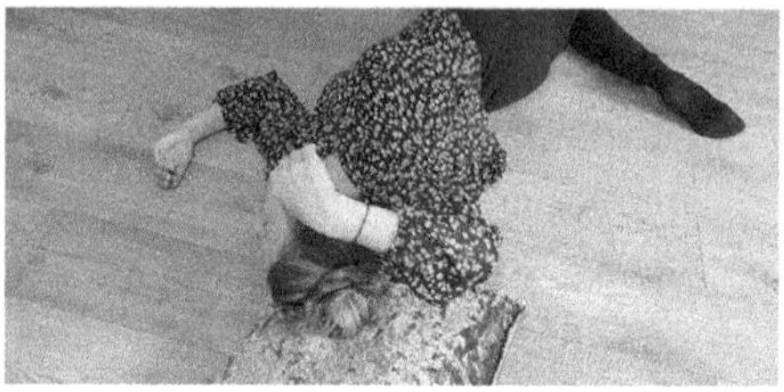

(l)

Sense–perceive your diaphragm and abdomen. Invite breath to take space in your abdomen. Good diaphragmatic breathing innervates the vagus nerve.

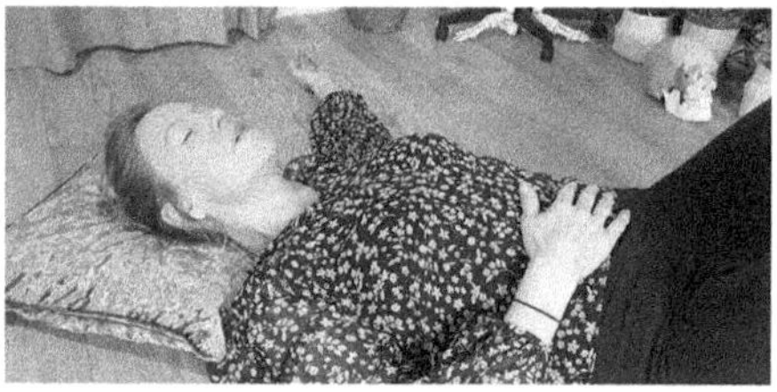

(m)

Breath into your thorax and diaphragm.

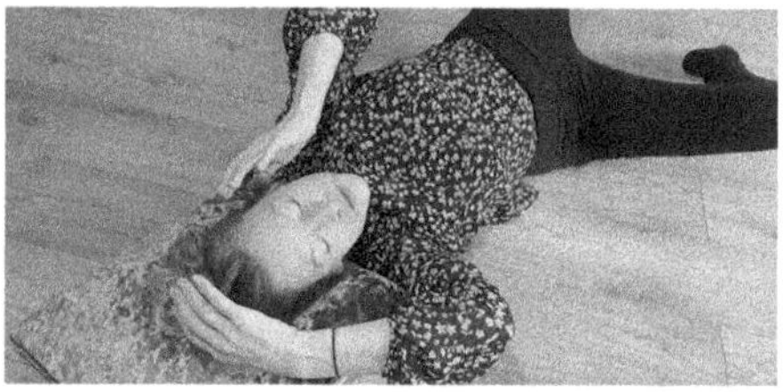

(n)

Invite sensory awareness of the brainstem back into your awareness.

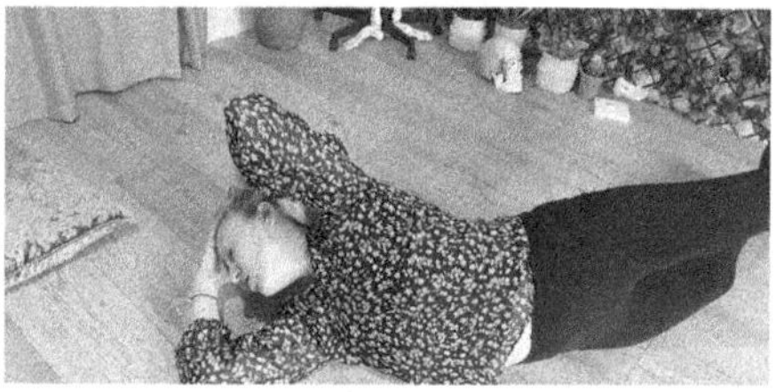

(o)

Curl and uncurl, initiating movement from the brainstem and occipital bone. Keep the rest of the body soft and responsive, following movement initiated from your vagus nerve.

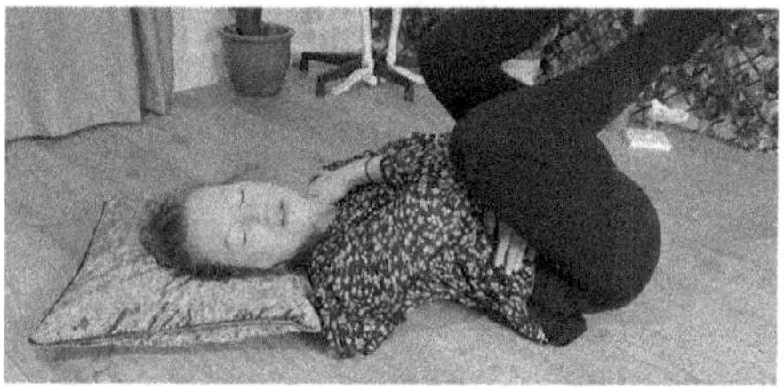

(p)

Sense–perceive your abdomen filling with nutritious breath. The vagus nerve creates a pathway all the way into your abdomen, supplying your stomach, oesophagus and your small and large bowel. Within your intestines, the vagus nerve continues, regulating the smooth muscles. Offer self-touch and massage all around the abdomen, acknowledging the living presence of the vagus.

FIGURE 2.3A–R: Amanda Williamson. Photographer: Scott Closson. (*Continued*)

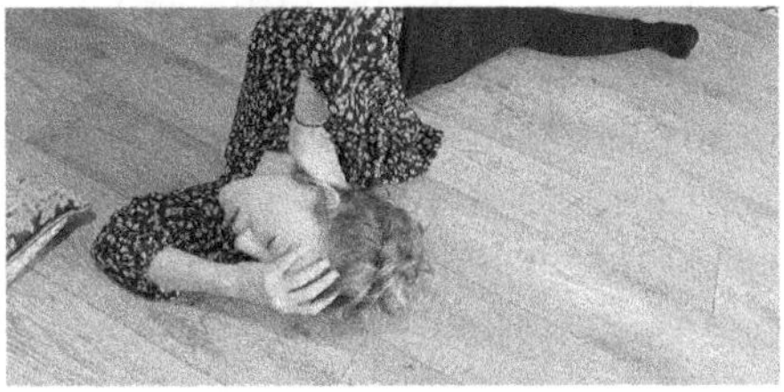

(q)

Invite movement to gently emerge from the brainstem and occipital bone again; invite the cervical, thorax, lumbar and sacral spine to follow. Notice your heart and abdomen following.

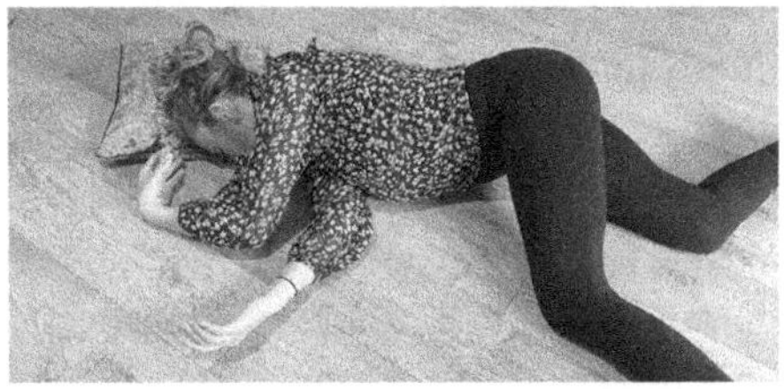

(r)

Roll onto your tummy and massage the vagus nerve into ground. Somatically play, and spiral, between supine and prone. Use self-touch whenever you feel you need sensory support. Listen to the tissues that call for self-touch.

FIGURE 2.3A–R: Amanda Williamson. Photographer: Scott Closson. (*Continued*)

Sense–perceiving the geography of the craniosacral and thoracic–lumbar divisions

It is important to share how to touch and sense–perceive the geography of the ANS. This part of your nervous system is a physical reality, living within you. It is easy to read about the ANS in physiology books, but in practice, we can actually attune to the physical locations of the ANS. Both sympathetic and parasympathetic nerve fibres can be sense–perceived through touch and self-regulatory movement. These locations are extremely important to know about objectively and subjectively. This knowledge can inform touch-based work and self-regulatory movement in manifold ways. In short, this knowledge provides a landscape that practitioners can use to craft and shape therapeutic processes in the studio.

The parasympathetic nervous system is often referred to as *the craniosacral division*. This is because the parasympathetic division begins from four paired cranial nerves in your cranium: these are *the oculomotor nerve*, *the facial nerve*, *the glossopharyngeal nerve* and *the vagus nerve*. Parasympathetic nerve fibres also arise from three paired nerves in your sacrum, specifically the sacral nerves of S 2, 3 and 4. Therefore, and shared briefly in Chapter 1, the caudal–cranial axis (head–tail) is the rather gorgeous emanating location of your parasympathetic nervous system. In stark contrast, the sympathetic division starts from the spinal nerves along your vertebral column between T1 and L2. Hence, the sympathetic division is often referred to as the *thoracic–lumbar division*. The spinal nerves that move out of each side of your vertebrae in your thoracic and lumbar regions are thus the radiating location of the sympathetic division. This rather lucid and beautiful geography offers somatic movement dance practitioners an excellent landscape to craft and offer therapeutic practice. In short, one can attune to the parasympathetic through moving the caudal–cranial axis or attune to the sympathetic division through moving the thoracic–lumbar vertebrae and easing the tissues in the thorax and lumbar–thoracic regions, and expressing energy out through the limbs. Before we move into practice, let us take a further look at sympathetic arousal and how it affects the tissues in your body.

> When we face a threat to our survival, there is a surge in the activity of the entire sympathetic chain, spreading the fight-or-flight response to mobilize the resources of the entire body. This response is immediate and total, which is appropriate if we are threatened or in danger. The muscles tense to prepare for movements needed to fight or flee; this is described in weightlifting circles as getting pumped-up.
>
> (Rosenberg 2017: 26)

> In a sympathetic state, the heart beats faster, which supplies more blood to the muscles. The muscles tighten ready for action. One's blood pressure also increases, so blood can be pumped into the muscles in preparation for fight or flight. Notably, the liver releases stored-up sugars into the blood to make extra energy available for the muscles to burn. The survival stress response from the sympathetic chain causes the muscles of the airways to open to the maximum, improving our breathing capacity and taking in the maximum amount of oxygen, in order to be fully mobilized to fight or run. At the same time other organs are slowed or stopped – particularly those to do with digestion.
>
> (Rosenburg 2017: 26)

Ideally, sympathetic and parasympathetic innervation should work together to maintain balance. After a period of stress, the parasympathetic nervous system should calm the body down. However, this is often not the case. In our pressurized world, the sympathetic response often overrides the parasympathetic.

This is because there is little time to slow-down, relax, take solace and just 'be'. As Dispenza notes,

> the fight or flight response has become maladaptive in our current global society. When the lion was chasing our ancestors, the stress response was doing what it was designed to – protect them from the outer environment. That's adaptive. But if for days on end, you fret about your promotion, overfocus on your presentation to upper management, or worry about your mother being in hospital, these situations create the same chemicals as though you were being chased by a lion.
>
> (Dispenza 2012: 100)

Although sympathetic neurons emerge specifically from the spinal cord between T1 and L2, the sympathetic chain reaches far beyond its points of emergence and thus affects your entire organism. This is why your entire body feels tense and agitated when you are sympathetically aroused. The sympathetic chain extends beyond T1 to L2 and moves,

- up the chain to the head
- up and out to the arms
- straight out to the periphery
- down the chain and out to the legs.

(Attlee 2012: 370)

The sympathetic nerve fibres start their life in the spinal cord but after leaving form what is termed the *sympathetic chain*. The sympathetic chain extends from the base of your skull to your coccyx. Therefore, there are other locations of *plexi* related to the sympathetic chain that are of profound significance in practice. Notably, they are areas where you might feel anxious, uneasy and emotionally upset. Your heart might beat faster, and you might feel nervous and upset in your solar plexus. Thomas Attlee refers to these places as energy centres. They are physical locations, made of bundles of nerves. They are,

- the cardiac plexus which innervates the heart; it is sometimes called the heart chakra
- the coeliac plexus which innervates the solar plexus – commonly referred to as the solar plexus.

(Attlee 2012: 371)

Example of practice: Sense–perceiving the geography of the craniosacral and thoracic–lumbar divisions

Because the sympathetic nerves emerge from your thoracic or lumbar regions, touch-based work along the vertebra between T1 and L2 (and from cranium to tail) can release sympathetic holding, as well as self-regulatory improvisational processes of unwinding the nerves between each vertebra, and expressing trapped energy out through the arms and legs. Relieving stress and tension in *thoracic–lumbar division* through softening and unwinding between T1 and L2 is a particularly effective way of reducing sympathetic arousal. Contacting the caudal–cranial axis, where the parasympathetic nerve fibres emanate (your head–tail), is another way of inviting the parasympathetic to override sympathetic arousal. On pages 60–62 I offer a process that helps participants locate the physical geography of their craniosacral and thoracic–lumbar divisions – sensed within the landscape and living tissues of their body. I always invite students to draw or write after moving. This helps participants to further attune to these important locations through symbolic visualization. I usually allow one hour for this self-regulatory process.

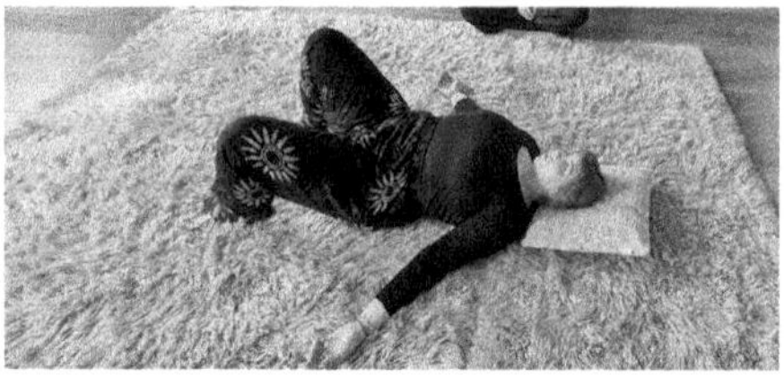

(a)

Invite participants to soften into the floor, releasing the weight of their cranium onto a cushion. Move awareness from the frontal lobe to the occiput. Sense breath.

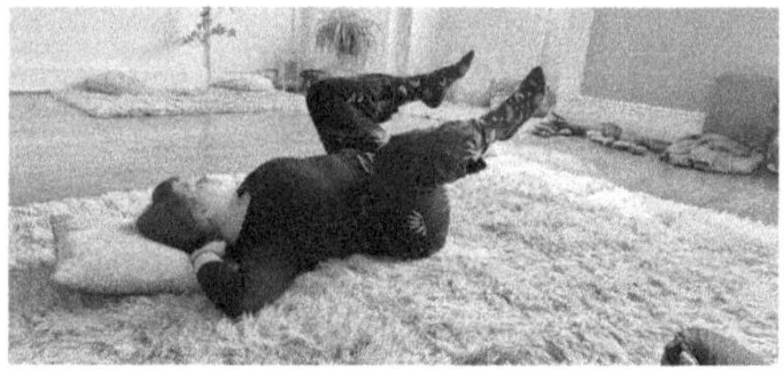

(b)

Invite the weight of body to drop: sense the cranium, scapulae and sacrum releasing into ground. Settle along your midline, softening the vertebral column into gravity.

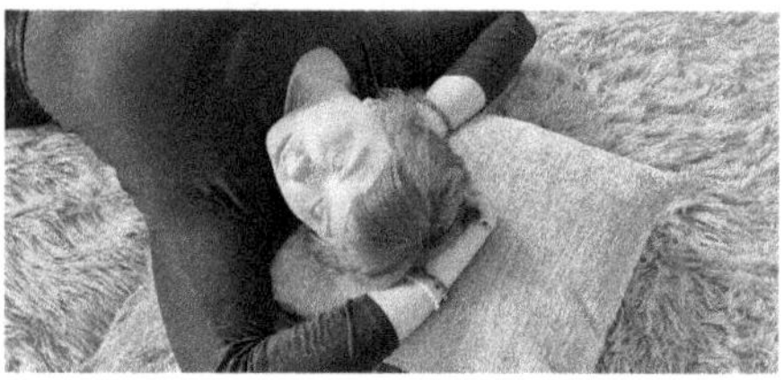

(c)

With breath awareness, invite participants to gently tip and pour the weight of their head from side-to-side, sense–perceiving their brainstem and releasing around the sub-occipital triangle. There are four paired parasympathetic nerves that emanate from the brainstem: the oculomotor nerve, the facial nerve, the glossopharyngeal nerve and the vagus nerve.

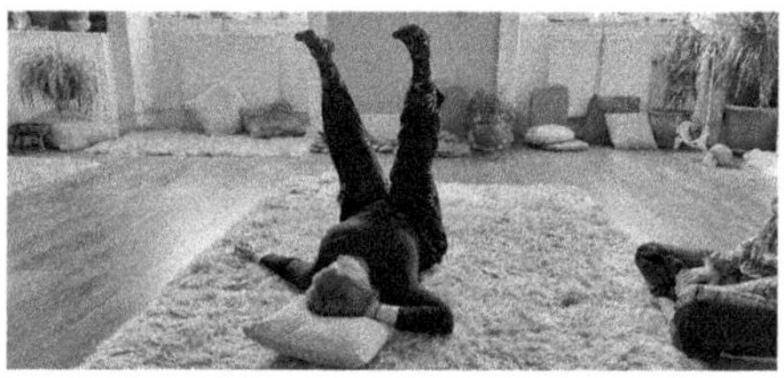

(d)

Invite participants to drop their awareness into their sacrum. Tip, pour, roll and soften the sacrum into the ground. Some participants like to place one hand, palm face down, under their sacrum and then soften the weight of their sacrum into their hand. Remember parasympathetic nerves also emanate from S 2, 3 and 4. These lovely nerves move out through the sacral foramina and down into the legs. Initiate movement gently from the sacral region, inviting the vertebral column to follow and unwind. Invite participants to loosen and ease the sacral region, noticing areas that need to rest, and areas that call for gentle compressions, decompressions and release. Enjoy resting awareness in the sacrum.

FIGURE 2.4A–J: Natalie Austin. Photographer: Scott Closson.

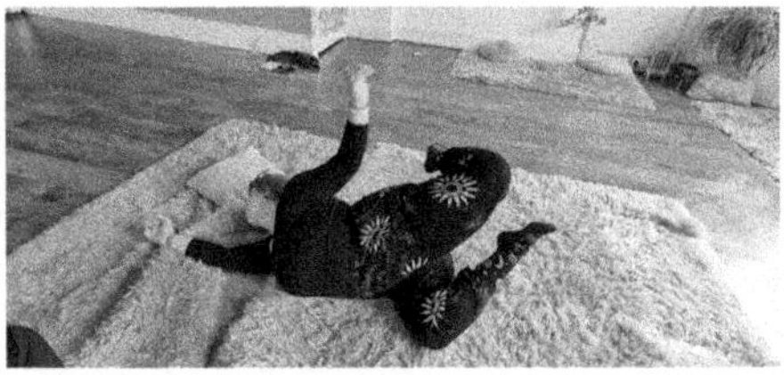

(e)

Invite participants into gentle slow-time movement initiations between their cranial and sacral regions. Here they are sense–perceiving their caudal–cranial axis, the craniosacral division. Play between the caudal–cranial axis, noticing the vertebral column spiralling and unravelling in between.

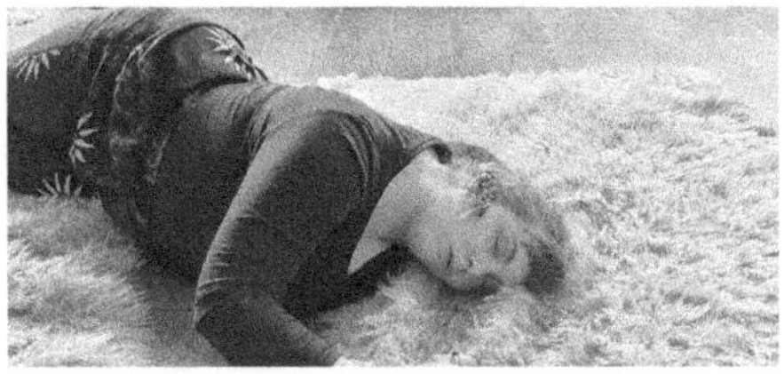

(f)

Invite participants to direct their awareness along their midline, sensing the vertebral column and thorax. Bring awareness to T1 and L2, the sympathetic thoracic–lumbar division. Breath into this area, remembering that the sympathetic chain emerges from this location. Notice any restrictions and places that feel tight or strained. Ease and breathe the fascia along the midline.

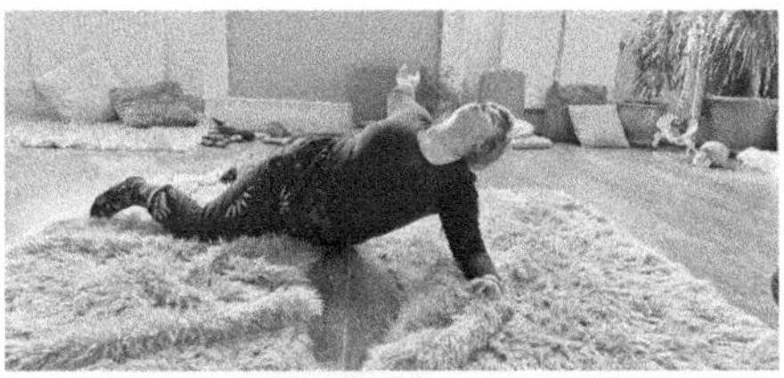

(g)

Invite movement to emerge from the thoracic and lumbar region, sense–perceiving the sympathetic chain. You may notice movement expressing through the ams, legs and head, as participants sense the directionality and energy of the sympathetic chain.

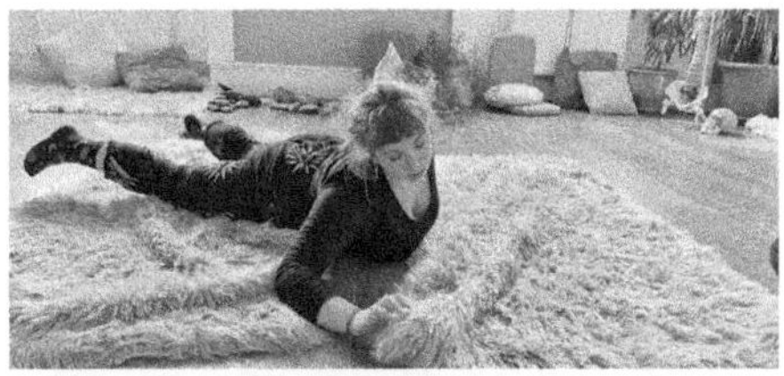

(h)

Tip, pour and roll on to your sides, and then invite the thoracic and the lumbar spine to express and unwind. Push, stretch and reach, inviting the sympathetic chain into expression.

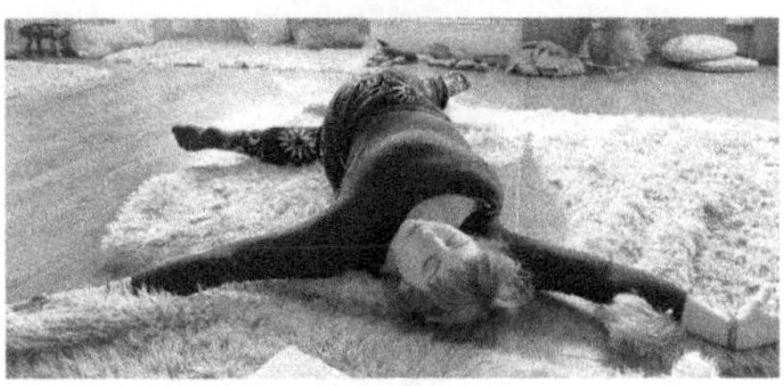

(i)

Invite the entire vertebral column to gently curl and uncurl in gravity, easing out places of restriction.

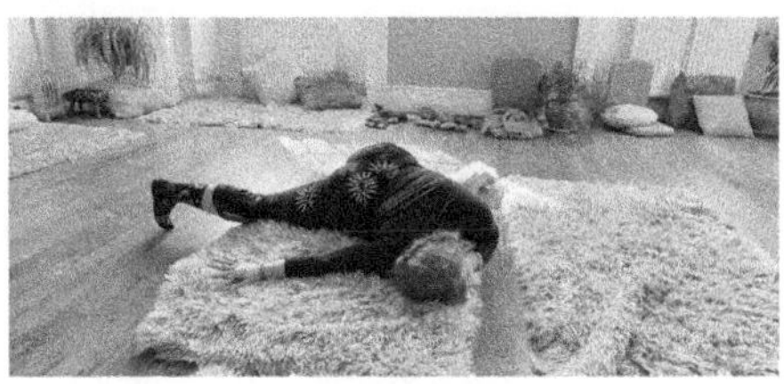

(j)

Let go of the parasympathetic/sympathetic framework and move into self-regulatory movement, following movement pathways that feel delicious and pleasurable.

FIGURE 2.4A–J: Natalie Austin. Photographer: Scott Closson. (*Continued*)

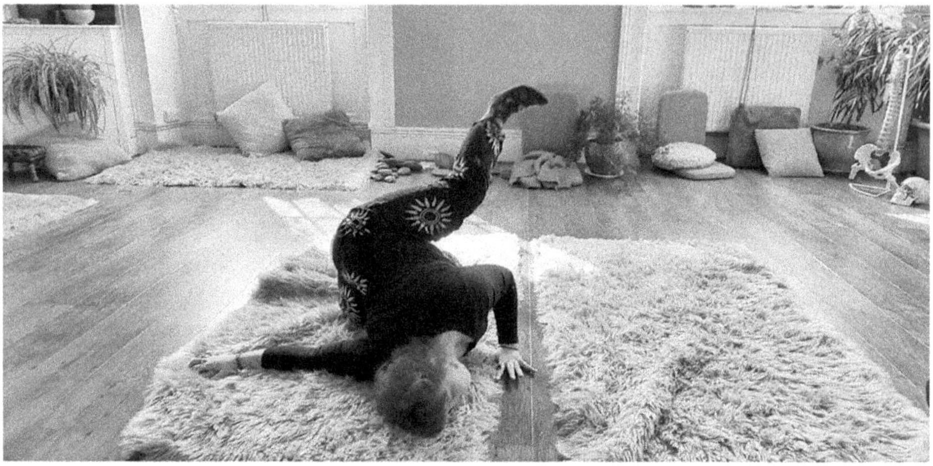

FIGURE 2.5: Natalie Austin. Photographer: Scott Closson.

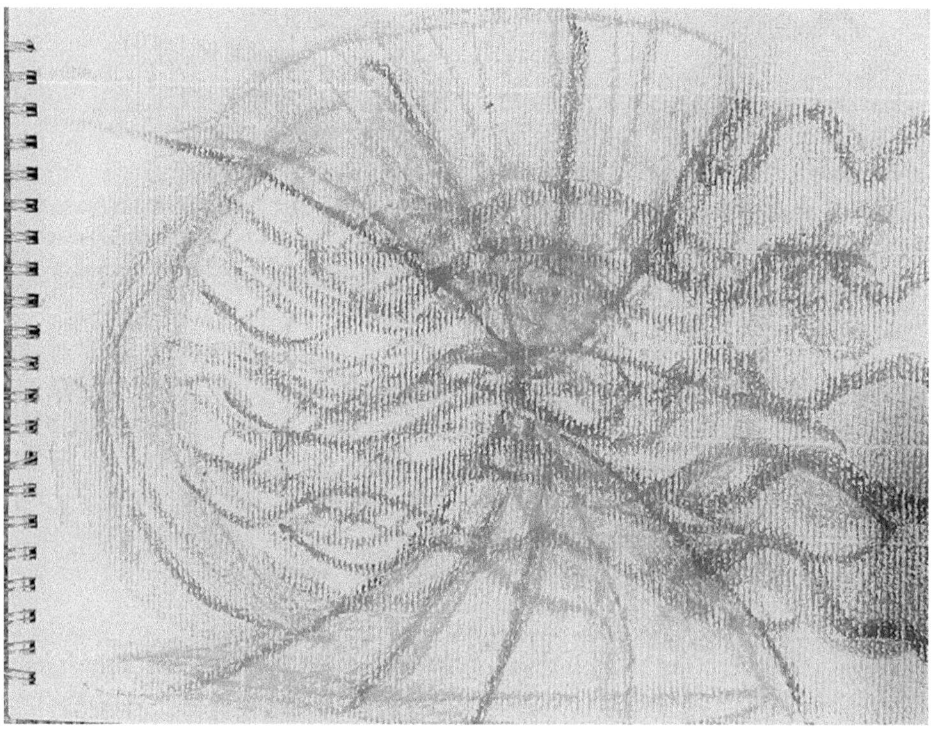

FIGURE 2.6: A student's painting after moving through the above process. Natasha Martin. Photographer: Amanda Williamson.

> Learning about this geography made no sense until I started to acknowledge these nerves in practice. I understand myself more. By listening to the living presence of these nerves I realized how lonely my body must have been. When I am angry, upset or worried, I feel more compassion for myself. Now I have a movement dialogue with these very nerves, a part of me previously unknown. After this practice I feel balanced and much fuller as a person. More of me has integrated.
>
> (Alison Blanche)

Through drawing and writing, we are inviting subjectivity to dance with objectivity. This is the beautiful balance between western anatomy and first-person subjective sensory experience. This is a key teaching tool, and an integrative part of the process.

Releasing sympathetic holding in the vertebrae through somatic touch

In addition to easing out the tension in the nerves and tissues between T1 and L2, it is wonderfully enlivening to experientially explore specific vertebral levels and neurological outpourings related to the sympathetic chain. The sympathetic nerves passing through the vertebra between T1 and L2 often become over excited through stress or fear. Offering additional support to the sympathetic chain through somatic touch can further calm and soothe these nerves, as well as release the fascia around these nerves. Before we move into practice, below are some important neurological outpourings related to the sympathetic chain. These neurological outpourings can be soothed by offering somatic touch, opening out into self-regulatory movement.

The thoraco-lumbar junction

The transition between T12 and L1 is called *the thoraco-lumbar junction*. 'It is the transitional area between the thoracic spine and lumbar spine below' and 'consequently it is an area of postural stress' (Attlee 2012: 379). The thoraco-lumbar junction also has incredibly important neurological outpourings and is the 'area of major sympathetic nerve outflow to many of the surrounding viscera, including the kidneys, the adrenals, the bladder, the small intestine and the large intestine (colon), and also the uterus, ovaries, prostate, genitalia and other pelvic organs' (Attlee 2012: 380).

T9: The apex of the thoracic curve

T9 is part of the thoracic spine.

> From a mechanical point of view, T9 is the apex of the thoracic curve and is therefore subject to strain due to anterior-posterior postural imbalances. More significantly, it is the vertebral level most associated with the solar plexus and the coeliac ganglia of the sympathetic nervous system.
>
> (Attlee 2012: 380)

Further, T9 'is therefore particularly significant in conditions of prolonged stress and pressure involving excessive stimulation of the sympathetic nervous system, excessive secretion of adrenaline and excessive activity within the solar plexus' (Attlee 2012: 380).

T4: The root of the neck

> From a mechanical point of view T4 vertebra is the root of the neck. While anatomically one might think of the neck as finishing at the base of the cervical spine, with C7, functionally the neck extends down to the T4 vertebral level.
>
> (Attlee 2012: 381)

Additionally, T4 'is also the level associated with the heart chakra and cardiac plexus and is therefore intimately involved with their associated anxieties and stresses. It is common to have points of agitation and restriction around T4' (Attlee 2012: 381).

L5–S1: The lumbo-sacral region

When L5 transitions into S1, it is referred to as the lumbo-sacral junction. It 'is a particularly vulnerable part of the vertebral column' because 'it is the junction between the mobile vertebral column above and the more solid foundation of the pelvis below' (Attlee 2012: 378–79). 'It is one of the principal sites of outflow for the sciatic nerve (whose roots emanate from L4, 5 and S, 1, 2, 3)' (Attlee 2012: 378)

Further,

- T1 and T4 has neurological outpourings which go to the heart
- T5 and T8 has neurological outpourings which go to the lungs
- T9 has neurological outpourings which go to the stomach
- T10 has neurological outpourings goes to the kidneys.

(Rosenberg 2017: 25)

Example of practice: Releasing sympathetic holding in the vertebral column

In this practice I am not correcting or manipulating, but rather inviting the participant to self-regulate, releasing their vertebral holdings via sense-perceiving specific areas, enhanced through touch.

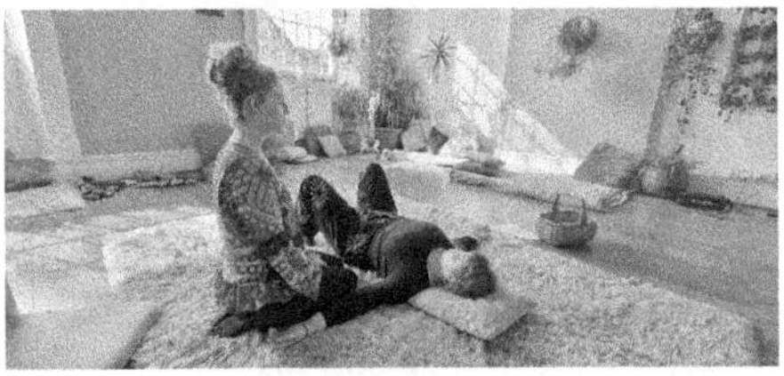

(a)

Invite the participant to settle into the floor, sensing the ground underneath them. Contact breath together, relaxing the oral cavity and softening the jaw. Invite them to sense–perceive their thorax expanding and releasing – rising and falling. Invite them to sense their diaphragm breathing them, taking space in their tissues.

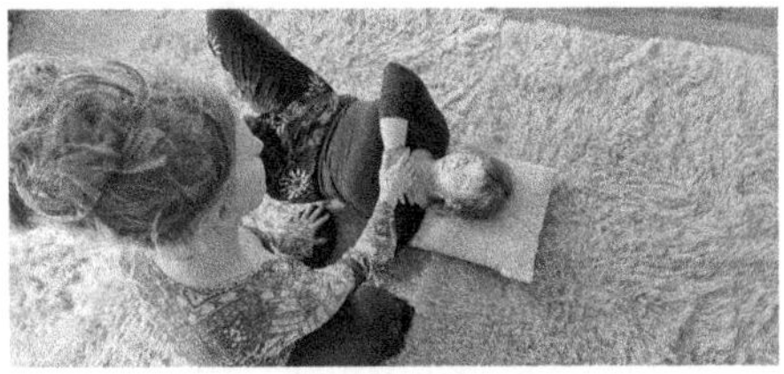

(b)

Invite them to contact their heart, sensing breath. Place one hand on their heart space, over their hand. Practitioner and client sense their breath and hearts together. This is the most important inroad into the parasympathetic.

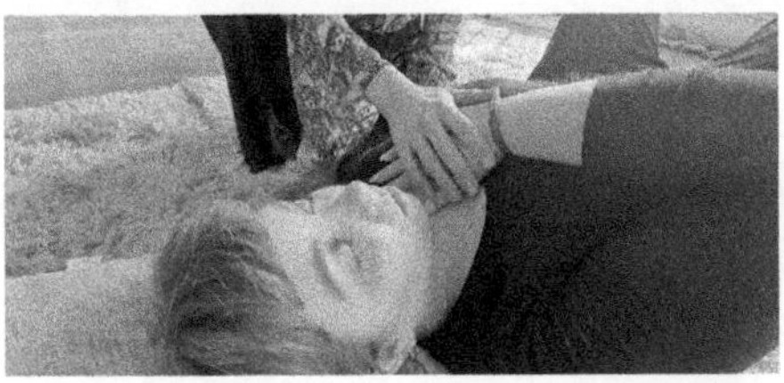

(c)

Place one hand on their heart space. Invite the participant to sense their living tissues breathing into your hand.

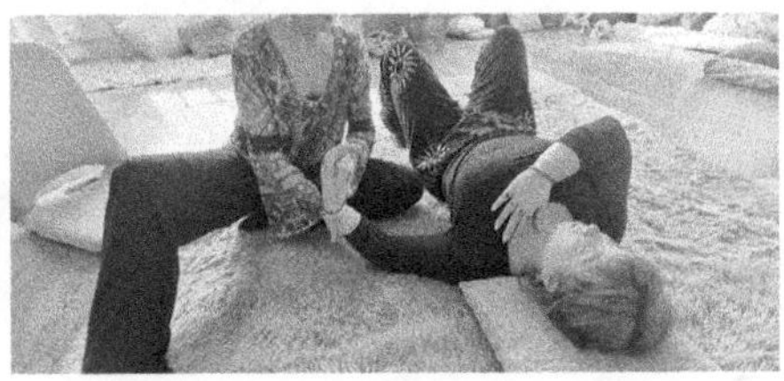

(d)

Invite the participant to release the weight of their arms.

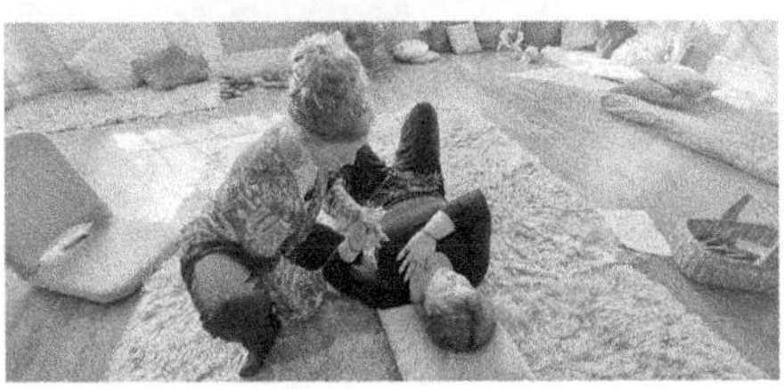

(e)

Invite the participant to slowly tip, pour and roll onto their side. Initiate the movement through their synovial joints. Encourage the movement initiation by folding through the fingers, wrists, elbows, and shoulders, resting one hand on their scapula.

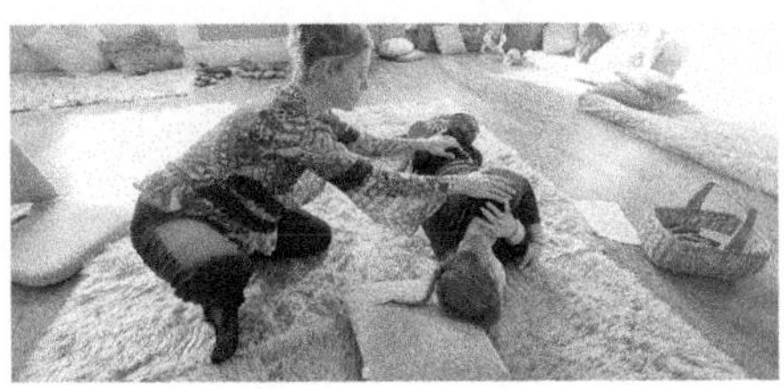

(f)

Simultaneously, support their tipping by inviting their knees to fall to one side, encouraging their pelvis to follow. Place your other hand on their ilium, supporting them to roll onto their side.

FIGURE 2.7A–Y: Natalie Austin and Amanda Williamson. Photographer: Scott Closson.

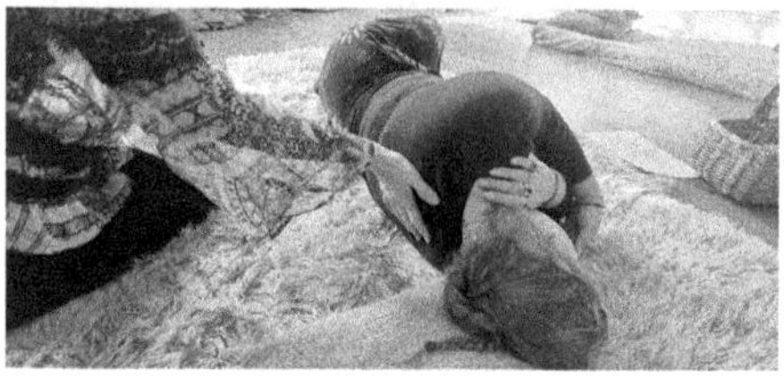

(g)

Invite the participant to soften, pour and roll back into your hand. Invite them to soften their weight into your hands. As they pour, place one hand gently under T4 (T4 lives between the scapulae). Your hand will be supporting their upper thoracic spine.

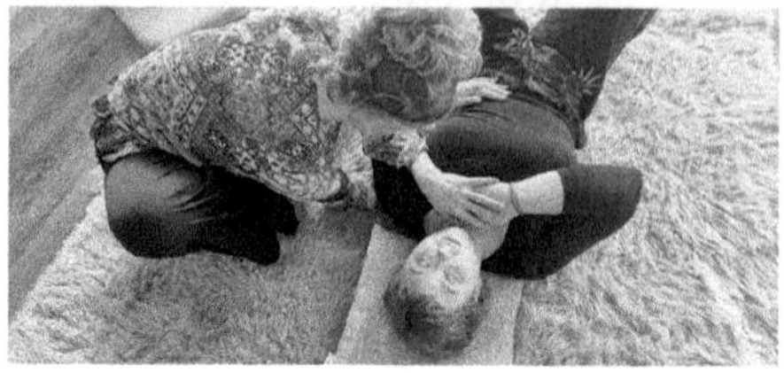

(h)

Invite the participant to pour their weight and soften their thoracic vertebra into your hand. Keep one hand underneath T4 between the scapulae and place your other hand on their heart space. Remember T4 is the neurological outpouring to the heart.

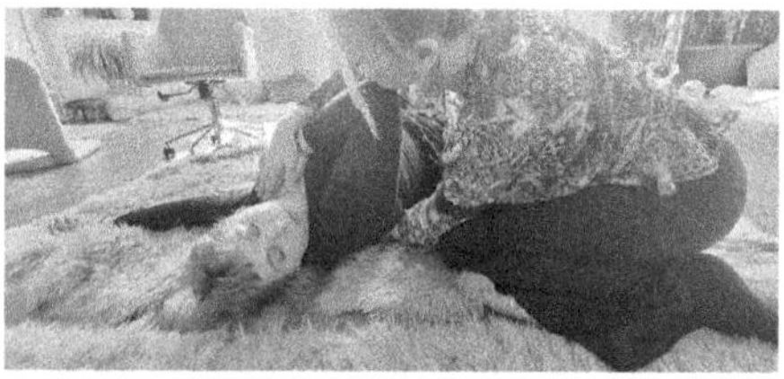

(i)

Invite the participant to soften their thoracic vertebrae into your hands and rest in breath in T4. Rest in breath together, sensing the tissues breathing between both hands. Sense heart and breath together.

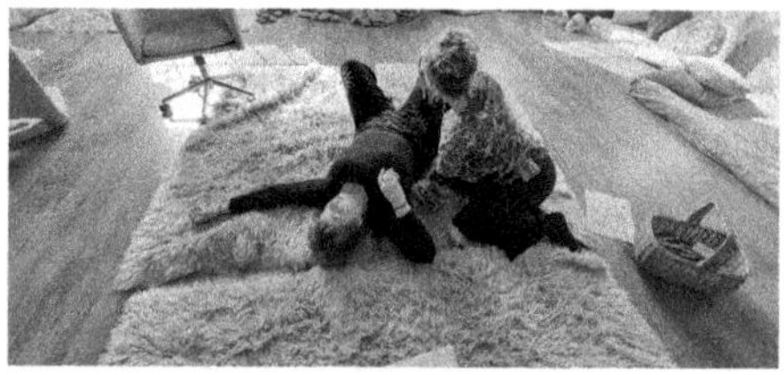

(j)

Invite your participant to use your hand like a fulcrum, encouraging them to initiate gentle compressions, decompressions and releases in their thoracic vertebrae.

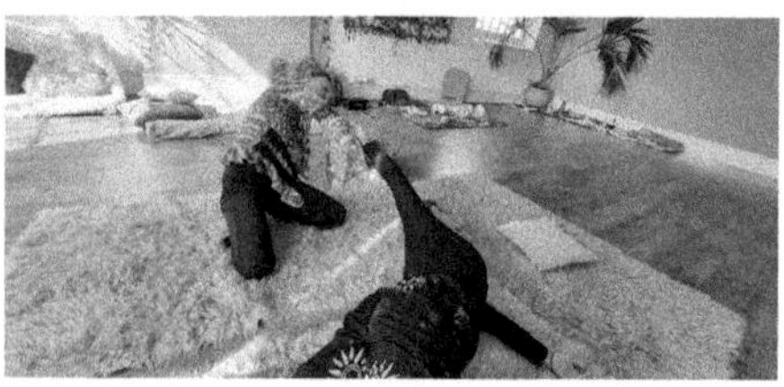

(k)

Invite the participant into their own movement response, encouraging their whole body to respond and express from T4 in particular. You will notice movement often extends through the arms.

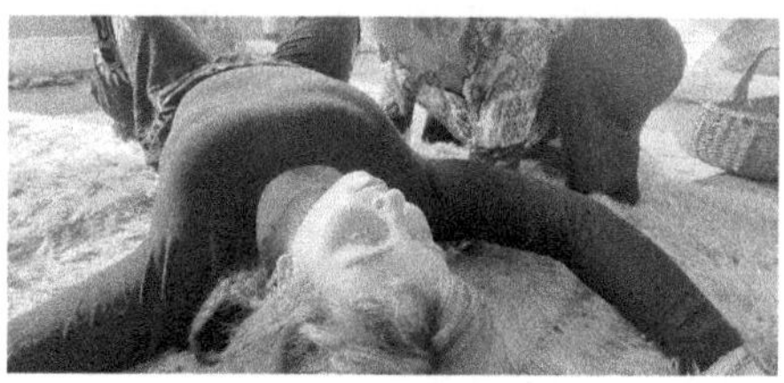

(l)

Invite the participant to tip and roll away from you again; as they pour back into your hands, place your hands gently under T5–T12 (the lower thoracic spine).

FIGURE 2.7A–Y: Natalie Austin and Amanda Williamson. Photographer: Scott Closson. (*Continued*)

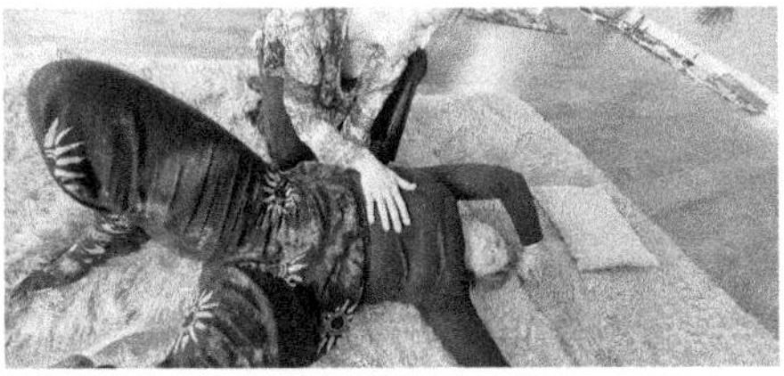

(m)

Invite them to soften their tissues and release their weight into your hand, relaxing the lower part of their thoracic vertebrae. Encourage a movement response, while sense–perceiving the thoracic spine.

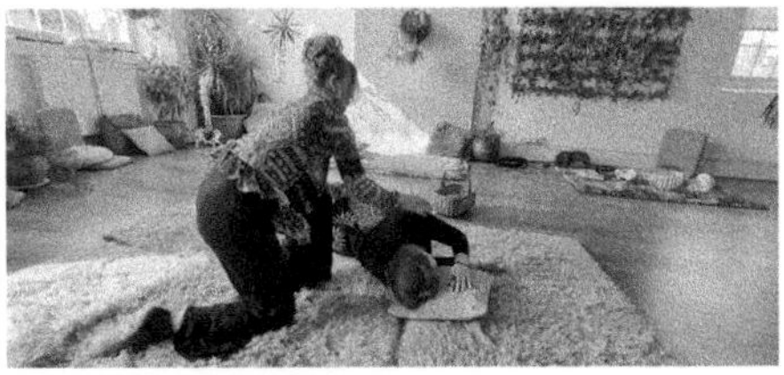

(n)

Invite them to tip and roll away again. As they roll back, place your hand under T9. Invite them to pour back into your hand and soften into T9, settling their thorax into your hand.

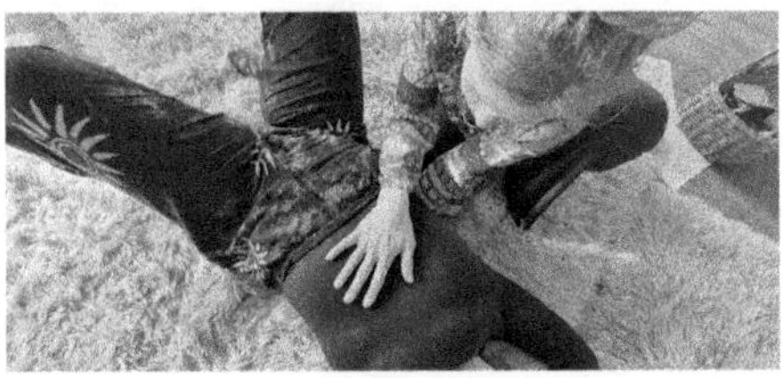

(o)

Place one hand on their solar plexus and the other underneath at T9 (connecting T9 with its neurological outpourings to the solar plexus). Rest together in breath, listening and attending to the solar plexus. Invite the participant to sense–perceive and rest in their solar plexus.

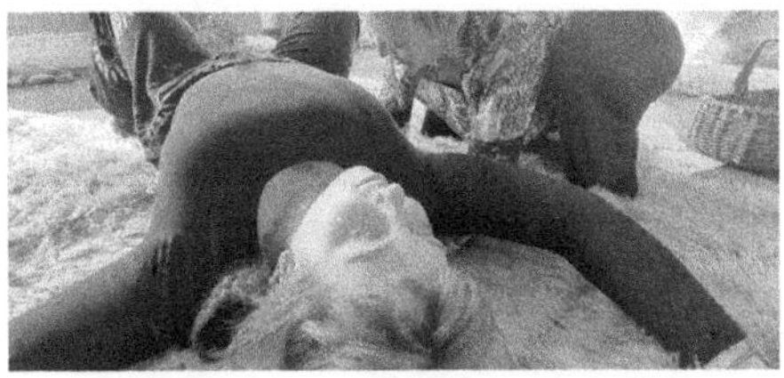

(p)

Invite them to tip and roll away from you again; as they pour back towards you, gently find the transitioning place between T12 and L1. This is the thoraco-lumbar junction with its sympathetic nerve outflow to the kidneys and the adrenals.

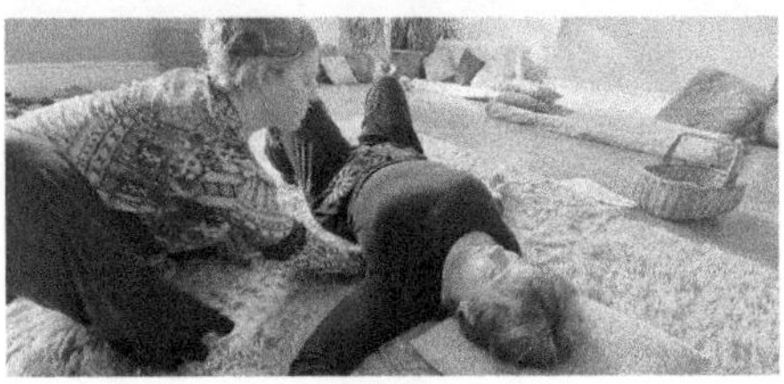

(q)

Invite the participant to soften and release their weight into your hands again. Again, invite them to use your hand as a fulcrum; sometimes resting and softening, and at other times compressing and decompressing. Rest together in breath, sense–perceiving thoraco-lumbar junction, and its neurological outflows to the kidneys and adrenals.

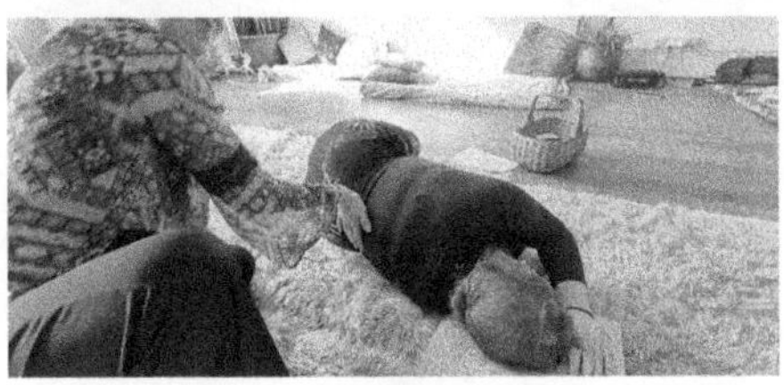

(r)

Invite them to roll away again; as they soften back towards you, place your hands around L5 and S1. This is the lumbar–sacral junction. Remember, this area provides the neurological outflow for the sciatic nerve (the roots of these nerves emanate from L4 and 5 and S 1, 2 and 3).

FIGURE 2.7A–Y: Natalie Austin and Amanda Williamson. Photographer: Scott Closson. (*Continued*)

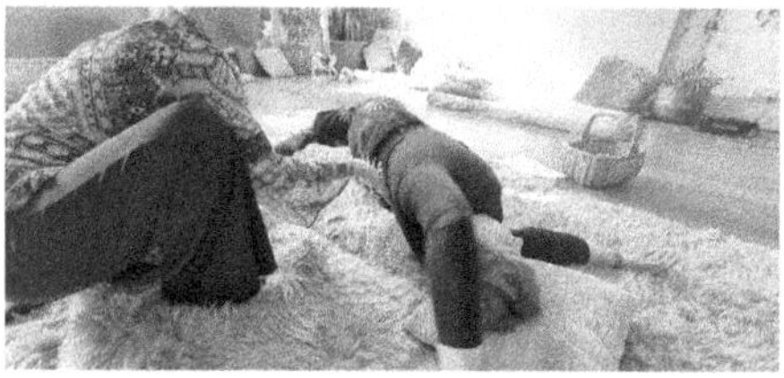

(s)

Invite them to pour back into your hands, softening and resting. Encourage them to initiate gentle attuned movement from L5 to S1.

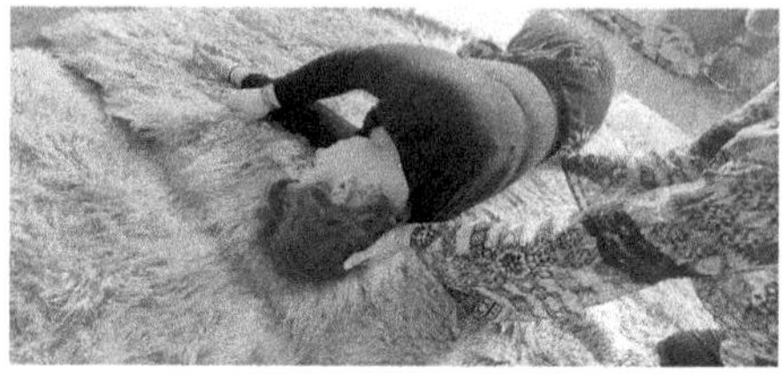

(t)

Invite them to tip away again; this time as they roll back towards you, place one hand under their occiput and the other under their sacrum. Here you are contacting the craniosacral division.

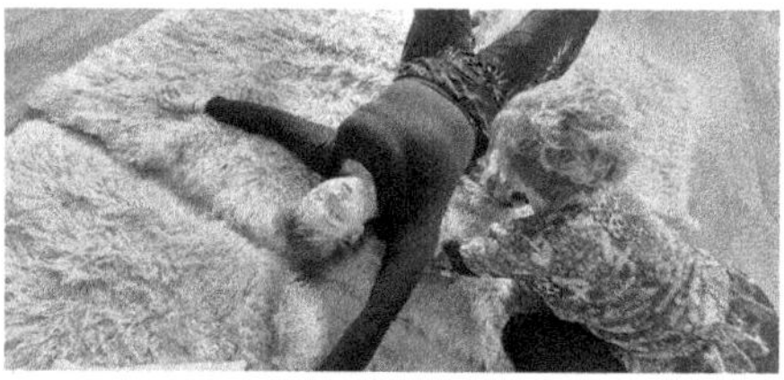

(u)

Invite them to simultaneously soften their occiput and sacrum into your hands. Encourage self-regulatory movement from these two distant, but related areas.

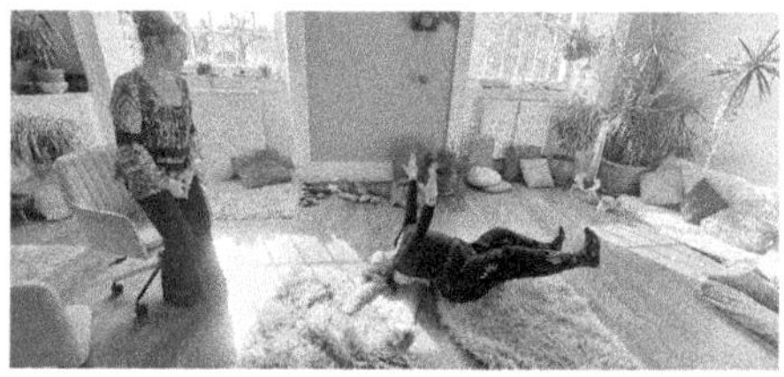

(v)

Encourage the head–tail connection, with the vertebral column unwinding in between.

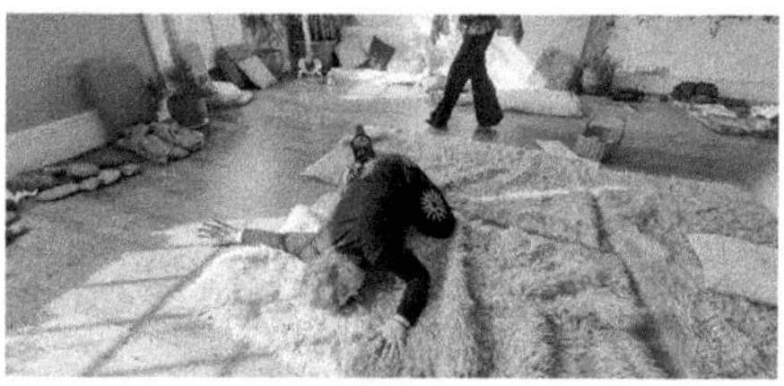

(w)

Invite them into a movement expression, sensing–perceiving the head–tail.

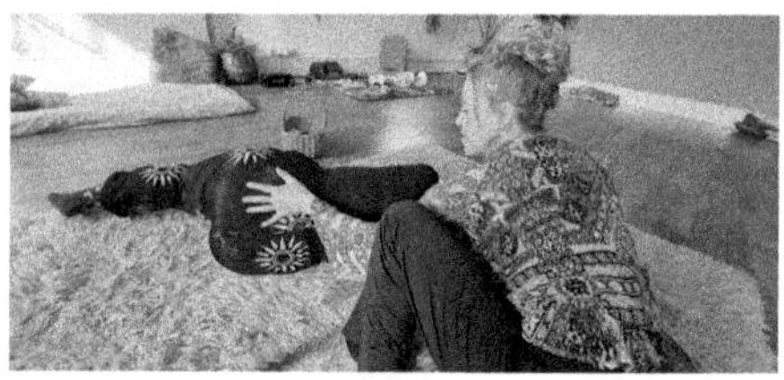

(x)

Invite them to tip and roll; as they pour back each time, place your hands underneath different parts of their thoracic, lumbar and sacral spine, inviting integrative awareness throughout the vertebral column, from the occiput all the way to the sacrum.

FIGURE 2.7A–Y: Natalie Austin and Amanda Williamson. Photographer: Scott Closson. (*Continued*)

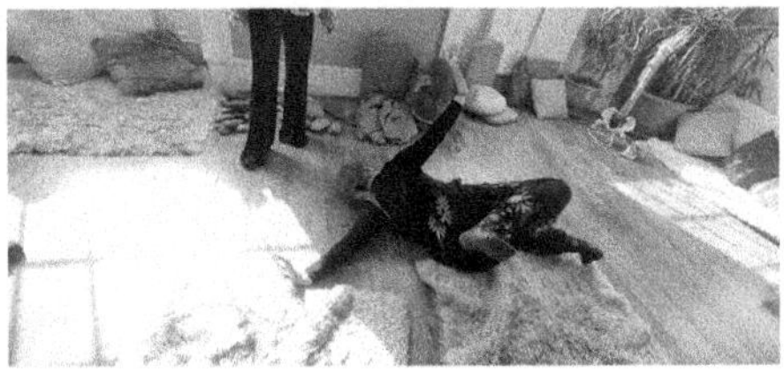

(y)

Move away and invite a movement response, emerging from the touch and bodywork – at times support the participant through soft touch, enhancing their movement expression.

FIGURE 2.7A–Y: Natalie Austin and Amanda Williamson. Photographer: Scott Closson. (*Continued*)

Polyvagal theory

In Chapter 1, we briefly touched on Polyvagal. In this section, I would like to take a deeper look at this theory and apply it to practice. Polyvagal theory is a ground-breaking theory developed by Stephen Porges (2017). Stephen Porges's research scientifically challenged the traditional divisions of the ANS. After the advent of Polyvagal theory, it is now widely accepted that the vagus nerve has two neural pathways – *the ventral branch* and *the dorsal branch*. Polyvagal theory still focuses on the incredible vitality of the vagus nerve, but underscores that the vagus nerve has two branches that behave rather differently. Notably, the two branches of the vagus nerve 'arise at different places and have very different functions' (Rosenburg 2017: 19). Below is a little information about where they arise and where they terminate.

> The ventral branch, for example, originates in the brainstem, at the top of the spinal cord, under the brain. Its function is rest and repair. Note, that the ventral branch of the vagus is sometimes referred to as *the supradiaphragmatic vagus*, because its pathways terminate in the organs above the diaphragm. In general, the ventral vagal circuit supports social engagement behaviours. Here we feel relaxed, open and engaged with others and the activity at hand.
>
> (Porges 2017: 5, 7)

> The dorsal branch originates in a fluid filled space – called the fourth ventricle, surrounded by cerebral spinal fluid. Its function is slowdown and total shutdown.

> Note, that the dorsal branch of the vagus is sometimes referred to as *the subdiaphragmatic vagus* because its pathways terminate below the diaphragm. In general, the dorsal vagal circuit supports immobilized defensive behaviours. Here we feel frozen, depressed, enclosed and dissociated from the activity at hand.
>
> (Porges 2017: 5, 7)

Noted earlier, a chronic state of sympathetic activity (stress) is common in our culture and society. In this state, people's muscles are often tense, and the spinal nerves and sympathetic chain are highly active, preparing for fight or flight. Many participants that come to sessions are in a sympathetic state of chronic holding, but some people express towards what is termed *a dorsal vagal feeling state*. You might notice that a participant is particularly withdrawn, quiet, dissociated from the group, depressed and unable to socially engage. Their muscle tone and tissues might express lethargy or a frozenness. Can you remember a time you felt like this? In this case, the person's dorsal vagal circuit is activated. Some people are open, relaxed, socially engaged and present in the space. In this case, it is likely their ventral circuit is activated. In terms of Polyvagal theory, there are three states, or circuits of the ANS, rather than two. They are:

> The dorsal branch of the vagus nerve – 'slowdown, shutdown, and depressive behaviours'
>
> The ventral branch of the vagus nerve – 'positive states of relaxation and social engagement'
>
> The sympathetic chain – 'fight or flight'.
>
> (Rosenburg 2017: 29–30)

Polyvagal theory thus 'describes three primary circuits that provide neural regulation of the ANS; these states are selectively regulated by the ventral vagal, dorsal vagal, and sympathetic pathways' (Porges 2017: 5). Below is additional information that might help you perceive your own, or another person's state:

> *The sympathetic chain* – Activity supported by the spinal sympathetic chain enables us to fight in order to meet a threat or run away in order to avoid it. This is because hard, tense muscles allow us to move the entire body more quickly. Higher blood pressure is also needed to get the flow of blood into the muscles that are tense and hard.
>
> (Rosenburg 2017: 29–31)

> *The dorsal branch of the vagus nerve* – Low levels of muscles tonus are found when the dorsal vagal circuit is activated, when there is no need to tense the muscles to fight or flee (or in some cases of extreme danger, when the body's survival response

> is to shut down). Low blood pressure is sufficient to get the blood into soft, limp muscles.
>
> (Rosenburg 2017: 29–31)

> *The ventral branch of the vagus nerve* – Normal blood pressure is appropriate for muscles that are neither tense nor flaccid – muscles that feel just right. In states of social engagement, there is generally no threat or danger in our environment. Our nervous system registers this fact, so we do not have to do anything; we can truly relax and enjoy being with others.
>
> (Rosenburg 2017: 29–31)

Further,

> The ventral branch of the vagus nerve relates to positive emotions of joy, satisfaction, and love. In terms of behaviour, it expresses itself in positive social activities with friends and loved ones. The state of enjoyment supports social behaviours in which we support and share with other people. Cooperation with others usually improve our chances for survival – we talk together, sing together, dance together, share a meal, cooperate to complete a project, teach and nurture.
>
> (Rosenburg 2017: 34)

> The second of the ANS's neural pathways is the spinal sympathetic chain, which is activated when our survival is threatened. If we mobilize our body in this response, we can make an extra effort to help respond to the threat. The state of 'mobilization with fear' arises when we are not safe, or do not feel safe. The spinal sympathetic chain relates to emotions of anger or fear, which can express themselves in behaviours such as fighting in order to overcome the threat or fleeing to avoid a threatening situation.
>
> (Rosenburg 2017: 34)

> The third neural pathway is the dorsal branch of the vagus nerve. This pathway is activated when we face an overwhelming force and imminent destruction. When there is no point of fighting or running away, we conserve what resources we have – we immobilize. Activation of this pathway fosters feelings of helplessness, hopelessness, and apathy, manifesting in withdrawal and shutdown. This state can be described as 'immobilization with fear'.
>
> (Rosenburg 2017: 34)

The dorsal branch is the older of the two branches and exists 'in all classes of vertebrates, from boneless fish up to and including human beings and other mammals. It is sometimes referred to as "the old vagus"' (Rosenburg 2017: 41).

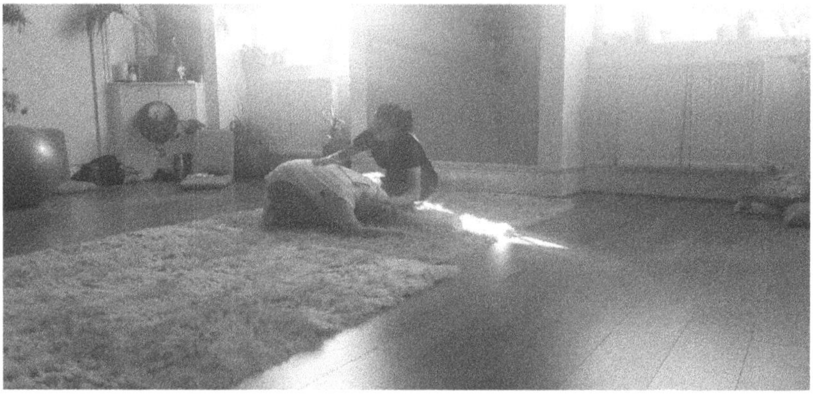

FIGURE 2.8: Miranda Henderson and Vanessa Tucker. Photographer: Amanda Williamson.

Further, 'the dorsal vagus, acting on its own brings about a state of metabolic shutdown. It enables animals to reduce the activity level of their vital functions, thereby conserving energy' [...] 'this is described as immobilization with fear' (Rosenburg 2017: 41). When we are in a dorsal vagal state, that is chronic, but not a total shutdown, the 'emotional correlate is characterized by depressive feelings' (Rosenburg 2017: 41). However, Porges's model does not reduce the ANS to only three states. He proposes two more, thus five states. These are:

1. Chronic sympathetic neural expression (fight or flight).
2. Ventral vagus (relaxation and social engagement).
3. Dorsal vagus (total shutdown).
4. 'Immobilization without fear': A hybrid state where the dorsal circuit works with the ventral circuit. In this hybrid state, you have slowed down, but still feel socially engaged because the environment is safe and calm. This state typifies the somatic studio, where participants are invited into slow-time meditative movement, but in the presence of a non-judgemental witness and supportive group. Thus, the environment is safe enough to relax, let go and enter a dream-like state. In the somatic studio, we slow down and thus the dorsal circuit is activated, but because the environment is safe, the ventral circuit is simultaneously activated.
5. 'Mobilization without fear': A hybrid state where the sympathetic nerves are active, and the ventral circuit is activated. This is referred to as stimulating activity combined with safety. Again, this state is often cultivated in the somatic studio. We might be exploring fast dynamic movement, using different speeds and qualities. On the one hand, the sympathetic chain is activated, but

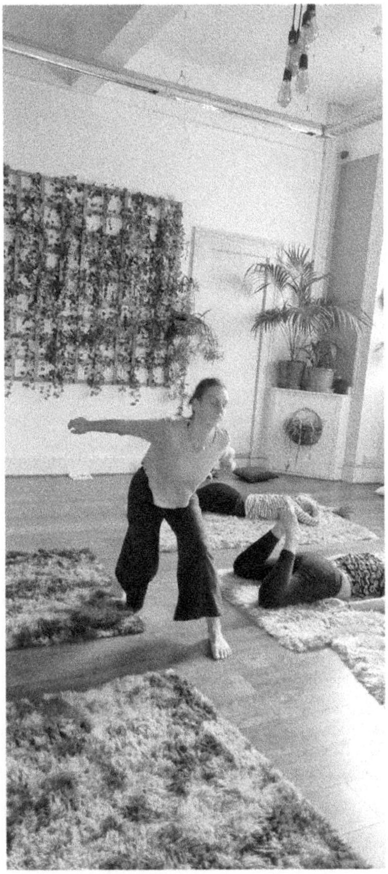

FIGURE 2.9: Jessica Cotton. Photographer: Amanda Williamson.

> because the environment is safe and non-judgemental, the ventral branch is also engaged. There is a lovely balance and healthy innervation of the ventral vagus and the sympathetic nerves. In the somatic studio we often speed up and play, moving through different qualities, dynamics, planes of action, rhythms and tempos. Thus the sympathetics are engaged. However, because the studio is playful and non-judgmental the ventral branch of vagus is also engaged.

Stephen Porges's ground-breaking research drew attention to the concept of safety, demonstrating that if a person does not feel safe, it is extremely hard to feel socially engaged. In short, safety is essential and underlies our ability to feel socially engaged. Thus, we need environments where there is no danger – where there is no need to flee, fight or shut down. Let us take a look at these nerves in detail and explore how to innervate immobilization without fear and the ventral circuit in the studio.

Immobilization without fear: Deep parasympathetic ease-and-release

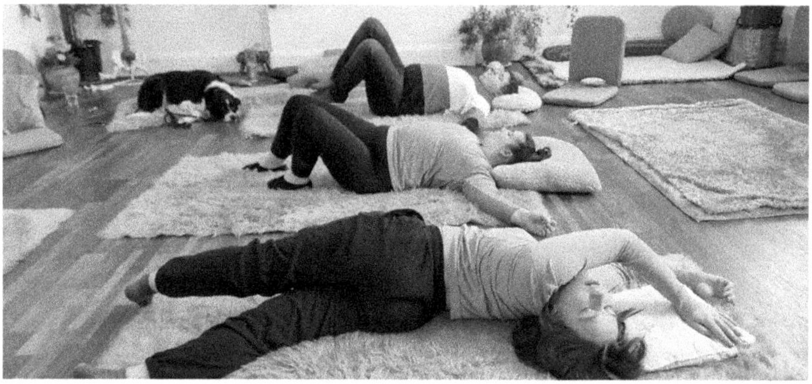

FIGURE 2.10: Movingsoma students: releasing into gravity. Photographer: Amanda Williamson.

Immobilization without fear is an important physiological state I explore in my work as a therapist. This does not mean a person is frozen, with no movement, but rather 'immobilization without fear' refers to feeling safe enough to slow down into a meditative state, supported via interoceptive awareness, and the co-regulatory presence of the non-judgmental (heart-felt) witness. Below I share students moving into a deep parasympathetic self-regulatory improvisational process. Within this process they are sense–perceiving the following tissues, which are essential to engaging the dorsal and ventral branches of the vagus nerve (immobilization without fear): gravi-ception, interoception (breath awareness and cardio-ception), cranio-ception, caudal-cranial-ception, soft-tissue-rolling and self-regulatory improvisational pathways of fascial release. Throughout I have shared reflections from students, post moving, after dropping into this physiological state of consciousness. Many of the sensory-perceptual movement processes I share below are revisited and physiologically deepened in the remaining chapters.

Gravi-ception is the sensory-perceptual ability to release into gravity. It is one of the most healing self-regulatory gifts we possess (the floor and gravity). I refer to this as *gravi-ception* in my practice. Releasing into gravity reduces the weight and pressure baring down on the fibrous, cartilaginous and synovial joints, and the entire vertebral column. All the tissues in the body have an opportunity to release tension, stress and neuromuscular holding.

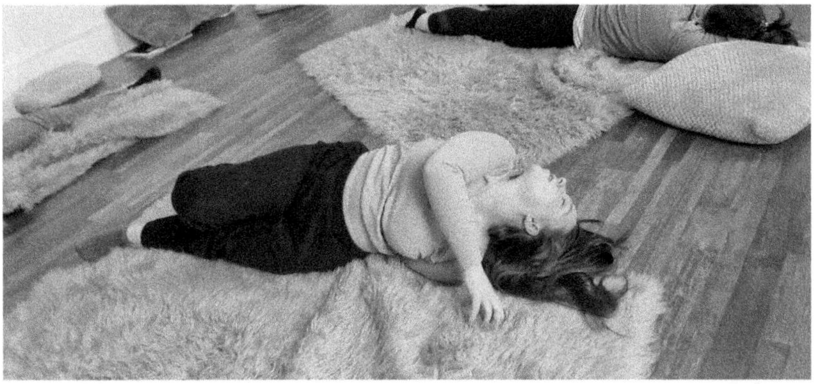

FIGURE 2.11: Natasha Martin: releasing her weight into gravity. Photographer: Amanda Williamson.

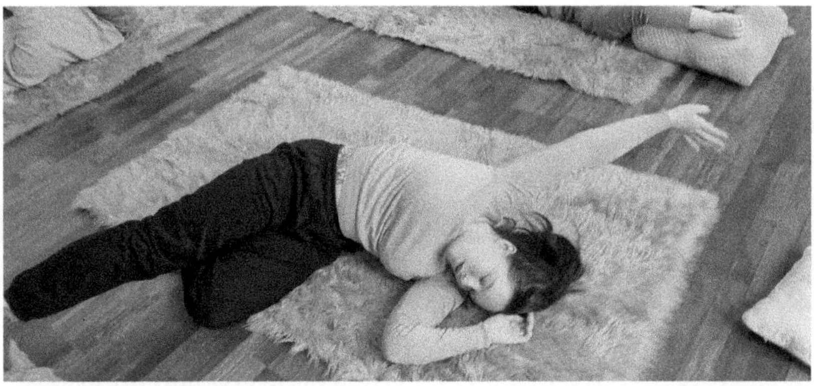

FIGURE 2.12: Natasha Martin: following her breath. Photographer: Amanda Williamson.

Misalignment and poor posture can also be relieved in gravity, and through curling and uncurling in particular (and head–tail movement initiations), gravitational play offers vertebral integration (cervical, thoracic, lumbar and sacral integration and fluidity). When lying and releasing into gravity, the cardiovascular system also slows down. Thus, the simple act of lying down, shutting your eyes and actively releasing into gravity slows the heart rate and supports a gentle shift in the nervous system towards parasympathetic ease-and-release.

> I had a great experience moving and easing my body in gravity, and excited to continue this journey. My mind tends to be quite energetic and not very relaxed but

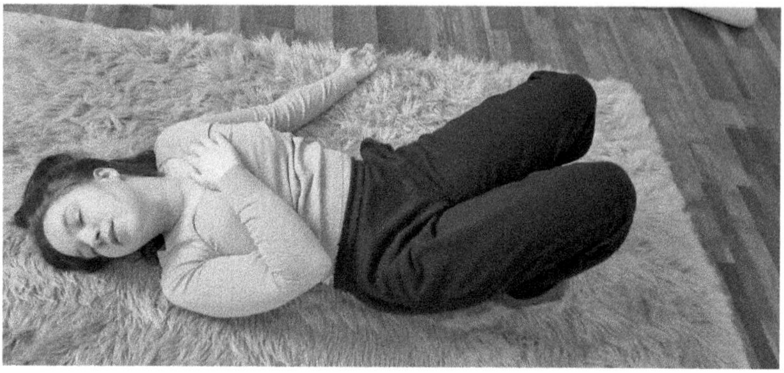

FIGURE 2.13: Natasha Martin: sensing her heart as she moves. Photographer: Amanda Williamson.

> coming here my mind and body feels a different kind of peacefulness which is unexplainable, but incredible. They came together in gravity. This way of moving gives you space to explore your body and mind as one. It helps me with pain, anxiety, depression and more. I always leave a session in a different state of mind than when I arrive (feeling much more calm and relaxed).
>
> (Ruby Gregory)

Interoception & breath flow: Sensing breath and how our tissues and bones move with the inhalation and exhalation invites the nervous system to shift from sympathetic arousal to parasympathetic release. Breath-sensing is the most powerful and efficacious inroad into the parasympathetic. Closing the eyes reduces exteroceptive overwhelm, supporting the gentle shift towards ease and restitution. Sensing the movement and aliveness of breath, filling and emptying, and in particular, sensing the diaphragm supports the vagus nerve to come into a state of health. Bringing awareness to breath, inviting breath to take space in the body and gently moving in response to the ebb and flow of breath, no matter how small, supports the nervous system to calm and induces a parasympathetic *state*.

> A chronic knee injury I've had for almost a year was relieved while moving in gravity and the pain is almost unnoticeable. After taking multiple different medications for this issuc to no avail, I finally feel a difference and would seriously recommend this over any other form of pain management. The session also allowed me time for myself, just to breathe and release the tension I've been holding for months. I came away feeling much happier and far more relaxed.
>
> (Lauren Williams)

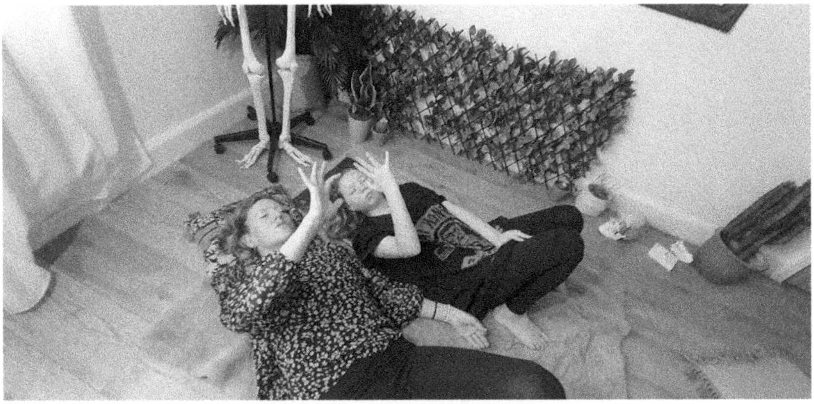

FIGURE 2.14: Amanda Williamson and Tala Closson: sensing their heart as they move. Photographer: Scott Closson.

Cardio-Ception: Noted above, sensing breath, closing eyes and releasing the weight of the body into gravity supports the nervous system to calm. Sensing the physical presence of the heart also supports the nervous system to calm, and thus sensing breath and heart (interoception) are vital pathways into the parasympathetic. I invite students to simultaneously move their awareness between breath and heart, or sense the heart moving with the diaphragm. Developing interoceptive awareness of the heart is, for me, the most essential ingredient in growth and compassion. 'Core heart feelings reduce the activity of the sympathetic nervous system and increase the activity of the parasympathetic nervous system' (Childre and Martin 1999: 23).

> When the facilitator asked me to bring awareness to my heart, I came to stillness. I had a profound stillness within me, a quietness and I could feel care for myself, like there you are, Lauren, and you need care. I give myself a hard time usually. This session changed the way I might feel about myself. In my heart I feel a connection to a deeper part of me. In breath and heart, I feel different about myself – perhaps I am not that bad. You know what I mean? Perhaps I need to care for myself more.
>
> (Lauren Henton)

> This way of moving allowed me to release emotions and physical symptoms manifesting within my body. It was a brilliant way of bringing calm to my body.
>
> (Elizabeth Ware)

Cranio-ception: Releasing the weight of the cranium and slowly tipping and pouring the head from side-to-side decompresses the cervical vertebrae and releases the

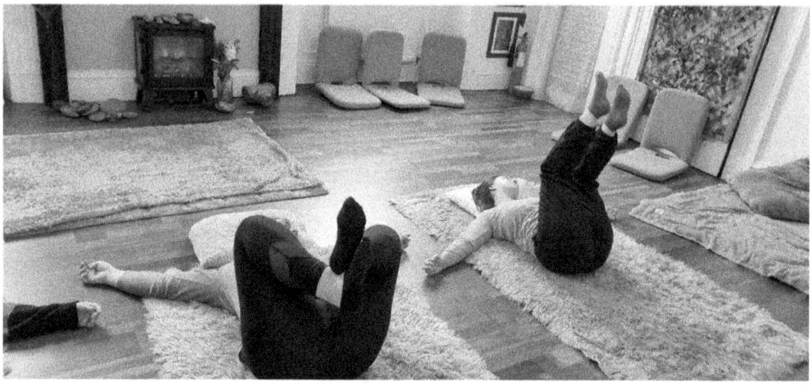

FIGURE 2.15: Natasha Martin and Celine Parsons: sense–dwelling in their sacrums. Photographer: Amanda Williamson.

tissues that pass through or around the sub-occipital triangle. The head weighs approximately 10 pounds and is the heaviest part of the human body. Releasing the weight of the head decompresses the cranial nerves, particularly the spinal accessory nerve, vagus nerve and glossopharyngeal nerve. These nerves drop through the jugular foramina (two holes between the occipital bone and temporal bones). They then move into the mouth and the soft tissues of the neck. Releasing the head also takes pressure off the vertebral artery that runs between the C1 and the occipital bone, supporting arterial flow. Additionally, the sub-occipital muscles may have the opportunity to release. Unwinding the many tissues that surround, attach to, or originate on the occipital bone and temporal bones supports the tissues in the neck to soften. Softening the muscle tissues that are connected to the shoulder girdle and the aforementioned cranial bones offers tremendous release. The sympathetic chain that is active in the neck is calmed through softening these tissues. Thus, releasing the head is one of the most important processes in entering parasympathetic ease-and-release. It is particularly the decompression of the vagus and spinal accessory nerves that support parasympathetic restitution. Additionally, all the sutures between the cranial bones can ease and soften, supporting cerebral-spinal fluid to flow.

The caudal–cranial axis: Sense–dwelling in both the cranium and sacrum also invites the parasympathetic into expression. Sense–perceiving the caudal–cranial axis helps participants to relax because parasympathetic nerves emanate from both locations. Sense–dwelling in the sacrum and cranial bones and moving with awareness of location and sensation, also invites participants into a deep parasympathetic state. Dwelling in afferent sensation and softening the thoraco-lumbar fascia is particularly calming and *delicious*.

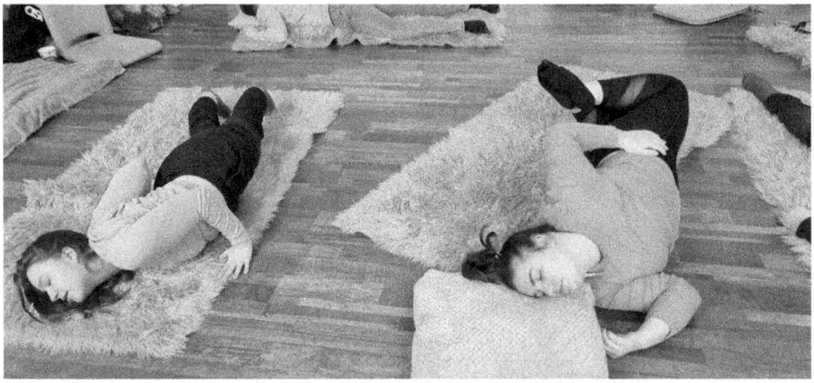

FIGURE 2.16: Natasha Martin and Celine Parsons: sense–perceiving the caudal–cranial axis. Photographer: Amanda Williamson.

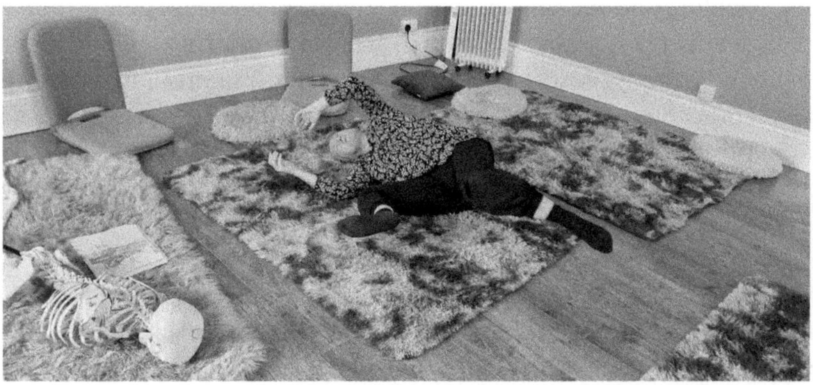

FIGURE 2.17: Karin Rugman unwinding her myofascial tissues through self-regulatory improvisation in gravity. Photographer: Amanda Williamson.

> The separation of body and self is closing, and I am knowing myself as an alive sensory organism always in process. Pain and illness are relieved, and I am more compassionate towards self and others. I am so grateful to have found this way of moving. It has the ability to offer solace and provides life-enhancing support for me and for our communities in these challenging times.
>
> (Vanessa Tucker)

Self-regulatory improvisational pathways and fascial release: Using the hard floor as a fulcrum to release sympathetic stress in the myofascial tissues is an

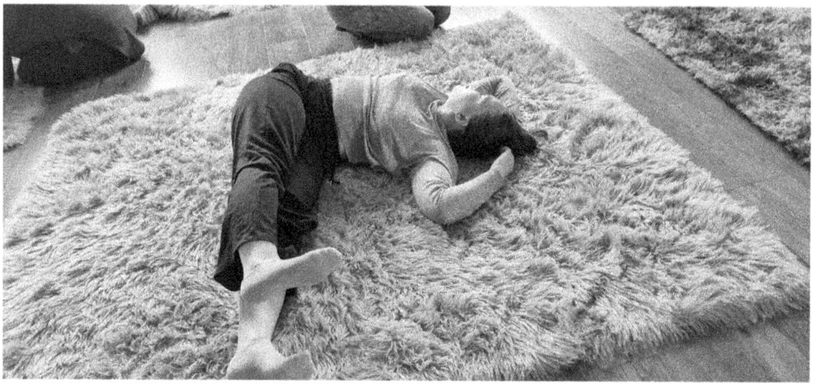

FIGURE 2.18: Natasha Martin: exploring asymmetry. Photographer: Amanda Williamson.

extremely important practice that supports relaxation. Releasing, tipping, pouring, yielding and melting, as well as pivoting, pushing, pulling and twisting into asymmetry – as well as stretching, reaching, rocking and shaking – invites the viscosity of fascia to change. Fascia holds emotions and responds to stress – this type of process offers deep tissue release and enhances a parasympathetic state. Improvisational self-regulatory pathways of fluidity and loosening unwinds the myofascial tissues, opens the myofascial meridians and releases energy.

> This way of working encompasses and honours the interrelationship of physiology and emotionality, offering a therapeutic process which can unwind and release these deep traumas. Bringing interoceptive awareness into my living body, through an in-depth understanding of anatomy and physiology, accessing the parasympathetic nervous system and through sense–perceived, heart-centred, creative and expressive processes, it is allowing my body to gradually heal, release tensions, torsions, traumas and express my true Self. Finding a therapeutic practice of self-regulation which I can continue beyond a facilitated session has given me the most powerful resource of all [...] the ability to heal myself.
>
> (Emma Harte)

> After a lifetime of trauma, accidents and chronic pain and a lifetime of searching for relief, I am deeply moved by how such a seemingly 'simple' practice offered me such a profound and life changing experience in such a short space of time. My physical body (and so all of me!) felt so happy, so relaxed, so connected to my innate self and so in tune with, well, the unified field, or Source.
>
> (Sara Martin)

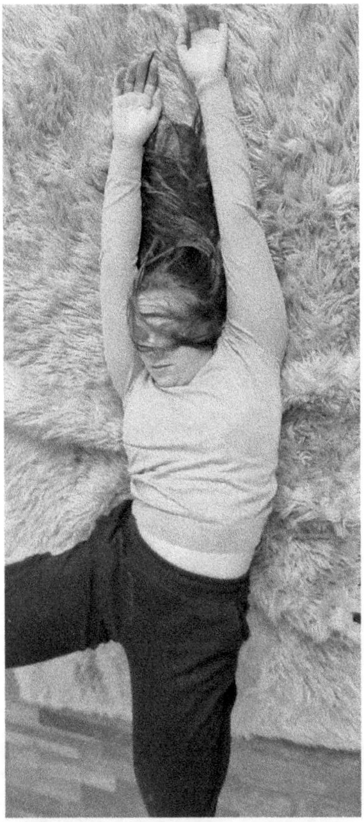

FIGURE 2.19: Natasha Martin: finding ease in tissues in gravity. Photographer: Amanda Williamson.

Proprioception: Sensing-perceiving your synovial joints in gravity and inviting them to float is a deeply relaxing way to engage the parasympathetic. Engaging your limbs and proprioceptive floating creativity, while in gravity, releases the pressure on these joints that are rich in proprioceptors. Floating the limbs and inviting the long bones to fall and suspend in their post-Newtonian synovial fluid is deeply relaxing.

> This knowledge and approach to moving brings more space and fluidity into my being and I am releasing decades of held tension. Embodying myself in this way is also a portal for connecting to my creativity, something that has felt blocked for a long while. It further supports my mental health.
>
> (Louise Barbara)

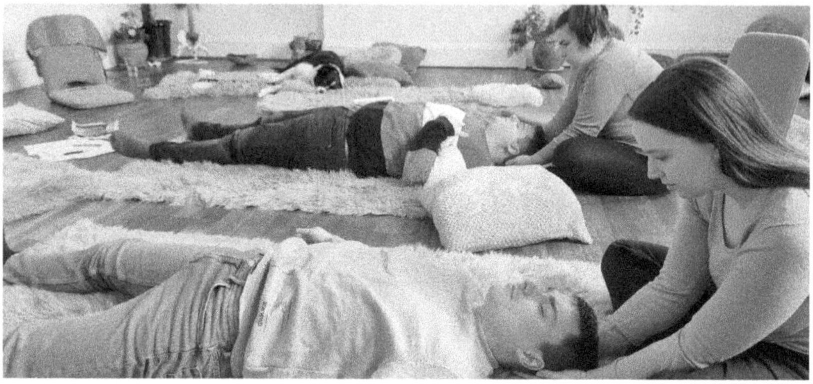

FIGURE 2.20: Movingsoma students: releasing the cranial nerves. Photographer: Amanda Williamson.

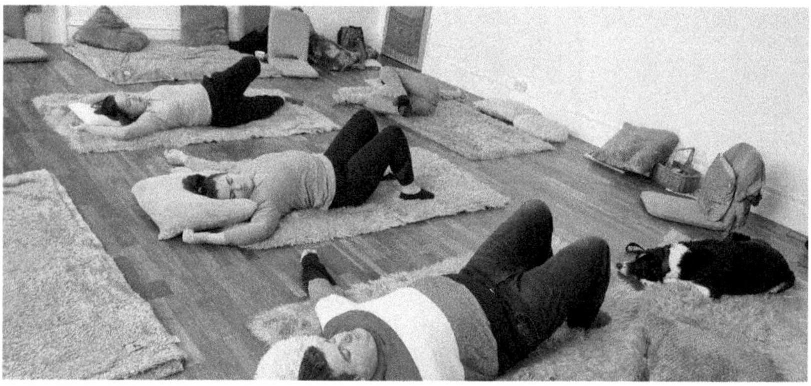

FIGURE 2.21: Movingsoma students: releasing the trapezius and the soft tissues between the occiput and scapulae. Photographer: Amanda Williamson.

Openhearted social engagement: The ventral vagus

Dropping peacefully into a deep parasympathetic state where both the ventral and dorsal branch of the vagus nerve are engaged enables participants to soften and relax. After supporting such deep parasympathetic relaxation (immobilization without fear), I offer processes that support a state of social engagement, where the ventral branch of the vagus nerve is engaged. Social engagement encompasses the aforementioned processes that contact the vagus nerve, but additionally focuses on releasing tension in, or stimulating the muscles in the face, easing tension in the jaw, and unwinding the neck and shoulders with greater attention. If your facial tissues are flat, or holding anger and fear, your shoulders are tense, and your jaw is tight it will deregulate not just you (therapist), but those around you (clients). There are five cranial nerves involved in social engagement: *the trigeminal nerve (V)*, *the facial nerve (V11)*, *the glossopharyngeal nerve (CN 1X)*, *the vagus nerve (X)*, and the *spinal accessory nerve (X1)*. Most of these nerves start life from the brainstem and thus, noted throughout this book, sense–perceiving the occipit and releasing the sub-occipital triangle is an especially important stimulating pathway, engaging the ventral branch of the vagus nerve.

> The ventral branch of the vagus nerve, together with the other four associated cranial nerves, promotes rest and restitution, ensuring that the physiological prerequisites are present for optimal physical and emotional health, friendship, cooperation, mutual support, parent-child bonding and loving relationships.
>
> (Rosenberg 2017: 40)

'When the ventral branch of the vagus nerve and the four associated cranial nerves function properly, human beings and other mammals enjoy a desirable state of social engagement' (Rosenburg 2017: 141). Caring for these five nerves and bringing conscious awareness to their presence is an important aspect of practice that can help to unravel malfunction in these nerves and bring you into a healthy state of social engagement. The face, throat, neck and shoulder girdle play an important role in social engagement. As we drop the weight of our body into ground (earth) and bring awareness to breath, we can also bring awareness to the five cranial nerves involved in social engagement. These nerves receive vital sensory information about whether the environment is safe, but as Porges notes, they are often damaged by fear in the first place. He calls this 'faulty neuroception' (2017). In short, fear and lack of safety deeply affect these nerves, and therefore it is often hard for people to socially engage. Our face may lack energy and droop through sadness, and our jaws often hold incredible amounts of tension/anger, and the muscles in our neck are often in a chronic pattern of sympathetic holding. For example, as Rosenburg notes, and somatic movement therapists are well versed in also, the trapezius and scapulae are often tightly pulled in or up, with the shoulders elevated, edging towards the ears – a significant pattern of fright (Rosenburg 2017: 141). The neck for example, might be retracted in a pattern of fear, and the sternocleidomastoid and trapezius asymmetrically held or twisted. Our organisms cannot escape the pressure, suffering and pain of human life and thus the ventral branch of the vagus nerve may be severely damaged by our lived experience in society and culture. 'There can be countless reasons for faulty neuroception. 'Our perception might be blinded by anger, fear, jealously, or apathy, or we might be locked into a traumatic memory. We may be fixated in a state of shock' (Rosenberg 2017: 63).

Therefore, these nerves, and the tissues they move with, are especially important to sense–perceive and ease in practice. Below I describe a little more about these nerves and offer photographic images of students exploring social engagement.

The ventral vagus

> Contacting breath is good when you are vertical, but much more effective when you are horizontal, dropping your weight and spreading your mass into ground and gravity, sensing the movement of breath in the thorax and diaphragm, and even the subtle movement of bones, ribs, clavicles, sternum and soft tissues throughout the neck, up to the cranium. Somatic practitioners are well versed in observing and resolving (through touch and moving meditations) breathing patterns that reflect fear, stress and indicate sympathetic holding. It is important to invite the diaphragm to take its full expression, motion and space within you. 'Good diaphragmatic breathing is an important element of social engagement' (Rosenberg 2017: 63).
>
> (Rosenberg 2017: 63)

The ventral branch of the vagus originates in your brainstem at the top of your spinal cord. These nerves travel out of your cranium through two small holes, called the jugular foramina, between your occipital bone and temporal bones. Soft-tissue-rolling the cranium and massaging the cranial bones (particularly the sutures between the occipital and temporal bones), as well as releasing the sub-occipitals, with breath awareness, is essential to flossing these nerves into health. Invite participants to release into gravity and gently tip, pour and roll

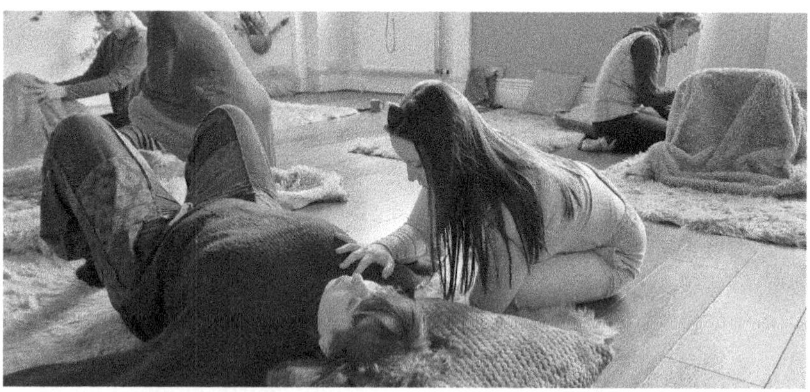

FIGURE 2.22: Movingsoma students: resting, releasing and softening their trapezius in gravity. Photographer: Amanda Williamson.

the weight of their head from side-to-side, massaging the sutures and the tissues between top of the neck and the occipital ridge. Here you can release the cranium, direct your awareness to the brainstem (where the cranial nerves are emanating) and unwind the vagus nerve as it moves from the cranium into the soft tissues of your neck. In this process, both the accessory nerve and the ventral vagus can unwind together and floss into health. Just by 'sensing our own bodies and staying grounded' helps to engage the ventral vagus (Rosenberg 2017: 63).

> I am learning a tremendous amount about the physical body, the nervous system and somatic bodywork practices. It is deeply nourishing for myself. I was able to receive the therapeutic benefits of the work while learning how I could offer it to others. I experienced a deep state of calm and clarity which felt like respite from the otherwise busy and highly stimulating world we live in.
>
> (Sam Nassbite)

> This is a space to learn that supports self-expression and authenticity, as well as a genuine sense of safety which invites participants to try new things.
>
> (Rachel Erickson)

The accessory nerves: Softening the trapezius and sternocleidomastoid

The accessory nerves innervate your trapezius and sternocleidomastoid. Note that these nerves also start from your brainstem and travel out of your cranium together with the vagus nerve, through your jugular foramina. These nerve fibres weave into the trapezius and sternocleidomastoid. Thus, releasing both these

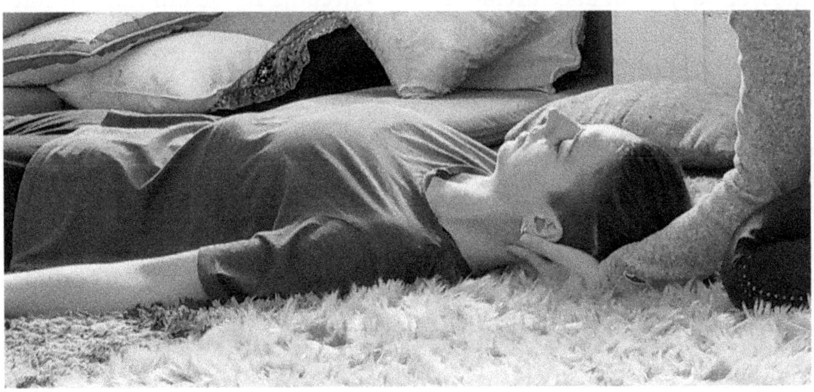

FIGURE 2.23: Staff at movingsoma teaching sub-occipital release. Photographer: Scott Closson.

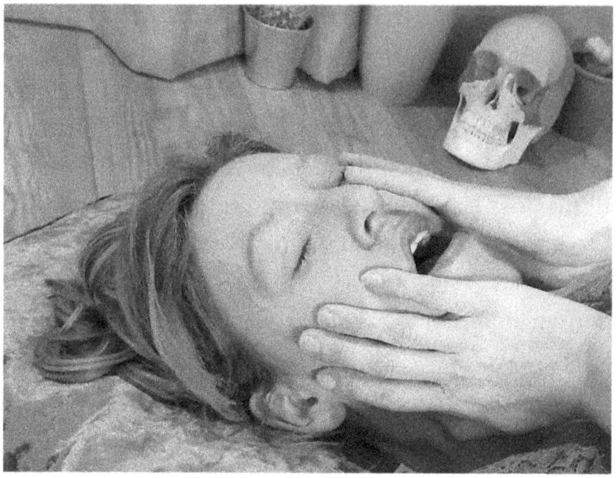

FIGURE 2.24: Amanda Williamson: softening in her face and jaw. Photographer: Scott Closson.

muscles is essential when supporting participants to feel socially engaged. Invite participants to soften the tissues of their trapezius into ground. Invite the weight of the cranium to pour from side-to-side with breath awareness, loosening and easing the sternocleidomastoid and trapezius (both attach between the shoulder girdle and neck). Remember these muscles are innervated by the accessory nerve, one of the five cranial nerves involved in social engagement. Holding the cranium, when trained in methods of sub-occipital release, is an especially important and efficacious way to decompress these nerves and floss them into health.

The glossopharyngeal and fascial nerves: Softening in the mouth, jaw and face

The glossopharyngeal nerves start life in your brainstem. They travel through the jugular foramina, with the vagus and accessory nerve, reaching your mouth, mucous glands, palatine tonsil and the base of the tongue. Along with the vagus, the glossopharyngeal forms the *pharyngeal plexus*, supplying the palate and throat (larynx and pharynx). The pharynx is part of the throat behind the mouth and the nasal cavity and the larynx is the voice box. The glossopharyngeal nerve supplies parasympathetic fibres that aid the body with rest and digestion and innervate the salivary glands. Thus, softening in the mouth and throat (particularly the stylopharyngeus muscles), as well as *sounding and singing* is a wonderful way to support these nerves enlivening into social engagement. Invite participants to hum, sound and tone as they move, sense–perceiving the movement and vibration of sound in their tissues. 'The ventral branch of the vagus nerve innervates many muscles of the small muscles of the throat, including the vocal cords, larynx, pharynx' and 'activity in this circuit has a calming, soothing effect, and promotes rest and restitution' (Rosenburg 2017: 34). Sounding, humming, toning and singing innervate the ventral vagus, supporting social engagement (Porges 2017).

The facial nerve is responsible for your facial expression and plays a vitally important role in your ability to communicate and socially engage. As Porges notes, our faces are often flat with trauma (2017). The facial nerve starts from the pons in the brainstem and exits the cranium through a different hole, in the temporal bone, called *the stylomastoid foramen.* Releasing the deep muscles in the face, and the pterygoids, unwinding tension and repatterning neuromuscular holding, as well as stimulating the flat muscles above and around the eyes, is especially important in supporting a ventral state.

The trigeminal nerve: Releasing and softening the jaw

The trigeminal nerve is responsible for the sensation in your face and your muscles of mastication. These nerves innervate the muscles you use to chew and bite. Thus, releasing tension in your jaw is particularly important. Invite the face and jaw to unwind. Often people are afraid and embarrassed to open their jaw and unwind their faces through unusual asymmetrical stretches and releases. Model this for your participants to give them permission to explore wildly. Invite the muscles in the face to stretch, lengthen, contract, release, soften and unwind. Invite the jaw to release tension.

> The studio is a sanctuary that holds a safe space, full of light and nature where I can unfurl and begin settle into a slower more natural rhythm, drop to gravity and come home to my body. As someone without a dance background I've found this process very liberating. Both the space and my experiences during our sessions have been profoundly nurturing and healing. Its helped me to develop a deeper awareness of my joints, tissues and nervous system and gain new perspectives. I am also grateful for the opportunity to witness and connect with other like-minded people and reengage with my creativity and the natural world and movement.
>
> (Sally Picken)

Stimulating the ventral branch of the vagus, as well as supporting deep release through immobilization without fear are two physiological states of embodied consciousness often experienced in the somatic movement studio. Most practices across the field innervate the nerves pertaining to social engagement, especially modalities that use sound, toning, relational touch and fascial unwinding. Sense–tracking the journey of breath through the body is a hallmark of

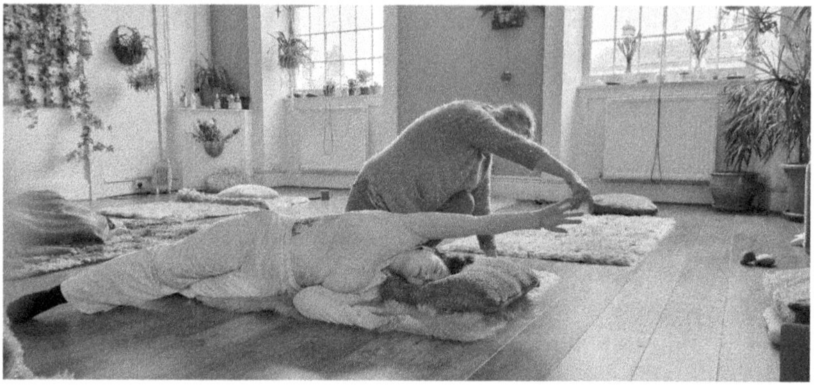

FIGURE 2.25: Karin Rugman and Natasha Martin: sensing breath. Photographer Amanda Williamson.

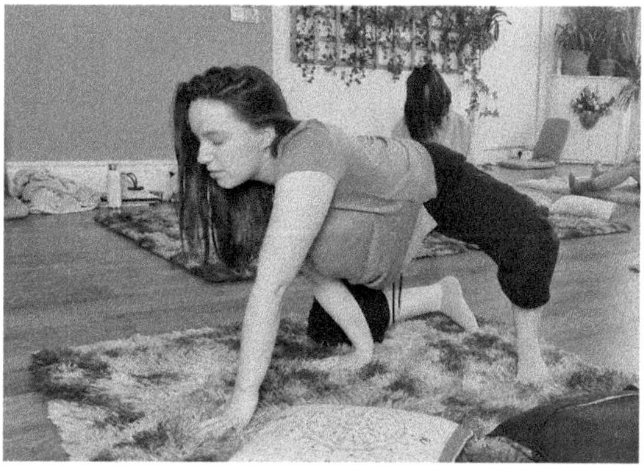

FIGURE 2.26: Natasha Martin: starting to push away from the floor. Photographer: Amanda Williamson.

somatic movement dance practices. In many modalities, participants are invited to soften and open their airways. We might, for example, invite participants to sense the air passing over their lips, moving into the pharynx and larynx, down the trachea and into lungs. Participants are invited to sense their breath and on the inhalation and exhalation, sound and tone. Attending to the movement of the thorax and indeed the diaphragm underpins many processes offered in the somatic studio. We experientially explore how the diaphragm invites breath and breathes us.

Relaxing the jaw, softening in oral cavity, sounding and toning are key aspects of international practice. Shutting the eyes, sensing breath, following fluid movement pathways of ease and inviting sound to arise from the sensory-perception of breath and the vibrations felt in tissues are extremely important aspects of practice. Just this process alone invites vagal health. Processes of breathing, moving, sounding and toning can last for over an hour with an experienced group. Laughter and the joy of free play, somatic touch and connection with Self and Other all support social engagement.

There are many more ways that somatic movement practices share common ground with Porges's research. The very fact we work with our eyes shut for long periods of time, breathing, sounding and toning, and notably unwinding and liquefying the tissues through fascial release in gravity will quite naturally innervate the nerves underpinning social engagement and immobilization without fear. Hence, practitioners are often attending to these healthy physiological states, even if they are not focussing on these nerves explicitly. Shutting the eyes for long periods of time (it can be up to an hour with an experienced group) is a very welcome break from constantly receiving the exterior public world through exteroception. Our faces, jaws and shoulders (and whole body) start to release as we attend to our internal world of breath and living tissues.

There are many other aspects of practice that stimulate the ventral and dorsal curcuits: perhaps the most obvious is what I term somatic touch and fascial unwinding. I attend to this area in-depth in Chapter 5, but for now let us hold in our awareness that somatic touch supports participants to enter a socially engaged state or a deep parasympathetic state. Somatic touch when offered with the right intention and attention releases restrictions and hypertonicity in the myofascial tissues (discussed in Chapter 7).

Rounding up

It is extremely interesting to note that scientists have measured sympathetic and parasympathetic states and now know that deep relaxation does indeed create altered states of consciousness. Parasympathetic states created by deep relaxation techniques (and somatic movement is a deep relaxation technique) cause the brainwaves to slow from beta to alpha to theta. Thus, the parasympathetic has been measured and it appears that deep relaxation techniques slow the brainwaves to alpha (8–13 cycles/second) and theta (4–8 cycles/second) (Dispenza 2012). Altered states of consciousness are a gift we possess but are often relegated to the esoteric, new age or simply considered wacked-out. There is nothing more wonderful and kinder than sharing with people how to shift from a sympathetic stressed-out state to parasympathetic ease-and-release, where they can balance their nervous system, breathe, rest, let go, dream, reflect, feel pleasure and take solace from the harsh landscapes of the exterior world. A large part of the healing process in somatic movement is altering one's embodied state of consciousness and enjoying the expansive parasympathetic realms of alpha and theta. In my practice I align alpha, which is a relaxed but alert state of being with social engagement. Additionally, I align and empirically investigate theta with deep parasympathetic release (immobilization without fear), where participants explore improvisatory landscapes underpinned by breath, heart awareness and soft tissue release for long periods of time. Such processes release participants from the mundane and expand one's awareness, and I add, help one to sense Self beyond the socio-economic world that constricts our sensuality and confines us to a one-dimensional barren consciousness.

In this chapter, we explored

- how to sense–perceive, stimulate and move with awareness of the vagus nerve;
- how to sense–perceive and move with awareness of the geography of craniosacral and lumbar–thoracic divisions of the autonomic nervous system;
- how to release sympathetic holding in the sympathetic chain and contact the neurological outflows of the sympathetic nerves to the heart, solar plexus and adrenals;
- how to engage the cranial nerves involved in immobilization without fear (engaging both curcuits of the vagus nerve);
- how to innervate the cranial nerves involved in social engagement (the ventral branch of the vagus nerve).

The practices I shared in this chapter are just four examples out of many ways that creative practitioners can educate and offer therapeutic practice in relation to the ANS. Our world is fraught with dangers and our institutions cause incredible stress through their bureaucracy, technocracy and focus on production and consumption, at the expense of understanding how humans need balance, restitution, safety and peace. Let us move on to Chapter 3, where we revisit some of the anatomy and physiology presented in this chapter in far more depth, as well as discern a number of other tissues that support rest, ease and release. Below I round up by offering some key learnings from this chapter.

Key offerings and learnings

- The vagus nerve is one of the most important nerves in the body.
- Engaging the vagus nerve helps to restore an over sympathetically charged nervous system.
- The tissues and pathways of awareness that help to engage the vagus are: interoception, cardio-ception, gravi-ception, cranio-ception and breath awareness (good diaphragmatic breathing).

- Deep tissue release supports emotional holding to express, discharge and liquefy. Different degrees of pressure and energy engage the parasympathetics and change the viscosity of fascia.
- The ANS has a physical geography in the body that somatic movement practitioners can craft practice around (the craniosacral and thoracic–lumbar divisions).

3

Fulcrums of Support and Soft Tissue Reorganization

I slide my fingers under my clavicles
and rest my open hand on my sternum.
I feel the rise and fall of my breath
and sense into my heart space.
A gentle wave of motion passes through me,
swaying me gently side to side, back and forth.
A warm, soft summer breeze blowing through the tall grasses,
Each stem quietly being lulled by the wind.
A sense of expansion and release fills my attention.
A flower opening its petals to greet the sun,
a warm smile fills my heart.
This positive attentiveness invites my thymus
to bathe in love and light.
Tips of fingers lightly sense the thyroid glands,
delicate and fragile.
I feel my neck soften into my hands,
sending gentle waves that invite my head
to rock and sway.
This sense of lightness and softness
eases my burdens.
My neck releases and head floats.
I feel an effortless motion,
a sense of peace.

(Karin Rugman, writing after directing
her awareness into living tissues)

In Chapters 1 and 2, I referred to the occipital bone and the temporal bones a number of times, with reference to why releasing the soft tissues surrounding the occiput, temporal bones and the cervical spine aids relaxation and parasympathetic release. In the first part of this chapter, I take a deep dive into these areas again, but through a closer anatomical reading and reflection. The occipital bone and temporal bones are primary fulcrums of self-regulatory support, especially when we settle into gravity at the start of sessions. These bones offer incredible structural support and a fulcrum (a pivotal place) to recognize the soft tissues that originate from, or attach to them, such as the trapezius, suboccipitals, levator scapulae and sternocleidomastoid. The scapulae are also primary fulcrums of structural and reorganizational support. For example, when we lie in gravity, contacting and easing the scapulae, we can reorganize the soft tissues that lie between the cranial bones and the shoulder girdle, particularly the trapezius. Further, we can ease the soft tissues that beautifully cross the glenohumeral joint, connecting the scapulae with the humerus, such as the rotator cuff. Additionally, when we ease the tissues surrounding the scapulae, we can bring self-regulatory health to extensive tissues, such as the latissimus dorsi, that grows out of the thoraco-lumbar fascia, hitches a ride on the inferior angle of the scapulae, and then reaches out so fluently to the humerus. Further, the sacrum is a major fulcrum of structural and self-regulatory of support. For example, when we soften, tip, pour, roll and ease the myofascial tissues snuggly surrounding the sacral region and pelvic bowl, deliciously compressing and decompressing the myofascia, we can reorganize the thoraco-lumbar fascia, the gluteus maximus, and the tensor fasciae latae. All these beautiful fulcrums are pivotal areas (islands of support) in our inter-connected wholeness, but often feel strained, compressed, twisted, and may have hard tonus. Softening into these fulcrums is emblematic of my practice,

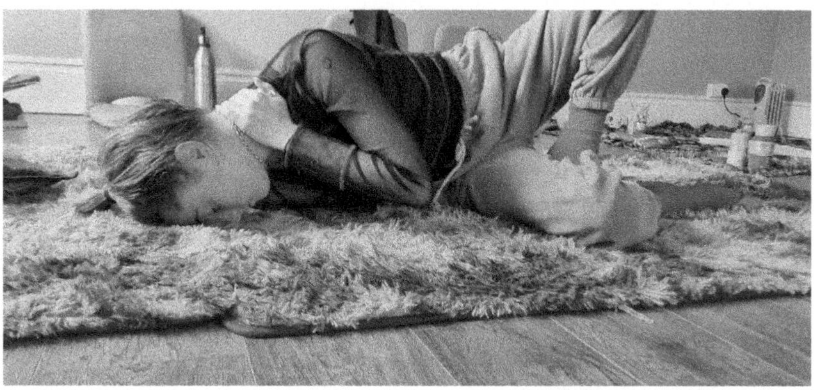

FIGURE 3.1: Movingsoma students exploring their fulcrums. Photographer: Amanda Williamson.

especially at the beginning of sessions. In this chapter, I unearth and unpick in detail why sense–perceiving these fulcrums and reorganizing the tissues that enfold and surround them has an advanced anatomical and physiological rationale; in short, there are very good reasons why somatic movement dance practitioners spend so much time sensing the occiput, tipping, pouring and rolling the cranium, in turn releasing the soft tissues between the cranial bones and shoulder girdle, melting the soft tissues surrounding the scapulae, rippling health and fluency throughout the arms, throughout the vertebral column, and all the way to the sacrum, pelvis and legs.

This chapter is not for the faint-hearted. It is long and complicated, paying attention to many small but highly significant details that underlie why practitioners offer so many processes in gravity, releasing the head, and unwinding and liquifying tissues. It is the most in-depth chapter in this book, in terms of anatomy and physiology. It is not a chapter one can read on a sunny morning from beginning to end, without pause and digestion. It takes intellectual work. This is not bad a thing, for the aforementioned fulcrums have many deliciously fluid secretes that are key to health and can be augmented into fluency through self-regulatory movement. I have divided this long chapter into the following distinctive parts.

Part 1: 'The occipital bone as a fulcrum of support and tissue reorganization'

Slow-time sensing-perceiving the occipital bone, the atlantoaxial joint and atlantooccipital joints.
Releasing the vertebral artery.
The foramen magnum.
The jugular foramina: the accessory, vagus and glossopharyngeal nerves.
Soft tissues, nuchal lines and the posterior surface of the occiput.
Sensing the suboccipitals.

Part 2: 'The scapulae as a fulcrum of support and soft tissue reorganization'

The bony landmarks of the scapulae.
The glenohumeral, sternoclavicular, acromioclavicular and scapulothoracic joints.
The rotator cuff muscles.

The sternocleidomastoid and trapezius.

Part 3: 'The sacrum as fulcrum of support and soft tissue reorganization'

The sacroiliac joints and lumbar–sacral joint.
The sacral plexus.
The thoraco-lumbar fascia.
The parasympathetic nerves and the pudendal nerve.

Introduction: Fulcrums of support and soft tissue reorganization

The occiput, the scapulae and the sacral region are five fulcrums that naturally emerge as areas of structural bony support when participants rest, soften, release and yield in gravity. Somatic movement sessions usually start in gravity, and often in a supine position. When participants lie in a supine position and release their weight, these fulcrums, which are wonderfully bony places, offer a structural landscape that supports participants to feel their longitudinal axis (the caudal–cranial/head–tail axis) and bi-lateral width (lateralization across the scapulae and arms). It is important to bring these bony places of structural support into sensory-perceptual awareness because the tissues that surround and enfold these fulcrums are relational tissues – they extend beyond each fulcrum, and many tissues connect the fulcrums. If the tissues in these fulcrums are compressed, tense, tort or twisted, the entire organism is negatively affected.

Fulcrum support and soft tissue reorganization might appear a simple practice to the outside eye. Outsiders, for example, would observe participants lying in gravity, with their eyes closed and sensing their breath. They would observe participants inviting gentle compressions, decompressions and releases in the tissues surrounding these bony fulcrums. They would observe the outward expression of soft undulating, rippling and unwinding movements initiated from the occipital bone, scapulae and sacrum. They would observe participants slowly pouring the weight of their craniums from side-to-side (sometimes tipping, pouring and softening their cranium and facial bones into their hands and into the floor). Very often, they would observe the whole body following and responding, welcoming a movement impulse felt in a specific fulcrum to ripple out through the limbs – perhaps reaching, extending, spiralling, curling, folding, softening and yielding. While this process might look simple to the outside eye, complex physiological

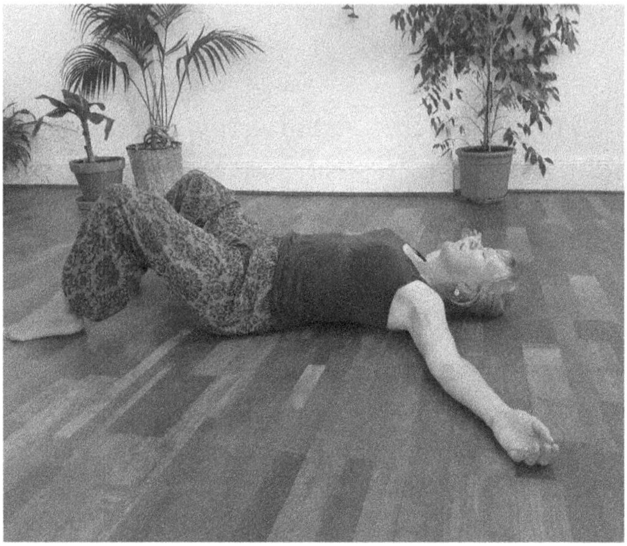

FIGURE 3.2: Karin Rugman: settling into her fulcrums of support. Sense–percieving her occipt, scapulae, sacrum and feet. Photographer: Amanda Williamson.

knowledge underpins my creative practice in the studio. I call this *micro physiological knowledge* – the incredible complexity underlying the apparent simplicity of somatic movement dance practice. Some of the physiological details I share in this chapter are so tiny, they would be imperceptible to the outside observer. Hence, to the outsider, it might appear participants are simply rolling around the floor, with no rhyme or reason. For example, decompressing and stimulating the occipital bone and temporal bones with awareness of *the jugular foramina* (the two little holes between the occipital bone and temporal bones that transmit the vagus, accessory and glossopharyngeal nerves) underlies part of the process I share in this chapter. This objective and subjectively sensed–perceived knowledge is of course miniscule, but deeply efficacious when embodied and empirically investigated by participants.

Many people who attend sessions express chronic neck and back pain, migraines and headaches, low mood, low self-esteem, a general feeling of unwellness, and high levels of stress. I have also felt these emotions and feeling states in my life – many times. Exploring fulcrum support and soft tissue reorganization can relieve sympathetic holding, bring symmetry to twists and torsions in the skeletal–muscular system and myofascial tissues, ease trigger points, and decompress fibrous, cartilaginous and synovial joints (supporting balanced posture in the vertical plane).

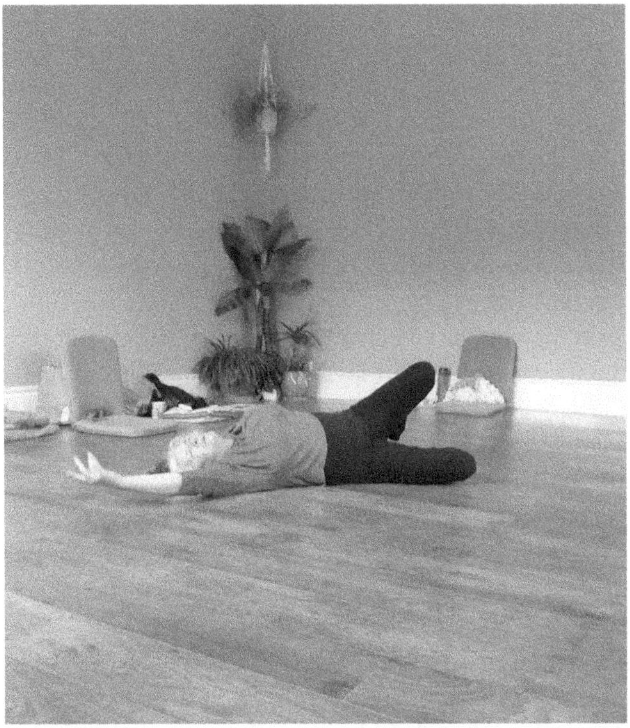

FIGURE 3.3: Heather Larkin-Joans: self-regulating the tissues around her scapulae. Reaching through the arms and compressing and decompressing the myofascial tissues on the lateral boarder of her scapulae. Photographer: Amanda Williamson.

Noted earlier, fulcrum support always starts by inviting participants to settle into the floor and close their eyes (initially starting in a supine position). They are further invited to release the weight of their body into gravity and invite their mass (living tissues) to ease and spread along the floor. Participants are further invited to notice how the ground is always there, meeting and supporting their weight, force and mass (the earth's ground reaction force). This process is always accompanied by the invitation to feel breath – to sense–perceive the movement of breath, to invite breath to flow through the tissues – to *still* and *rest* in breath. The invitation to close the eyes reduces the amount of information entering the central nervous system through the exteroceptive system. Thus, at the beginning of sessions the focus shifts from experiencing the world outwardly, through the exteroceptive system (the public and egoic world), to re-experiencing the world inwardly (our private world of source and life-energy, ebbing and flowing), through interoceptive awareness.

Participants are further invited to sense–perceive their primary fulcrums of support – how their occiput, scapulae and sacrum easily meet the ground. Here participants can begin to sense their bony structure, as well as the living state of the soft tissues that surround and enfold these fulcrums. By structural support, I specifically mean developing a sensory–perceptual relationship with the occiput, scapulae and sacrum – bony places where participants can land, ground and earth, compress and decompress. By soft tissue reorganization, I specifically mean releasing neuromuscular and myofascial holding felt in and around these fulcrums, through self-regulatory movement.

Many places in the body can be contacted as fulcrums of support and soft tissue reorganization – toes, feet, hands, hips, iliac crests and the acromion process, for example. When we work and play in gravity, we often intuitively contact a particular body part and start to pivot around this area, releasing and decompressing. Pivoting around fulcrums through self-regulatory movement is a defining feature of my work. Notably, most joints in the human body, no matter how small, can be explored as mini fulcrums of reorganization, especially when spiralling, extending, softening and bouncing in the post-Newtonian liquidity of synovial fluid. Fulcrums can be defined as pivotal places, where tissues orginate or attach, but often become disorganized through stress and strain. While there are many fulcrums in the human body, the occiput, the scapulae and the sacrum are macro fulcrums. These five macro fulcrums are places where considerable strain often accumulates, but paradoxically, these same places, when listened to, and moved with gentle attuned self-regulatory awareness, are superb locations of reorganization, release and flow (Williamson 2020a). Reorganizing the tissues that surround a fulcrum influences the health of the surrounding tissues, and the whole organism. Thomas Attlee refers to fulcrums as

> [a] fulcrum is a pivotal point around which a system operates – whether it be a simple mechanical lever, or a more complex system. Within the body structure there are countless fulcrums. Every joint – vertebral joint, knee joint, finger joint, any joint – acts as a fulcrum in relation to a localised activity. The body also operates as an integrated unit, with certain pivotal areas acting as fulcrums for the body as a whole.
>
> (Attlee 2012: 94)

These five macro fulcrums, while some distance apart, are deeply relational. When we soften, tip, pour, pivot and play in gravity between these fulcrums, there is a rippling undulating conversation between them. Thus, fulcrum support is always facilitated through a relational framework. The process is guided by a facilitator who languages, tones, sounds, supports and guides participants through the process. The process is self-regulatory and improvisational (underpinned by listening to how tissues need to unwind and follow nourishing movement pathways). In this chapter I dissect and analyse how sense–perception of these tissues can offer release and ease. This chapter is long. The actual process in real time might last for 40–60 minutes. The process invites participants to:

Release into gravity with breath awareness (attuning to interoceptive awareness).
Direct their awareness to these fulcrums one at a time, and sense–perceive the state of these living bones and tissues.
Listen to afferent information streaming in from these fulcrums through slow-time sensory-perceptual awareness and follow pathways of ease and fluency.
Initiate movement from these fulcrums, inviting the rest of the body to tenderly follow and respond.

For clarity, detail and illumination, in this chapter, I will explore each fulcrum individually, with attention to relationality where possible. Here, I am drawing attention to why these fulcrums are important and some key tissues that can be recognized through self-regulatory movement. Other practitioners might bring awareness to different tissues. For every tissue I differentiate in this chapter, there are many more. I have chosen particular tissues that are related to parasympathetic ease and social engagement, such as the suboccipitals, the trapezius, sternocleidomastoid and rotator cuffs, in order to build on the knowledge shared in previous chapters. This chapter begins with the occiput and moves to the scapulae and sacrum.

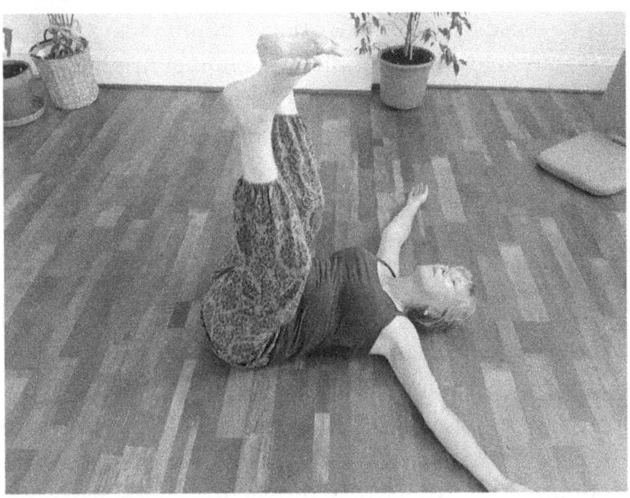

FIGURE 3.4: Karin Rugman: self-regulating her lumbar–sacral region and scapulae. Photographer: Amanda Williamson.

On a global note, before we begin to differentiate tiny tissues, when we rest in our primary fulcrums of support in a supine position, we can sense–perceive how the occiput, scapulae and sacrum are all connected to our midline (our vertebral column). Hence any movement initiated from a key fulcrum is also inviting the vertebral column to follow, respond and unwind. For example, initiating movement from the occipital bone invites the cervical vertebrae to follow and unwind. Initiating movement from the scapulae invites the thoracic spine and ribcage to follow and unwind. Initiating movement from the sacrum, invites the lumbar spine into fluency. Thus, fulcrum support and soft tissue re-organization is always inviting our midline into integrative awareness. Additionally, because we invite the rest of the body to tenderly follow and respond to fulcrum initiations, the limbs are always invited into expression and fluency.

I also note early that all the individuated tissues I mention in this chapter are surrounded by fascia. Fascia is the largest body-wide organ in the human body, found underneath the skin (the superficial or subcutaneous fascia), around every muscle (the epimysium), every buddle of muscle fibres (the perimysium), every cell and fibre (the endomysium), and indeed every bone (the periosteum). Fascia has ten times more sensory receptors and six times more pain receptors than muscle (Schleip 2017), and thus when you invite participants to sense individuated muscles or bones (as I do in this chapter), they are also receiving a wealth of information about pain and hypertonicity from the surrounding fascia. Hypertonicity is often felt in and around these fulcrums. Participants are invited to ease this via compression, decompression, different pressures, strectching and melting, softening, relaxation and rest. Thus, self-regulatory movement will naturally support students to sense hypertonicity, tigger points, scar tissue, and adhesions in fascia. Through melting, softening, sliding, gliding, tipping, pouring and yielding, compression and decompression, and resting, they are supporting damaged fascial tissues to heal. Additionally, as participants curl and uncurl, spiral, reach and stretch-out through their limbs, they are transmitting bio-tensional forces, opening, strengthening, and releasing kinetic energy through the myofascial fascial meridians, particularly the superficial front line (SFL), the superficial back line (SBL), the lateral line (LL), the spiral (SL), and the four front and back arm lines (Myers 2014). My main point being, sense–perception of individuated tissues in this chapter, will affect the fascia throughout the body.

Fascia is the topic of Chapter 7. However, it is really important to note early that sense–perceiving individuated tissues and moving within a self-regulatory improvisational movement framework will support the health and vicosity of fascia locally and globally. As participants gently sense–perceive individuated tissues and invite movement to ripple, emerge, swell, and spiral forth from a particular focus point, they are inviting more blood to reach and repair adhesions

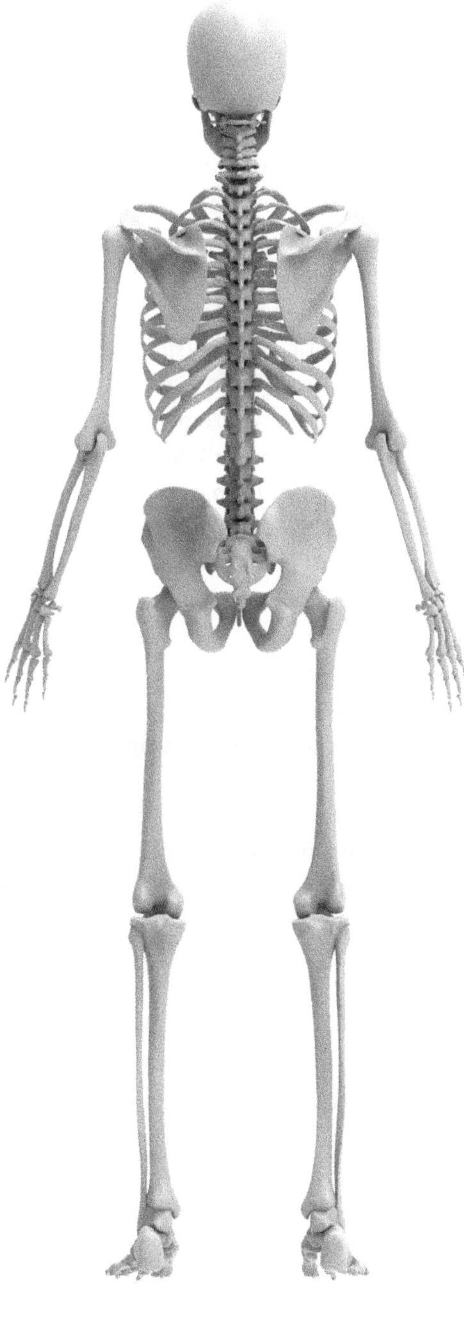

FIGURE 3.5: The human skeleton (posterior view). Notice the occiput, the scapulae, sacrum and ilium: places to land, rest, pivot and play.

and scar tissue caused by lack of mobility, depression, stress or repetitive movement. For example, in this chapter I focus on the scapulae. All the muscles and bones of the scapulae are covered by fascia. As participants compress, decompress, stretch and release in their scapulae, all the surrounding fascial tissues have an opportunity to remodel. Sense–perceiving and sense–dwelling in a localized area, starts the ripple effect out through the fascial matrix. Because fascia surrounds bones, muscles, nerves, cells and the vascular system, focusing on a particular area helps to free matted and restricted fascial tissues that are hindering blood supply and electrical charge. As such, while I invite our attention and awareness to dwell in specific tissues or through particular physiological pathways in this chapter, as movement arises and ripples forth, many systems are being cared for, such as the lymphatic, vascular and nervous systems also. Freeing the fascia supports neuro-excitability, and releases energy. Self-regulatory movement, by its nature, invites new and manifold neuromuscular pathways to open, and this supports the fascia also, especially because fascia is damaged by repetition. Improvisation can be the antithesis of repetition, and hence, self-regulatory movement is extremely important to fascial health. As Sanderson so importantly shares below:

> Movement is essential to the repair and maintenance of healthy fascial tissue. It provides direction for the disposition of collagen and encourages vascular regeneration. Movement also lubricates and hydrates connective tissues.
>
> (Sanderson 2021: 15)

Keeping this in mind, let us begin to differentiate some lovely tiny tissues that you can sense–percieve and improvisationally unwind in gravity. Let us start by exploring the secrets of the occiput.

Part 1: The occiput as a fulcrum of support and tissue reorganization

Across the field it is common to witness facilitators inviting participants to release their occiput into gravity, tip and pour their craniums from side-to-side and encourage the rest of their body to tenderly and receptively follow. In short, one's whole living organism is invited to respond to movement initiated from the occiput and cranium, with breath awareness. Releasing the weight of the cranium and soft tissue rolling in gravity is emblematic of much therapeutic work taking place internationally. Keeping the body soft and responsive is a key skill we teach in the studio. If the body can tenderly respond and follow the cranial bones, the tissues surrounding the suboccipital region can ease, loosen and unwind. Simultaneously, the tissues surrounding the cervical, thoracic, lumbar and sacral spine can soften

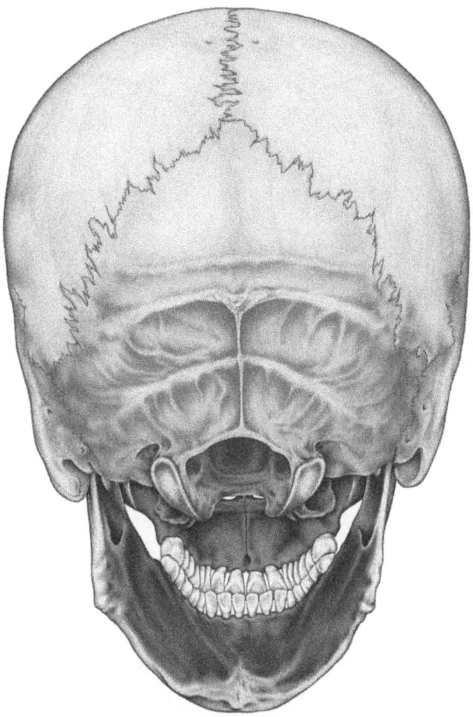

FIGURE 3.6: The occipital bone and foramen magnum: posterior view.

and liquify. Note, to the outsider this might look easy, simply playful, and perhaps silly. However, it is a skill we teach students and participants – and it is not an easy skill. This skill underlies safe practice. Keeping the body soft and responsive underlies safe practice, as well as supports sensing and playing with relationality.

When we invite participants to soften and rest in gravity, lying on their backs, notably the cranium, but much more specifically, the occiput meets the ground first. The cranium is the heaviest part of the human body. An adult head weighs approximately ten to eleven pounds or four and a half to five kilograms. While dancers often lie in gravity before or after class, languishing in their living senate and breath, imagine how novel it is to introduce a client who is not a dancer to rest and settle into the floor, release the weight of their head, and free the pressure baring down on their cervical, thoracic, lumbar and sacral spine. People who are not trained dancers spend most of their life moving in the vertical plane, usually working at a fast pace, sympathetically charged, with little time to rest. It is a huge relief for participants to rest their bodies and release their craniums in gravity. This reduces the load placed on the cervical spine (and the entire vertebral column),

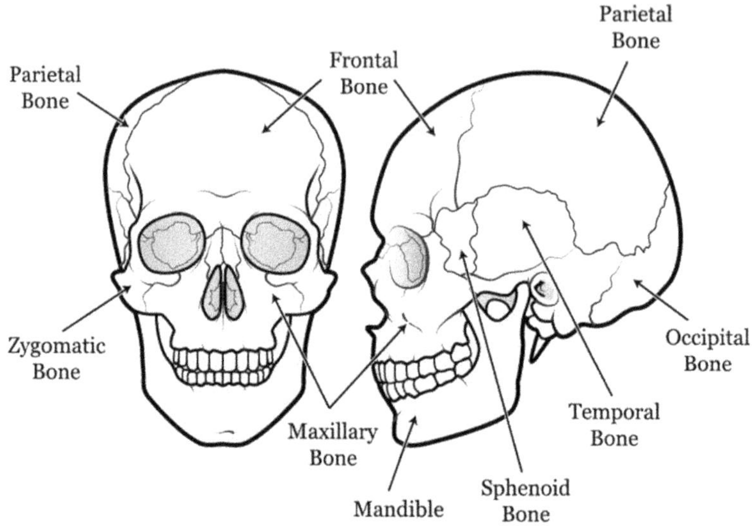

FIGURE 3.7: The occipital bone in relation to the other cranial bones and sutures.

every joint in the body, and indeed every muscle and fascial tissue under stress as you stand. Noted in previous chapters, but worth remembering, releasing in gravity also reduces the heart rate. The heart does not have to work as hard when you are lying and playing in gravity. Thus, gravitational play is also superb for the cardiovascular system, reducing the heart rate and aiding parasympathetic ease.

The occiput is the lovely curvaceous shaped bone at the back of your skull. It provides a very real fulcrum that supports your body as you explore releasing into gravity, sensing the earth calling you. On the one hand, it is a bony structural support, but it is also a fulcrum where you can reorganize many tissues that surround, pass near to, or move through the occiput, such as the vertebral arteries and veins, the vagus, accessory and glossopharyngeal nerves, the internal jugular vein, the suboccipitals, the sternocleidomastoid, the trapezius and the dural tube – to name only a small number. Hence, when we soften our occiput and start to pour the weight of our head in gravity a number of relational tissues can be eased and released. Some of these tissues are on the exterior surface of the occipital bone, such as muscles and fascia, while others are located within and behind the occiput itself, such as the brainstem, arteries, nerves and the dural tube. In short, releasing the cranium in gravity offers the opportunity to reorganize the tissues around the suboccipital region. This region is often under considerable strain, as we shall see.

The occiput curves under the skull rather like a seashell. In general anatomical literature, it is described as a saucer or trapezoidal in shape, curved under itself like a shallow dish. The occipital bone overlies many important structures and tissues.

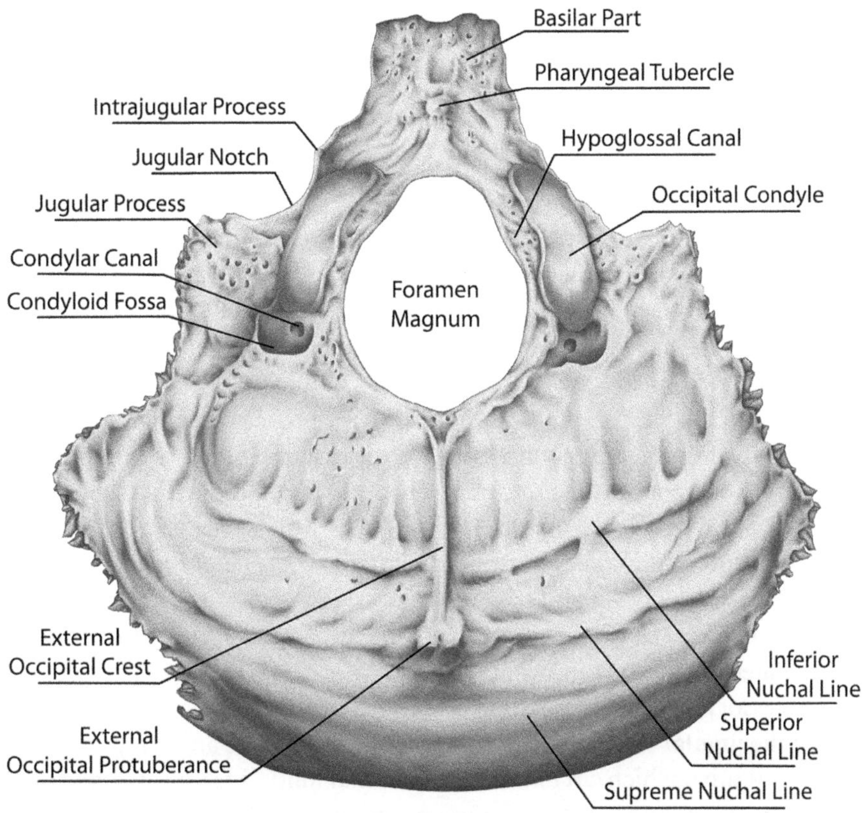

FIGURE 3.8: The curvaceous occipital bone. Notice the foramen magnum, the condyles and nuchal lines.

This information, normally hidden away in books on anatomy and physiology, is rarely shared with the general populous. When embodied and empirically investigated, this knowledge supports self-regulation, particularly the flow of arterial blood, venous drainage and the free flow of cerebral spinal fluid. This bone has many secrets that are key to self-regulatory health. In fact, it has so many remarkable secrets that the experiential study of the occipital bone is continued in Chapter 6. Unlocking the secrets of the occipital bone is a central offering in this book.

The occiput is rather beautiful, like a seashell formed over millions of years. In many ways, our life-force is transmitted and sustained by this bone, or more accurately, the foramen magnum (the large whole within the occiput) offers itself as an opening through which life can ascend and descend through neural, lymphatic, arterial and venous vitality. When we approach the occipital bone in the studio, we do so with quietness, gentleness, reverence and awe. This is because the occiput overlies and transmits many vital tissues that often become compressed and are under duress. To paint the rich scene for our long discussion, let us take a cursory glance at the list of vital structures that live near, are attached to, or move through the occiput:

- The occiput connects to the vertebral column through two synovial joints called the atlantooccipital joints, providing the meeting place between the top of the vertebral column and the cranium.
- The foramen magnum (the large hole in the occiput) provides the meeting place between the brainstem and the spinal cord; the top of the spinal cord meets *the medulla oblongata* just behind the occiput, which is the lowest part of your brainstem.
- The vertebral arteries, and the anterior and posterior spinal arteries pass through the foramen magnum, bringing oxygenated blood to your brain.
- Behind the occiput lies the brainstem, the part of your brain that regulates your breathing and heart rate.
- Behind the occiput also lies the fourth ventricle where cerebrospinal fluid flows out to cleanse the brain and spinal cord.
- The vertebral artery moves between the atlas and occiput bringing fresh oxygenated blood to your brain.
- The accessory, vagus and glossopharyngeal nerves pass down through two holes called the jugular foramina, between the occipital bone and temporal bones.
- The dural tube, which circulates cerebrospinal fluid, is firmly attached around the entire circumference of the foramen magnum (the large hole in the occiput).
- Many crucial muscle tissues originate or attach to the exterior surface the occiput, such as the suboccipitals, the trapezius and the sternocleidomastoid.
- The occipital bone connects to the sphenoid bone through a cartilaginous joint called the sphenoid-basilar joint, playing a vital role in the movement of cerebrospinal fluid.

Sensing the connectivity of the occipital bone

In western anatomy, the vertebrae are numbered and divided into the following parts: seven cervical (C1–C7), twelve thoracic (T1–T12), five lumbar (L1–L5), five sacral (S1–S5) and the coccygeal region. The first 24 bones are moveable, and the rest of the vertebrae (the sacrum and coccyx) are fused. In fulcrum support and soft tissue reorganization, we extend the normative geography of the western vertebral column to include the atlantooccipital joints, the spheno-basilar joint, and the many fibrous joints (sutures) between the cranial bones. We generally read *the atlantoaxial joint* (the AA joint) is the top of the vertebral column.

This is where *the atlas* (C1) and *the axis* (C2) articulate to form the most mobile joint in your vertebral column. As participants move their attention and awareness into their occiput and gently tip and pour onto to their temporal bones and parietal bones, they are inviting their atlantoaxial joint into awareness. Even though the atlas and the axis are incredibly important to sense–perceive, release and decompress in the studio, there are other joints in the cranium that are just as vital to integrated health. For example, above the atlantoaxial joint, we find *the atlantooccipital joints* (the AO joints). The occiput offers the curvaceous base of the cranium providing two condyles that articulate with the atlas, forming the atlantooccipital joints. Thus, shifting your awareness above the *atlantoaxial joint* to where the atlas articulates with the occipital bone brings sensory awareness to a higher part of your longitudinal midline. The atlantooccipital joints are incredibly special locations in the landscape of your body. It is worth spending time resting and sense–perceiving the atlantooccipital joints; not only do they connect your vertebral column with your occiput and cranium, they also lie laterally (on both sides) of your foramen magnum (the hole in the occipital bone, where CSF flows).

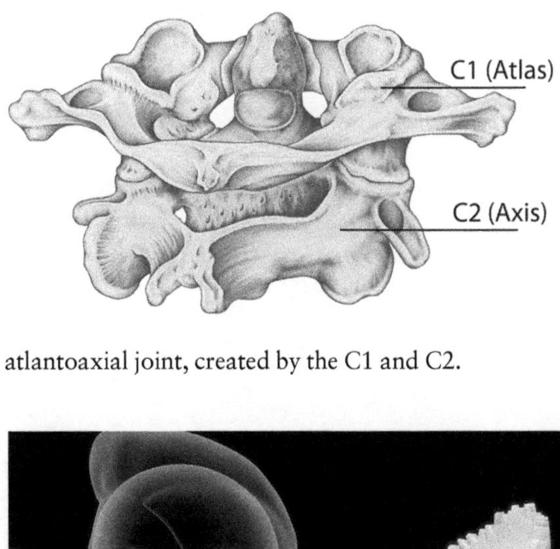

FIGURE 3.9: The atlantoaxial joint, created by the C1 and C2.

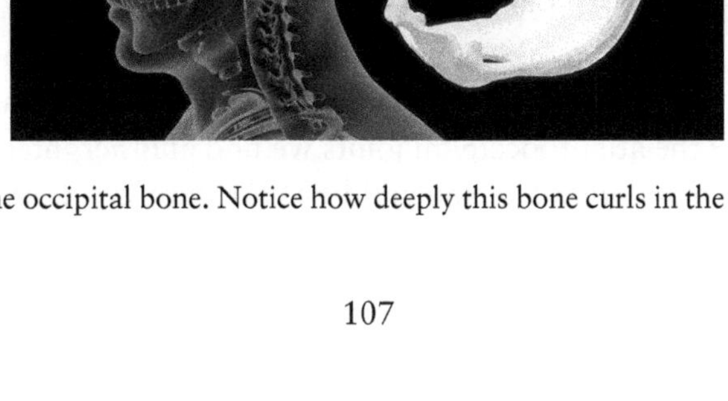

FIGURE 3.10: The occipital bone. Notice how deeply this bone curls in the cranium.

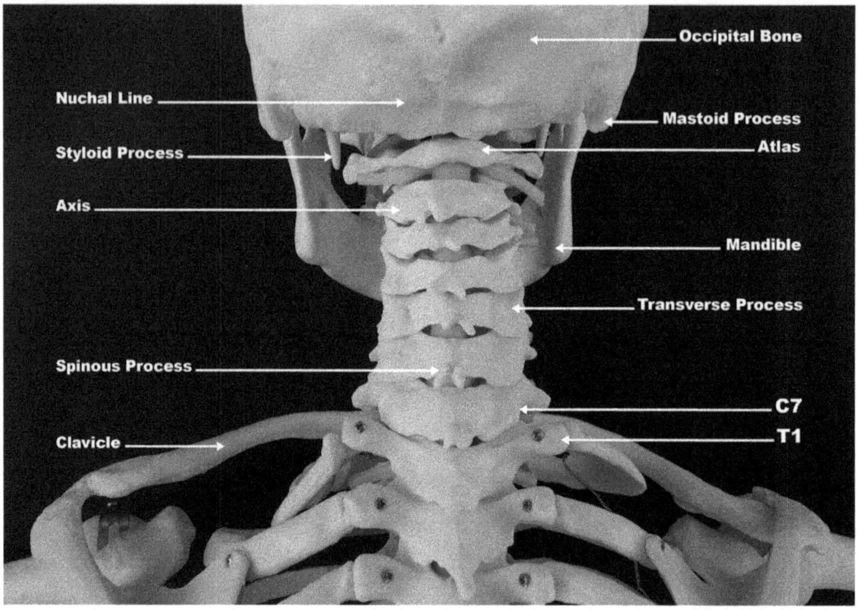

FIGURE 3.11: The cervical vertebrae meeting the occipit. Notice the atlas meeting the occipit.

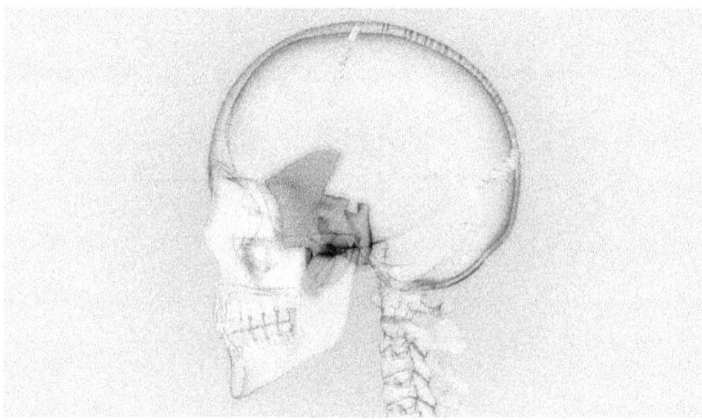

FIGURE 3.12: The sphenoid bone. Notice how deep this bone is within skull. This bones meets the occipit via the sphenoid-basilar joint.

Participants can begin to sense–perceive their atlantooccipital joints by gently nodding their head up and down, or from side-to-side. While these joints have far less mobility than the atlantoaxial joint, they are exceptionally important to sense–perceive. It is on these joints that the occiput can delightfully float and decompress. Moreover, above the atlantooccipital joints we find another integral joint, called *the sphenoid-basilar joint*. The sphenoid-basilar joint is a critically important cartilaginous joint. This joint is formed between the occiput and the sphenoid bone, and it is the 'pivotal fulcrum around which the whole bony craniosacral system revolves' (Attlee 2012: 180). This joint moves with internal motility (the internal flow of cerebrospinal fluid). Thus, you cannot move this joint so consciously, but rather can enhance its functioning through decompressing *and floating* all the cranial bones surrounding it. The significance of this central joint forms the topic of Chapter 6, but for now, let us hold in our awareness, that participants are likely to make sensory contact with their sphenoid-basilar joint without knowing it, as they gently initiate movement from their occipital bone, pouring their weight onto the surrounding cranial bones or learning to decompress their cranium and ease the sutures through gentle self-regulatory movement.

Additionally, the sutures surrounding the occiput and between all the cranial bones are fibrous joints, full of blood vessels, nerves and fascia. Thus, sensing into the occiput, tipping and rolling onto the other bones, provides the opportunity for participants to decompress all their cranial sutures. An in-depth exploration of the cranial bones is offered in Chapter 6 , where I share a great deal of anatomical differentiation about the health of the cranial bones. In preparation for Chapter 6, I will refer to the cranium in this chapter as *bio-tensile*, which means, contrary to traditional normative constructions of the human body, there is subtle movement between the cranial bones, at the level of millimetres, unable to be seen by the human eye. As we move through this chapter together, let us keep in mind, that releasing the occipital bone into ground, combined with soft tissue rolling around the cranium, offers the opportunity for participants to decompress all their cranial sutures.

When we invite participants to settle in gravity, release the weight of their occiput, and gently tip, roll, pour and yield their craniums into ground, they have the wonderful opportunity to release all the joints shared above. My main point being, this is one reason why rolling around on the floor and releasing the cranium is important, even if it looks rather haphazard and silly to an outside observer more familiar with the mechanistic paradigm.

The vertebral artery

Settle your awareness on Figure 3.14. You are viewing *the vertebral arteries (red) and vertebral veins (blue)*. The vertebral arteries are paired arteries located on both sides of your neck. They ascend through your cervical spine, bringing fresh blood to your brainstem (and other posterior regions of your brain, such as your occipital lobes and posterior fossa). These arteries run up through your cervical spine and through your foramen magnum. It is useful to note that these arteries enter

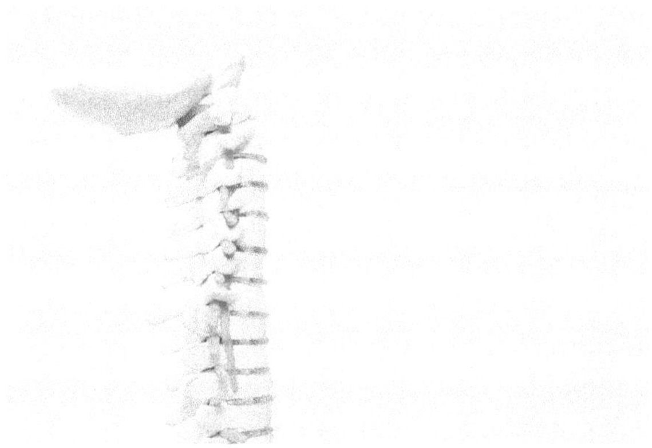

FIGURE 3.13: The vertebral artery. Notice how it moves between the C1 and the occipit, taking a sharp bend.

the cervical spine at C6 or C7. After moving over the atlas (C1), these arteries then move through the 'suboccipital triangle' and then into the foramen magnum. If the head is protracted or retracted, and thus misaligned, these arteries often become compressed. If your atlantoaxial and atlantooccipital joints, and cervical vertebrae are compacted with stress, cerebral circulation is impaired and compromised. Notice how these arteries ascend through the transverse processes (the little holes) of your delicate cervical spine. Can you imagine how misalignment of the occiput on the cervical spine, or compression in the cervical vertebrae might hinder and damage the flow of fresh oxygenated blood?

Bringing conscious awareness to the atlantooccipital joints is particularly vital because the vertebral artery often becomes compressed between the atlas and occiput. This is why it is so useful to offer slow-time sensing and release in this area. In Figure 3.13, notice how the vertebral arteries run vertically within the transverse processes of the cervical spine, but then suddenly turn a sharp corner to become horizontal. To paraphrase Thomas Attlee, these important arteries take a 'tricky awkward turn' between the atlas and occiput (Attllee 2012: 141). Therefore, it is particularly important to invite participants to sense–perceive their atlantooccipital joints and invite spaciousness between the atlas and occipital bone. This is one reason why across the field internationally you often hear language such as the following, 'invite your occipital bone to float on C1'. It is useful to use the image of the occipital bone floating on the top of vertebral column to invite gentle release and ease compacted tissues. As Attlee notes below, the vertebral arteries

> follow a tortuous, right angled, S-bend route over the atlas vertebra and in and through the foraman magnum, a pathway which renders them liable to

be compressed between the occiput and atlas. This can be a major contributory factor in reducing oxygen distribution to the brain and may be relevant to anyone who has suffered a head or neck injury or who holds significant levels of tension in this area.

(Attlee 2012: 141)

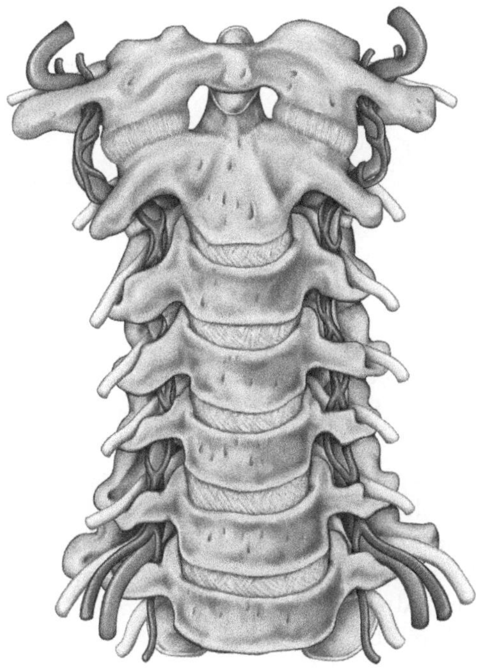

FIGURE 3.14: The vertebral arteries and veins. Notice how they run through the transverse processes in the cervical vertebrae.

Example of practice: Slow-time sensing: The occipital bone, the atlantoaxial and atlantooccipital joints

Slow-time sensing, feeling, perceiving and moving lies right at the heart of all somatic movement dance modalities and therapies. The slowness of the work often surprises people new to practice. Building an intimate relationship with living tissues takes time. I always invite participants to build a relationship with their cranial bones in gravity, sense–perceiving their occiput first. Using soft cushions that support the cervical spine, as well as the cranium, is essential, especially with people new to practice. The cushion should not be too high. If it is too high or low the occiput becomes misaligned. Use flattish cushions in the studio that enable participants to rest and unwind their cervical spine from T4 (the neurological outflow from the heart), to C7, through to C1 and to the occiput. The occipital bone takes on new meaning when participants sense–perceive its location, shape and relationality, feeling how this remarkable bone is a living and breathing part of their being.

Below is a brief example of slow-time sense–perception of the cranial bones and the aforementioned joints.

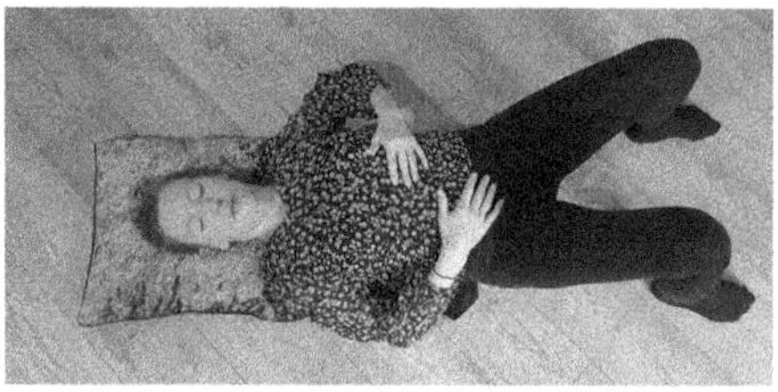

(a)

Invite participants to settle and land in their fulcrums of support: the occiput, scapulae and sacrum. Invite them to direct their sensory-perceptual awareness to their occipital bone, scapulae and sacrum. Offer constructive rest as an option so the lumbar–sacral region can release and soften into ground. Rest in these fulcrums of support, with breath awareness. Notice how these fulcrums bring support and provide a structure for all the soft tissues in your body.

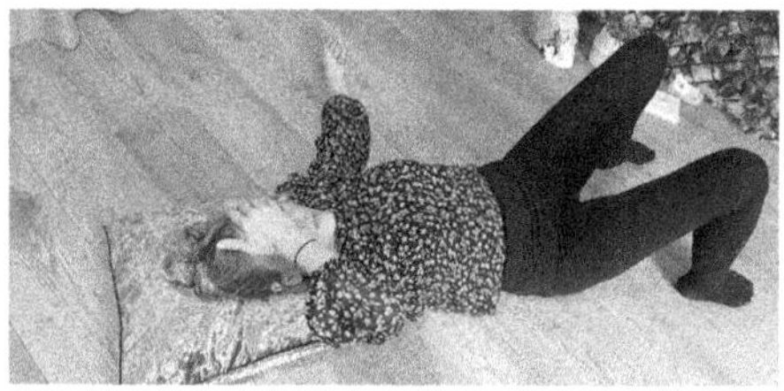

(b)

Invite a slow-time sense–perceiving in the frontal bone: feel a tiny space between your palm and the frontal bone. With the lightest of touch, invite the frontal bone to breathe and float towards your hands.

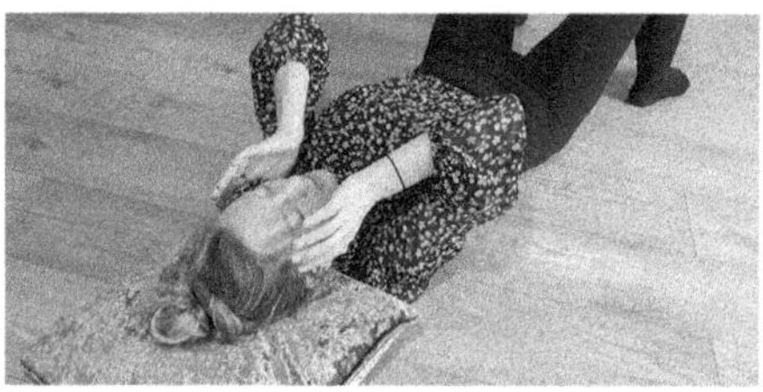

(c)

Sense into the temporal bones, with the lightest of touch. Breathe into the space between your palms and the temporal bones. Sense the living presence of these bones. Invite the bones to float.

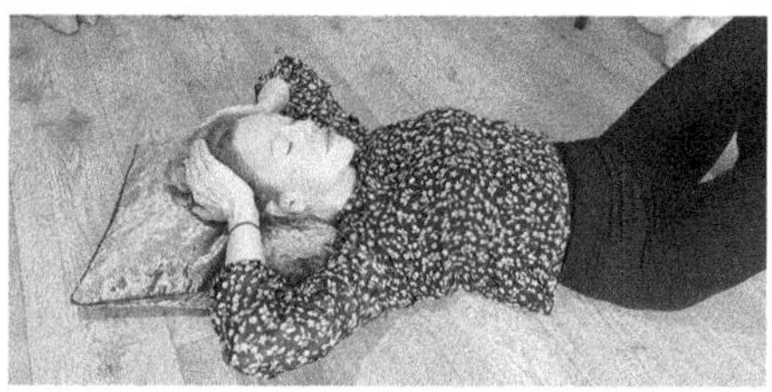

(d)

Sense–perceive the parietal bones. Notice their energy and sense–feeling. Do not push or prod. Invite the bones to breathe into your hands. Often these bones feel alone, and call for touch and connection.

FIGURE 3.15A–I: Amanda Williamson. Sensing her occipital bone. Photographer: Scott Closson.

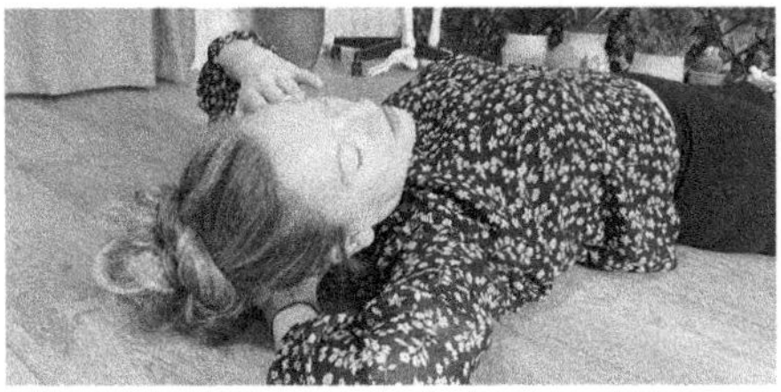

(e)

Sense into the sphenoid bone, with a very light touch. Invite this bone to flex and extend with breath. Sense into the occipital bone, and acknowledge the aliveness in this bone. These bones are connected by a cartilaginous joint called the sphenoid-baslier joint. (This connection is discussed further in Chapter 6.).

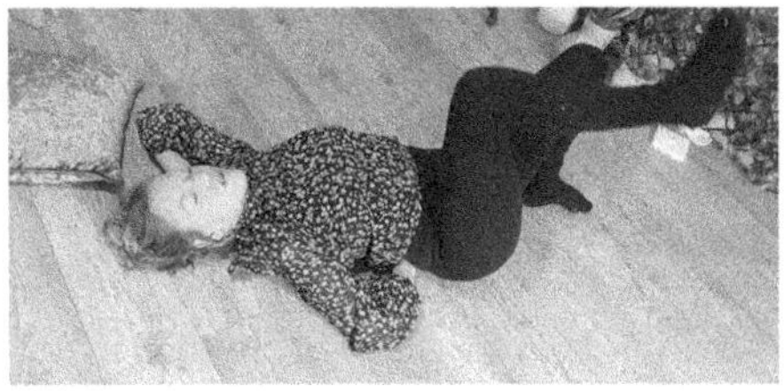

(f)

Sense–dwell in the occipital bone and sacrum, releasing your weight into your hands. Soften into these distant, yet connected fulcrums. (discussed in-depth in Chapter 6.)

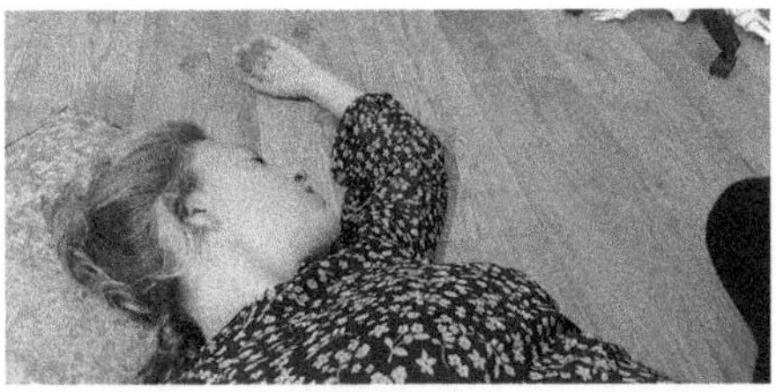

(g)

Invite participants to pour the weight of their cranium slowly from side-to-side, noticing the mobility in the atlantoaxial joint. This is the most mobile synovial joint in your vertebral column. You can sense–perceive this joint at the very top of your neck.

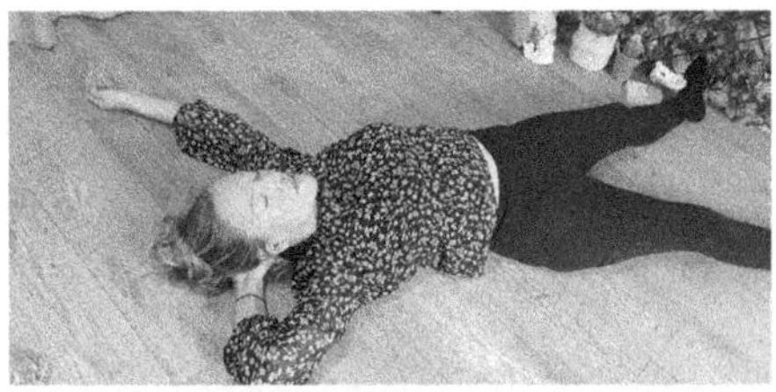

(h)

Invite participants to gently nod their head up and down, and ever so slightly from side-to-side, making sensory contact with the atlantooccipital joints. These joints are much harder to sense–perceive. They have far less mobility.

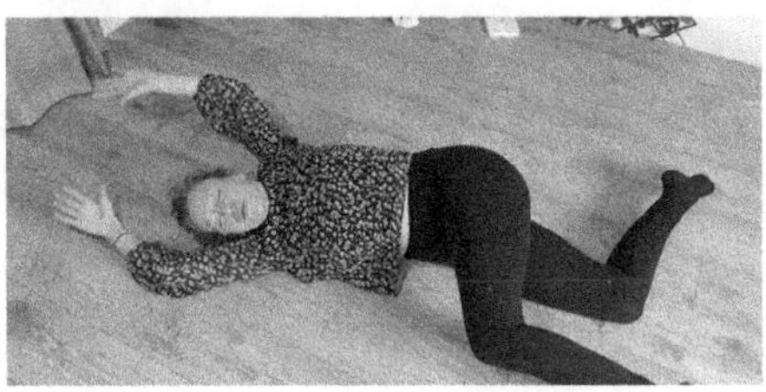

(i)

Invite participants to gently tip and pour their head, moving from and off their occiput onto their temporal bones and other cranial bones. Invite the rest of the body to tenderly follow.

FIGURE 3.15A–I: Amanda Williamson. Sensing her cranial bones. Photographer: Scott Closson. (*Continued*)

Example of practice: Initiating movement from the occiput and inviting the vertebral column to follow

I often then invite gentle movement initiations from the occiput pouring onto all the cranial bones, welcoming the rest of the body to receptively follow, spiral and respond. This practice experientially explores the fluid continuum between the vertebral column, the occiput and all the cranial bones, as well as releases the soft tissues between cranium and shoulder girdle. Rather than viewing the cranium as separate and disconnected from the vertebral column and the rest of the body, the cranial bones are viewed as a bio-tensile continuum, floating on the top of vertebral column.

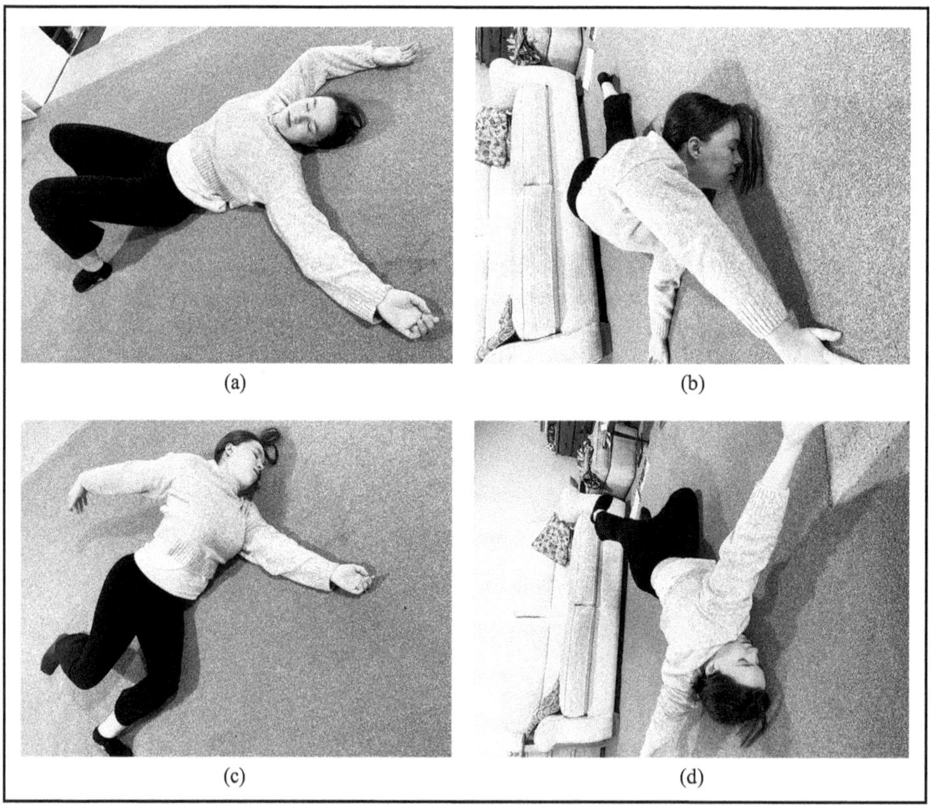

FIGURE 3.16A–F: Natasha Martin: releasing the weight of her head. Soft tissue rolling her cranial bones and easing the tissues that lie between the shoulder girdle and the cranium. Photographer: Amanda Williamson.

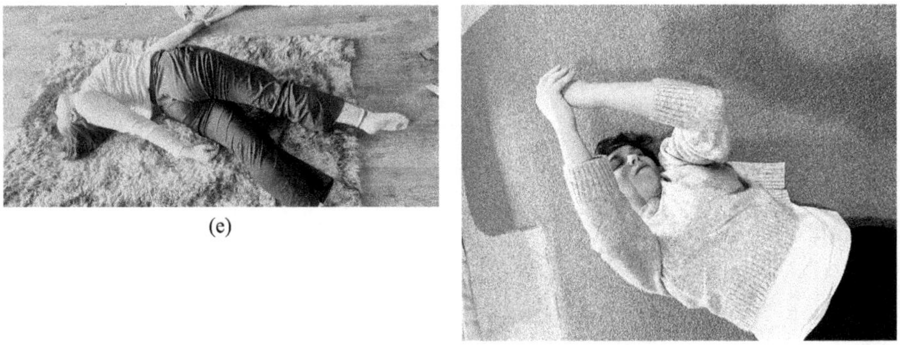

(e) (f)

FIGURE 3.16A–F: Natasha Martin: Easing her cranial bones, sensing her fluid continuum. Photographer: Amanda Williamson. (*Continued*)

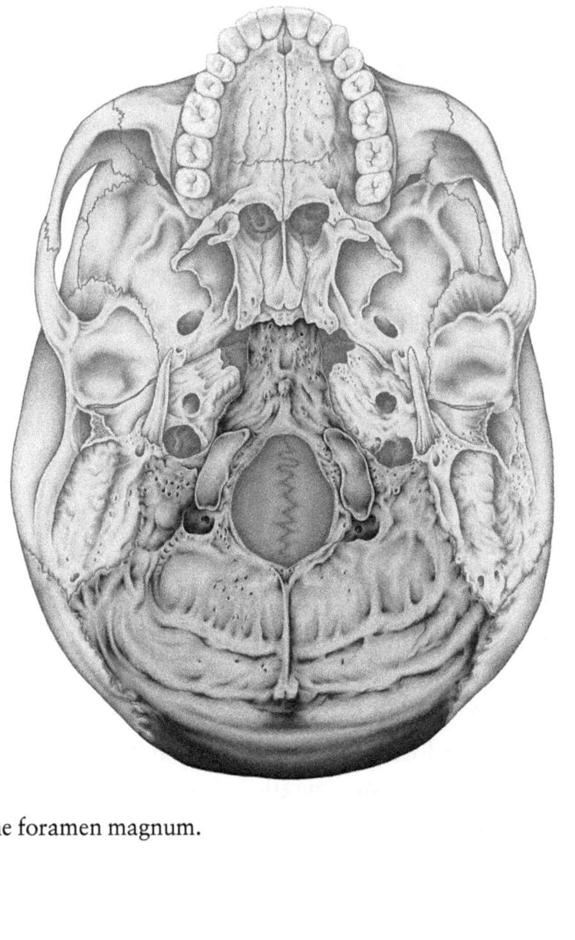

FIGURE 3.17: The foramen magnum.

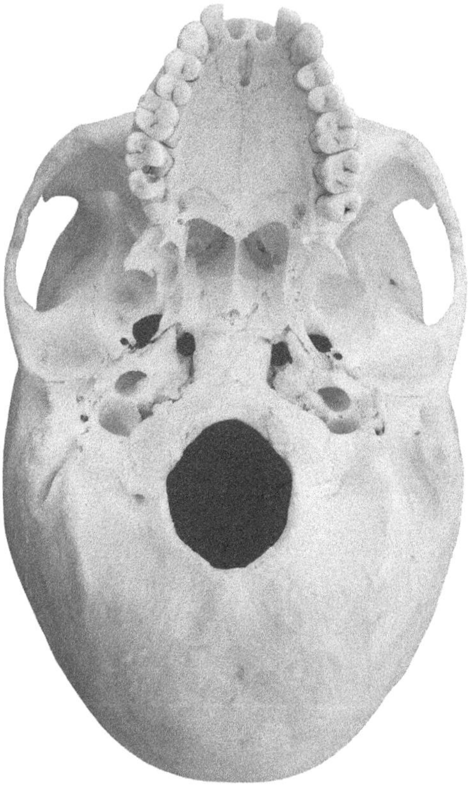

FIGURE 3.18: The foramen magnum.

The foramen magnum

Rest your awareness on Figures 3.17 and 3.18. You are looking at two inferior images of the skull. Notice, there is one large hole in the middle of the occipital bone. This large hole is called the *foramen magnum*. This simply means large hole in Latin. It is the biggest cave-like cavity you see in front of you. It looks to me, like a deep cave. Several vital structures and tissues flow through this hole. Of deep significance, the foramen magnum provides the meeting place between the brainstem and the spinal cord; the top of the spinal cord meets *the medulla oblongata* here, which is the lowest part of your brainstem. Additionally, the accessory nerves, the vertebral arteries, and the anterior and posterior spinal arteries pass through the foramen magnum. Noted above, but worth reiterating, arterial blood surges up through the transverse foramina of the cervical vertebrae and then through the foramen magnum. The foramen magnum is thus an incredible passageway of arterial flow, breath and fluid life.

Significant arteries that provide oxygenated blood to the brain, as well as important sinuses and veins that return deoxygenated blood and waste products to the heart move through the foramen magnum. For example, the vertebral arteries discussed earlier, are part of the vertebrobasilar system. These important arteries supply blood (nutrients and oxygen) to the spinal cord, brainstem, cerebellum and the posterior fossa of the occipital lobes (and other posterior parts of the brain). These important arteries unite in the skull to form one artery called the midline basilar artery. Therefore, a potent healthy flow of blood within these arteries is largely dependent on an easeful and released articulation of the cervical spine with the occiput.

The foramen magnum also provides the oval opening that transmits the flow of cerebrospinal fluid. This is the big topic of Chapter 6, but for now note, the dural tube is firmly attached around the entire circumference of the foramen magnum. This is where cerebrospinal fluid flows down and around the spinal cord. All these tissues and fluids become highly compromised when the occiput is misaligned and the tissues between the neck and occiput are restricted, particularly if the head is protracted or retracted in a pattern of neuromuscular holding, or tilted off to one side. If the occiput is misaligned with the cervical spine, arterial pulse and cerebrospinal fluid can become highly compromised, and notably, less oxygen can get to your brain. Sensing the foramen magnum is hard. Some anatomical texts say it is impossible to sense the foramen magnum. However, if you bring sensory awareness to the atlantooccipital joints that lie bi-laterally on both sides of the foramen magnum you can begin to sense its location. Additionally, bringing awareness to the squamous part of occiput (this is the big part of the occipital bone that lies behind the foramen magnum), the lateral condylar part of the occiput (this is where the atlantooccipital joints are), and the basilar part of the occiput (in front of the foramen magnum), helps to locate the allusive foramen magnum. Note, it is worth showing participants models and images of the foramen magnum to help them locate this deep and magnificent part of them.

Example of practice: Sensing the allusive foramen magnum

Sense–perceiving the occipital bone and the foramen magnum, and initiating movement from this area, can help to enhance the flow of cerebrospinal fluid, arterial pulse and venous drainage. It is hard to sense the foramen magnum; below I offer a few ways.

Using self-touch and enjoying releasing the weight of the occiput into your hand helps to sense–perceive the squamous part of the occiput. This is the big part of the bone behind the foramen magnum.

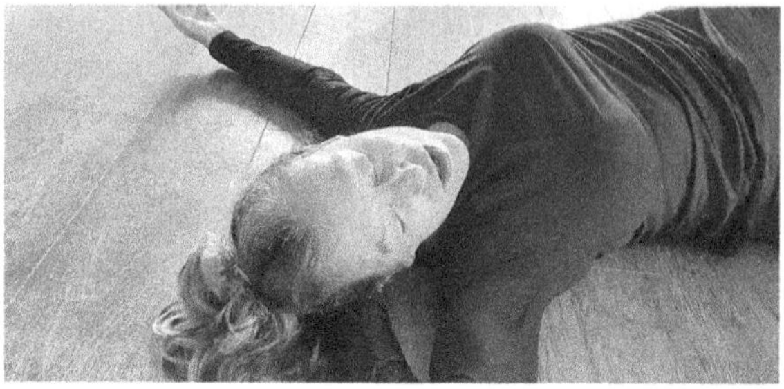

FIGURE 3.19: Amanda Williamson: sensing her foramen magnum via contacting the squamous part of her occipital bone. Additionally, moving her awareness to the basilar part of her occipital bone. Releasing the jaw and mouth helps to sense the basilar part of the occipital bone. Photographer: Scott Closson.

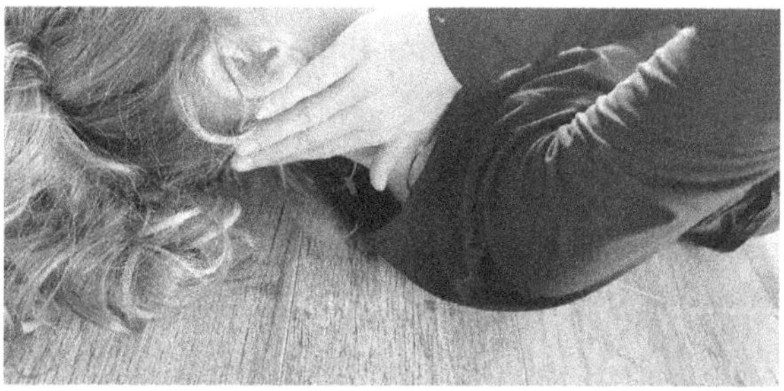

FIGURE 3.20: Amanda Williamson: sensing her foramen magnum via contacting the lateral condylar part of the occipital bone. Photographer: Scott Closson.

Invite participants to sense–perceive the basilar part of the occiput. This is hard. This part of the occiput lies in front of foramen magnum. Sense just in front of the occipital condyles – or atlantooccipital joints.

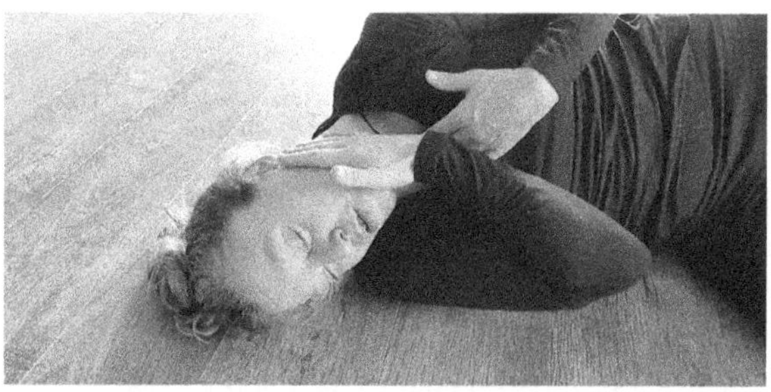

FIGURE 3.21: Amanda Williamson: sensing her foramen magnum via directing awareness to her atlantooccipital joints. Photographer: Scott Closson.

Invite participants to sense the atlantooccipital joints on either side of the foreman magnum. Release your mouth, open the neurocavity, and you may notice a fluid filled foreman magnum. Explore initiating movement from your sense–perception of the foramen magnum and atlantoocciptial joints. The movement will be tiny and incrementally small and gentle (likely to be snake like).

The jugular foramina: The accessory, vagus and glossopharyngeal nerves.

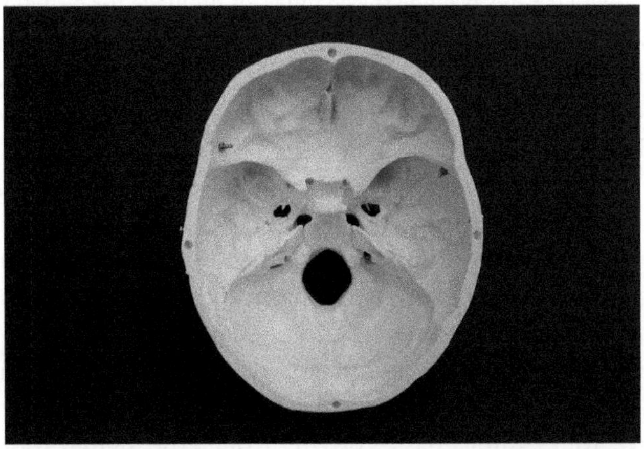

FIGURE 3.22: The jugular foramina.

In Chapters 1 and 2, I shared that the cranial nerves, particularly the vagus, accessory and glossopharyngeal nerves support parasympathetic release, vagal tone and social engagement, if they are supported into a state of health. If you rest your awareness on Figure 3.22, you will notice the skull has a number of foramina (holes). For our purposes here, note the two smaller holes called *the jugular foramina*. They are formed between two bones, the petrous portion of the temporal bone and the occipital bone. Sensing the location of the jugular foramina is extremely hard. Luckily, the jugular foramina are actually located just in front and lateral to the atlantooccipital joints. Thus, again we find another reason why building a sensory–perceptual relationship with the atlantooccipital joints is so important. The jugular foramina transmit *the accessory*, *vagus* and *glossopharyngeal nerves*. These nerves are involved in parasympathetic innervation and engagement of the ventral branch of the vagus nerve (our ability to be socially engaged). These incredibly important foramina, hidden from the human eye, are pathways of neural and venous vitality. However, these little holes (that hardly seem significant) often become restricted when our neck and craniums are impacted by, and compacted with stress. Thus, these little holes can become pathways of dysfunction, where our vitality becomes restricted and highly compromised (see Attlee 2012: 141–43). These two little holes also transmit the jugular vein and thus are involved in venous drainage. Restriction in these nerves and veins, as they pass through these little foramina can compromise venous drainage, leading to 'sluggishness in cerebral circulation' (Attlee 2012: 141–43). Attlee reflects this extremely important detail:

> The internal jugular veins provide the channels of drainage for virtually all venous blood from the cranium. They pass through the jugular foreman on each side of the suboccipital region. Restriction of these major veins may lead to venous congestion within the cranium, and stagnation of all fluids, including arterial blood and cerebrospinal fluid, around the brain.
>
> (Attlee 2012: 141)

The aforementioned nerves play an extremely important role in aiding rest and restoring balance to an over sympathetically charged nervous system. The importance of these nerves is so central to good practice that it is worth inviting participants to spend time sensing into the occipital bone and temporal bones and bringing presence to the jugular foramina and the tissues they transmit. The accessory nerve, for example, passes down through the jugular foramina supplying innervation to the sternocleidomastoid and trapezius muscles (I discuss these muscles further below). Releasing the occipital bone and temporal bones through soft tissue rolling, with awareness of the jugular foramina transmitting the accessory nerves influences the health of the sternocleidomastoid and trapezius muscles. Unwinding the soft tissues in the neck and around the base of cranium is a key stage when inviting the parasympathetic into expression. We noted in Chapters 1 and 2 that the vagus nerve is the longest parasympathetic nerve in the human body and travels with the accessory down through the jugular foramina supplying innervation to almost every organ in the human body. The glossopharyngeal nerve also travels through the jugular foramina supplying the mouth, the mucous glands, tonsils and the tongue. The glossopharyngeal nerve supplies parasympathetic fibres aiding the body with rest and digestion processes. Thus, softening in the mouth, while soft tissue rolling the cranium is super in inviting rest and repair.

It is extremely hard to sense–perceive the jugular foramina. Note, these holes are deeply located between the temporal and occipital bone. However, if you place your thumbs around the base of the occiput and your fingers gently on the temporal bones, feeling into how these bones are connected, you can begin to sense–perceive energy and vitality here. Directing awareness to the base of the occiput and near the atlantooccipital joints also helps to locate these little holes. As you sense into the jugular foramina, bring awareness (intellectually and subjectively), to how the vagus, glossopharyngeal and accessory nerves make their journey through these little holes, and then pass down into the tissues of your mouth and neck. Initiating movement from the occipital bone and temporal bones, inviting the neck and the rest of the body to tenderly respond, follow and unwind, is a lovely way to invite these nerves into expression and health. This micro sensory process acknowledges their living presence, decompresses and stimulates their pathways – and brings their nature into being (which can aid you in feeling well).

Further, deoxygenated blood drains from the brain, emptying blood into the internal jugular veins, that also pass through the jugular foramina (notice the internal jugular vein in Figure 3.23 and how it moves out of the jugular foramina). Equally, *the carotid canal,* which is another foramen in the temporal bones (see Figure 3.23) invites the internal carotid artery to enter the middle cranial fossa from the neck. If you look at Figure 3.23 can see just how vital it is to sense–perceive the temporal bones, as well as the occipital bone, inviting a free passageway of arterial blood up through the carotid canal. Thus, as we bring our attention and conscious awareness to an easeful articulation of the cervical spine in relation to the temporal bones and occipital bone, we are continuing

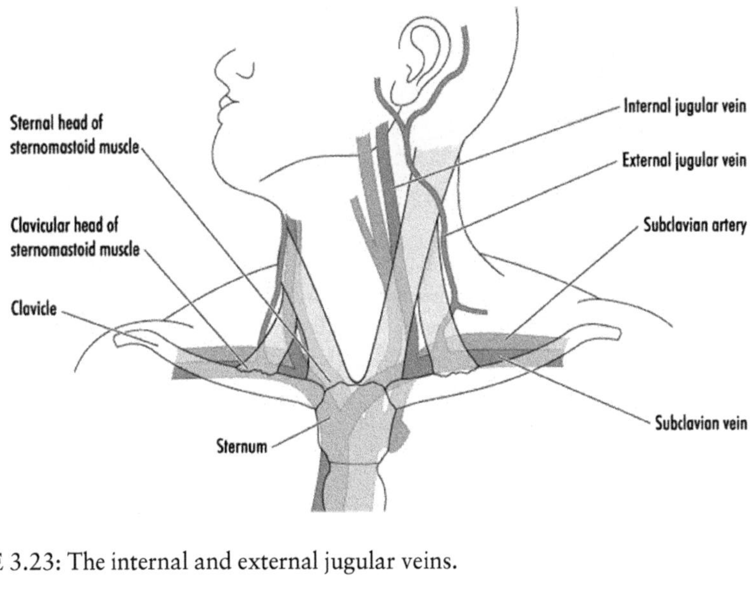

FIGURE 3.23: The internal and external jugular veins.

to support the flow of oxygenated and deoxygenated blood in the circulatory system. Compression of the arterial and venous system leads to a poor circulatory flow, as Attlee shares:

> With so many crucial structures present in such a specific localised area, it is clear that any injury, trauma or tension here could have widespread repercussions; and yet this is the area of the body most susceptible to trauma and tension, perhaps more than anywhere else in the body.
>
> (2012: 143)

Example of practice: Sensing the jugular foramina

Sense–perceiving the occipital bone and the temporal bones, with the soft tissues in the neck and shoulder girdle following and unwinding, decompresses the jugular foramina and the significant tissues passing through these holes. This is yet another reason why soft tissue rolling the cranium in gravity for long periods of time is offered in the somatic studio.

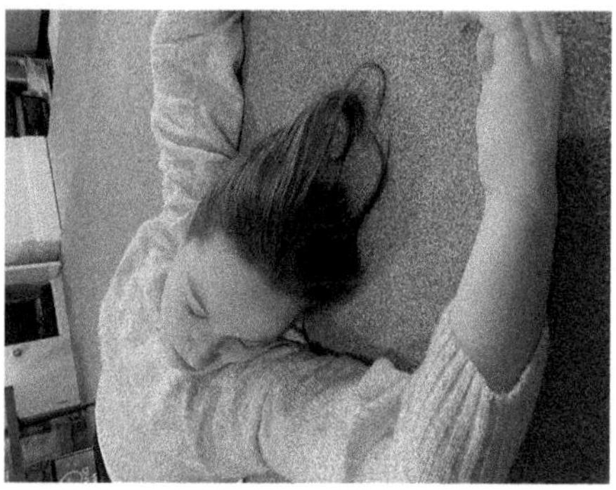

(a)

Trying to sense the jugular foramen is extremely hard. Invite participants to bring awareness to the mastoid process on the temporal bones. Find or sense the mastoid process and share that the petrous part of the temporal bone is just behind the mastoid process. The jugular foramina lie between the petrous part of the temporal bone and occipital bone.

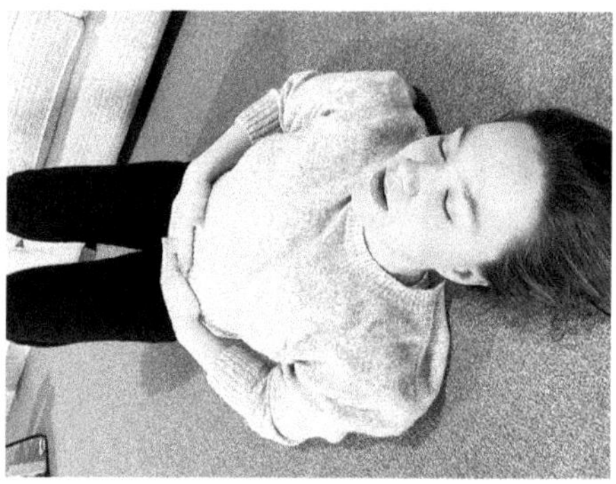

(b)

Invite participants to bring their awareness to their atlantooccipital joints, sharing how the jugular foramina are just in front and lateral to these joints.

FIGURE 3.24A–E: Natasha Martin. Photographer: Amanda Williamson.

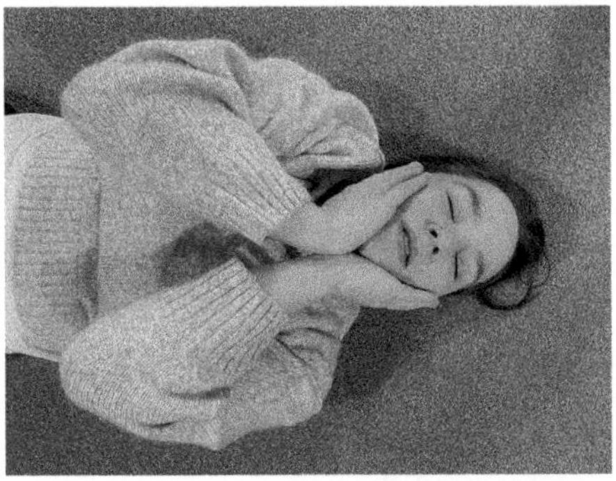

(c)

Invite participants to become aware that the vagus, glossopharyngeal and accessory nerves travel out of the jugular foramina and then move into the tissues of the mouth and neck.

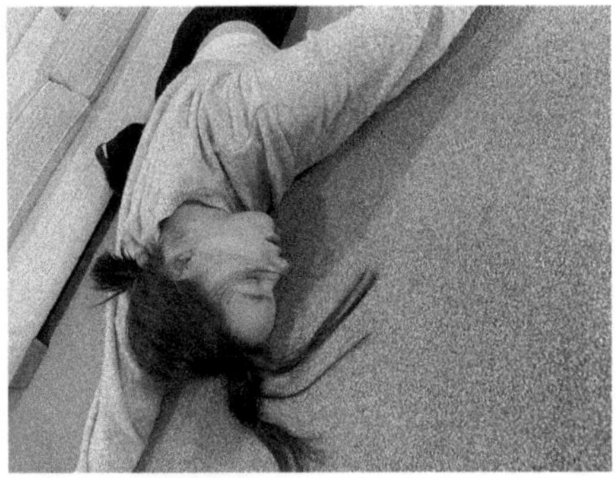

(d)

Initiate movement from the occipital bone and temporal bones, inviting the soft tissues in the neck and shoulder girdle to follow. The vagus and accessory nerves can unwind, find space and release restrictions. Releasing the oral cavity will help to bring awareness to the glossopharyngeal nerve.

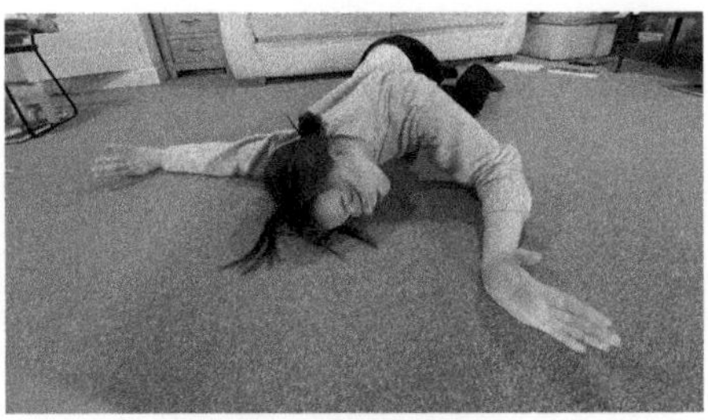

(e)

Enjoy soft tissue rolling from the occiput onto the temporal bones, with breath awareness. As usual, invite the rest of the body to follow. Never hold the body still. Softness, responsiveness and breath are keys to unwinding compacted tissues.

FIGURE 3.24A–E: Natasha Martin. Photographer: Amanda Williamson. (*Continued*)

Soft tissues, nuchal lines and the posterior surface of the occiput

Rest your awareness on Figures 3.25 and 3.26. You are viewing the posterior surface of the occipital bone. You will notice some lovely curvy lines or ridges; these are called *nuchal lines*. These curvaceous lines and protrusions provide the

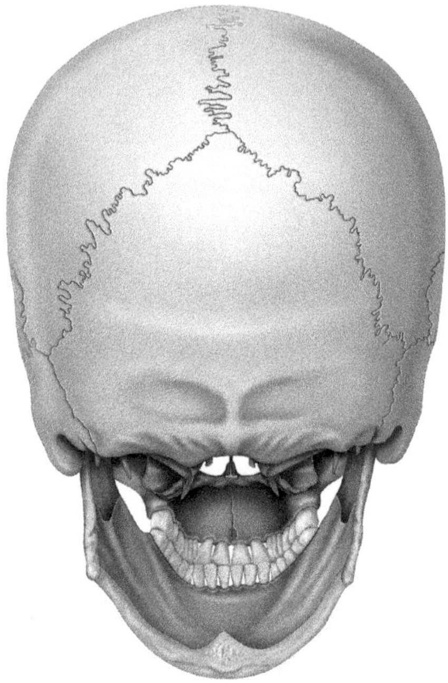

FIGURE 3.25: The nuchal lines.

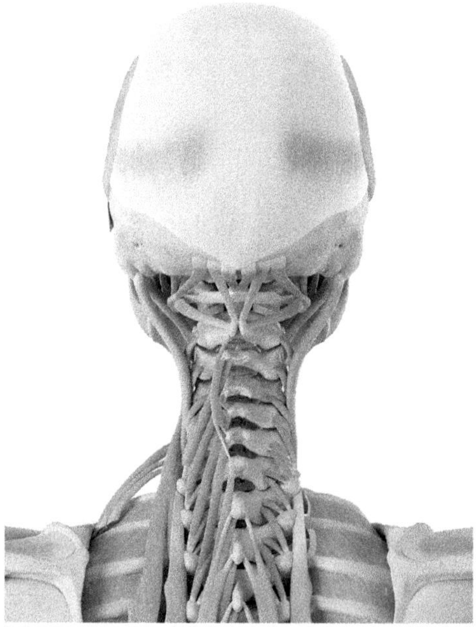

FIGURE 3.26: Suboccipitals.

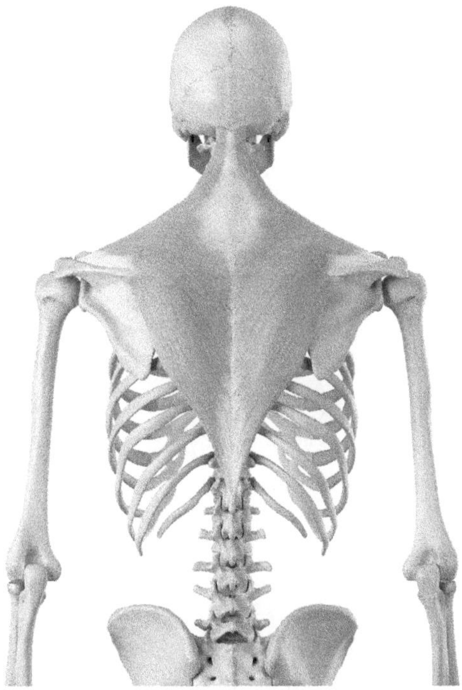

FIGURE 3.27: Trapezius.

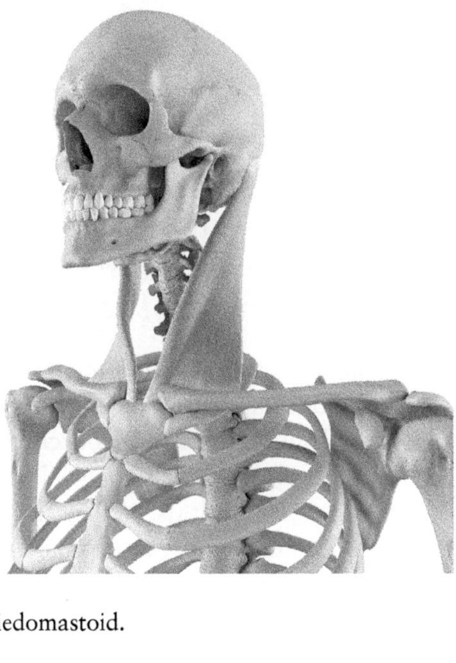

FIGURE 3.28: Sternocliedomastoid.

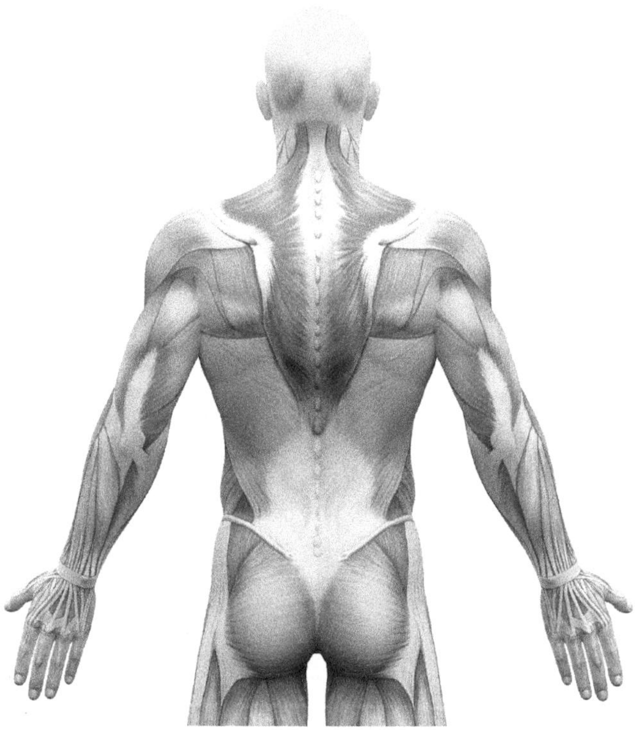

FIGURE 3.29: Trapezius.

landscape where significant muscle tissues attach or originate. These tissues live and breathe snugly right up against the cranium and are often tight and pain sensitive. When we soften the tissues around the occiput and temporal bones, we contact some very significant muscles attachments that play a critical role in our ability to feel safe and socially engaged; specifically, the trapezius, sternocleidomastoid and suboccipitals. Settle again on Figure 3.25. Bring your awareness to the four nuchal lines (curvy ridges). The highest point on the occipital bone is a protuberance referred to as *the inion*. Can you feel your own occipital protuberance? Melting, softening and yielding the skin and fascia surrounding the occipital bone (and all the cranial bones) is incredibly soothing and through this process we can particularly invite the trapezius, sternocleidomastoid and suboccipitals to begin to release.

There are three important muscles involved in social engagement, the trapezius, sternocleidomastoid and suboccipitals. When we are frightened these muscles tense, pulling our bones and joints out of place, and sometimes trapping nerves and arteries. Note, the trapezius originates on the occiput, and the sternocleidomastoid attaches to the temporal bones and the occipital bone. Both muscles connect the shoulder girdle, one anteriorly (the sternocleidomastoid) and the other posteriorly (the trapezius). Further, let us bring to awareness how the suboccipitals (Figure 3.26) weave among the atlas, axis and occipital bone, connecting the cervicle vertebrae with the occipit. Thus, you can see why compassionately and tenderly contacting the soft tissues enveloping the occiput and temporal bones, and softening the tissues around the ridge of occiput, and throughout the shoulder girdle, is so important.

Example of practice: Sense–perceiving the nuchal lines and easing out the tissues that live and breathe between the cranium and shoulder girdle

It is wonderful to invite participants to sense–perceive the soft tissues surrounding and enveloping the occiput and temporal bones, and then invite self-regulatory movement response. This is yet another reason why somatic movement practitioners offer soft tissue rolling around the occiput and cranial bones, inviting the soft tissues between the shoulder girdle and the cranium to release.

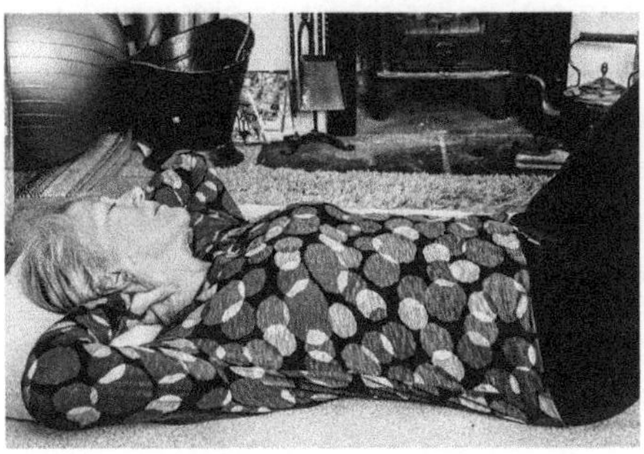

(a)

Rest and breathe in the soft tissues at the base of the occiput. Invite participants into sensory awareness of the posterior surface of the occiput and the temporal bones, noting that significant tissues originate or attach here, extending down to the scapulae, such as trapezius, or reaching up from the clavicle, such as the sternocleidomastoid.

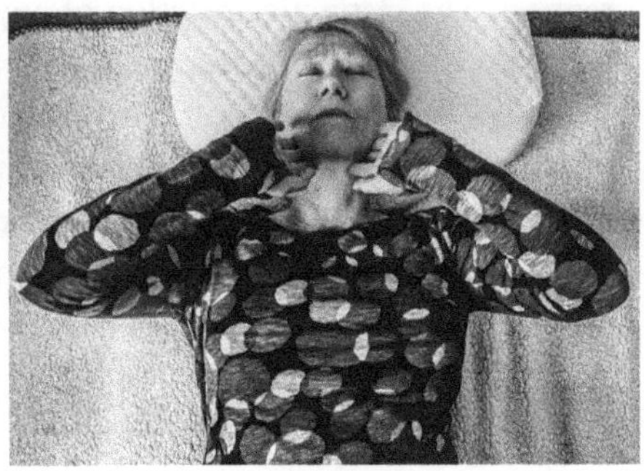

(b)

Invite participants to move in response to the soft tissues surrounding and enfolding the occiput, releasing the suboccipital triangle. Invite them to notice restrictions down the neck and throughout the shoulder girdle, and sense–perceive how tension and stiffness wants to unwind.

FIGURE 3.30A–D: Karin Rugman: gently and slowly bringing awareness to living tissues surrounding her cranium and those living between the shoulder girdle and cranium.

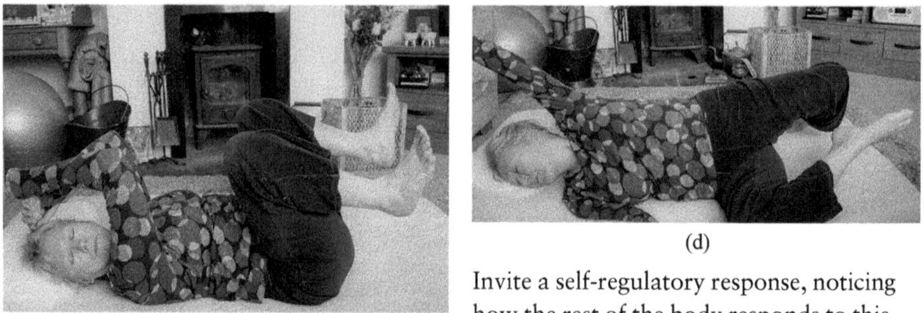

(c)

Invite participants to soften the tissues around the base of the occiput and the mastoid process of the temporal bones.

(d)

Invite a self-regulatory response, noticing how the rest of the body responds to this area.

FIGURE 3.30A–D: Karin Rugman: gently and slowly bringing awareness to living tissues surrounding her cranium and those living between the shoulder girdle and cranium. (*Continued*)

Sense–perceiving the suboccipital muscles

> The suboccipital region is one of the most common sites for the holding of emotional tension. The instinctive reaction of any mammal under threat or pressure is to contract in the suboccipital region, pulling its head protectively down into its neck. Consider, for example a cat reacting to a sudden loud noise. Similarly, humans under persistent stress tend to contract and tighten in this area as a matter of habit. Day-to-day tensions will readily accumulate here, but most significantly, chronic patterns of tension and pressure will create deeply ingrained patterns of restriction and blockage in this crucial region.
>
> (Attlee 2012: 143)

The suboccipital muscles are the intricate group of small muscles you can observe in Figure 3.26. You hear about these muscles in cranio-osteopathy, craniosacral therapy, in massage therapies and in many vitalistic therapies generally. They are a key group of muscles that somatic movers attune to through soft tissue rolling and releasing the head in gravity for long periods of time. These are the muscles that F. M. Alexander extensively explored in his modality, *The Alexander Technique*. Believe it or not, the state of these little muscles affects the whole vertebral column. Retraction in these muscles 'produces a forward movement of the occiput on the atlas and takes the O-A (atlantooccipital) joint into hyperextension' (Earls and Myers 2017: 198). As Earls and Myers note, such a retraction 'is a very common fear response' (Earls and Myers 2017: 198). While retraction is very common in these muscles, 'a unilateral shortness' also often occurs on one side, which rotates the spine, putting strain on the atlantoaxial joint (Earls and Myers 2017: 198).

> It is difficult to overestimate the effect that release of these muscles can have on the movement in the spine, release of the sacrum, diminution of headaches, release of vision, correction of head-forward posture, relaxation of the fear response and plain old head and neck mobility.
>
> (Earls and Myers 2017: 199)

Notably, 'these muscles have a high number of muscle spindles, and they are hard-wired to your eyes. As your eyes move, these muscles "listen" to that movement, and adjust the spine accordingly' (Earls and Myers 2017: 199). These muscles, working with the eyes, anticipate changes to your centre of gravity.

> This small group of muscles is hugely important for proprioception. They constantly monitor and assess the position and balance of the head on the cervical vertebrae, working to keep the eyes and ears orientated to the horizon or whatever else is engaging your attention, and contracting in anticipation of any change in the centre of gravity.
>
> (Earls and Myers 2017: 217)

It is important to share with participants that the suboccipitals are often under considerable strain, and they are related to the fear response. Of heightened note, these are the only muscles in the body that are directly connected to the spinal cord. One of these muscles called *the rectus capitus posterior minor*, 'propels connective fibres into the dura matter (a protective layer surrounding the brain and the spinal cord)' (Earls and Myers 2017: 216).

> Walking through life with your head a little in front of yourself puts extra strain on the tissues at the back of the head and necessitates extra tension, and eventually serious restriction, in the tissues around the base of the occiput.
>
> (Earls and Myers 2017: 216)

Rest your awareness on the images of the suboccipital muscles (Figure 3.26). Notice how the suboccipital muscles weave among the atlas (C1), the axis (C2) and the occipital bone. Thus, they connect the top of the cervical spine to the occipital bone. Three of these muscles attach to the inferior nuchal line of the occipital bone. Below are some details about where these muscle tissues originate and attach. Notice the lovely connection and intertwining tissue pattern between the occipital bone and the atlas and axis.

Obliquus capitis superior: observe how this muscle originates on the transverse process of the atlas (C1) and inserts between the superior and inferior nuchal lines of the occipital bone.
Rectus capitis posterior major: observe how this muscle originates on the spinous process of the axis (C2) and inserts onto the lateral part of the inferior nuchal line of the occipital bone.
Rectus capitis posterior minor: observe how this muscle originates on the tubercle of the atlas (C1) and attaches onto the inferior nuchal line of the occipital bone.
Obliquus capitis inferior muscle: observe how this muscle originates on the spinous process of axis (C2) and inserts on transverse process of atlas (C1).

As you soften around the base of the cranium and the posterior surface of the occiput, you can start to dialogue with these muscles sensorily. In most therapies, suboccipital release relies on the therapist releasing the client's suboccipitals for them. While I do teach suboccipital release in pairs, I often invite participants to explore releasing their own suboccipitals. Soft tissue rolling in gravity in a parasympathetic state will invite these muscles to release.

So far in this chapter I have differentiated some key tissues surrounding and passing through the occiput and temporal bones. However, it is impossible to talk about the occiput in isolation. The occiput has a profound and deep relationship with the cervical and thoracic vertebrae, and notably the scapulae – the topic of this next section. We have many intelligent muscle tissues that connect the cervical spine and thoracic spine to the cranial bones, and many that connect the scapulae to the cranium. In the next part of the chapter, I will

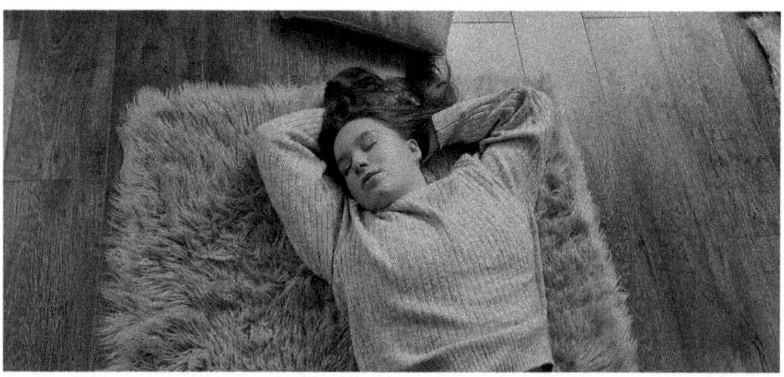

FIGURE 3.31: Natasha Martin: sense–perceiving and releasing her suboccipitals: Photographer: Amanda Williamson.

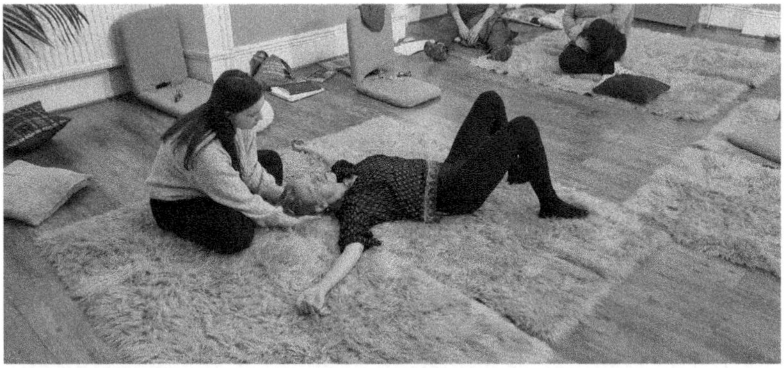

FIGURE 3.32: Movingsoma students: sub-occipital release into self-regulatory movement. Photographer: Sylvia Gregory.

zoom in on the scapulae, the shoulder girdle, the trapezius and sternocleidomastoid. However, before we move to the next section, let us round up key areas explored so far.

Key offerings and learnings

Developing a slow-time sensory–perceptual relationship with the occipital bone and temporal bones in gravity for long periods of time is important because:

- Bringing awareness to the occiput invites participants to sense–perceive and move with awareness of their atlantooccipital joints; awareness of these joints helps to free the vertebral artery that often becomes compressed between the atlas and occipital bone.
- Additionally, awareness of these joints supports participants to sense their cranial bones as a fluid continuum of the vertebral column.
- Bringing awareness to the occiput invites participants to sense–perceive and move with awareness of their foramen magnum, augmenting the flow of arterial and venous blood, as well as the flow of cerebrospinal fluid.
- Bringing awareness to the occiput invites participants to sense–perceive and move with awareness of the jugular foramina (the two holes between the occipital bone and temporal bones), helping to decompress, floss and unwind the vagus, accessory and glossopharyngeal nerves, as they move out of the cranium down into the mouth and neck. These nerves are involved in parasympathetic release and social engagement.

- Bringing awareness to the occiput invites participants to sense–perceive and move with awareness of the soft tissues that surround the occipital bone, helping participants to release their suboccipitals, trapezius and sternocleidomastoid.
- Releasing the occiput into gravity, tipping and pouring the cranium and inviting the rest of the body to tenderly respond is emblematic of my practice. This type of gravitational practice releases tissues that become compressed and compacted around the suboccipital region, and between the cranium and shoulder girdle.

Part 2: The scapulae as a fulcrum of support and reorganization

The scapulae are incredible fulcrums of sensory-perceptual support. When we lie down at the start of a session, we can sense the occiput easily and the next bony structural supports we meet are the scapulae. The scapulae provide a very landscape where you can land, rest, settle, ground, pivot, push, compress and decompress. When we lie in gravity, we can easily feel their bony landscape, especially their ridges, such as the medial boader, the lateral boarder, the spine of the scapulae and the acronium process. Approximately seventeen muscles either attach to or originate from the scapulae. Therefore, any type of gentle movement initiated from the scapulae, will affect and potentially change the vicosity of the myofascial tissues surrounding these bones. When participants pour the weight of their craniums from side-to-side, inviting the cervical, thoracic, lumbar and sacral vertebrae to follow in a spiral, the scapulae and thoracic ribcage follow. In doing so, gentle pressure is applied across the soft tissues surrounding the scapulae, such as the trapezius, rhomboids, levator scapulae, rotator cuffs and latissimus dorsi;

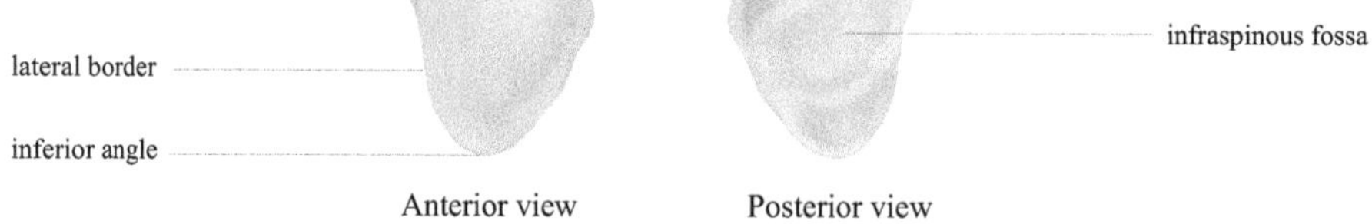

FIGURE 3.33: Scapulae. Notice the lovely bones, crests and ridges.

participants thus have the wonderful opportunity to release significant amounts of tension in these myofascial tissues.

Release-based dancers often have a heightened sense of their scapulae and shoulder girdle and the relationship of their shoulder girdle to their arms, and it is likely the myofascial tissues surrounding their scapulae will be in a good state of fluent glimmering health. However, non-dancers, often have little sensory awareness of their scapulae and the importance of integrating the movement in their scapulae with the movement throughout their arms and thorax. The scapulae are extremely important to sense–perceive and bring into a state of health because they bring structure, integrity and fluency to the shoulder girdle, as well support movement articulations throughout the arms. There are many important tissues that pass through, over or under these beautiful bones that are vital to integrated health. The list would be too long to share them all here. The following tissues are particularly relevant in supporting sensory awareness and fluid movement integration:

The bony landmarks and landscape of the scapulae.
The sternoclavicular, acromioclavicular, glenohumeral and scapulothoracic joints.
The trapezius and sternocleidomastoid.

When we lie in gravity, we can feel our scapulae meeting the hard floor quite effortlessly. However, when we direct our awareness into these bones and sense into the tissues surrounding them, we often sense incredible tension, trigger points, torsions, twists and emotional holding. The scapulae often reflect how we feel about ourselves and the world around us. We often pull these bones in or up in fear, or when under stress, straining the rhomboids and the trapezius, for example. These bones may feel tight and painful because the fascia sounding them is stiff and crystalized, impairing mobility. Everyone will have a different sense of their scapulae – their own living felt-sense – their own emotionality is held in these bones. Directing awareness to the scapulae and unwinding the tissues through self-regulatory movement can relieve enormous stress in the tissues surrounding the scapulae, the tissues between the shoulder girdle and cranium, and the tissues between the scapulae and the arms (humerus).

The scapulae are commonly referred to as the shoulder blades and sometimes the wing bones. They are wonderfully accessible bones, because they have so many bony ridges, sharp points, curves, crests and edges that can be contacted easily in gravity. Gentle compressions, decompressions and soft tissue reorganization around each scapula is particularly delicious. If you rest your awareness on the image above, you can view the wonderful landmarks of the scapulae. Note these landmarks, and like the bony edges on the posterior surface of the occiput, provide the ridges, curves and crests for the attachment and origination points of many important muscle tissues. For example, if you look at Figure 3.33, you will see bony landmarks called *the acromion* and *the spine of the scapular*. The trapezius attaches here. If you glance at Figure 3.33, you will see *the infraspinous* and *subscapular fossa*. These are lovely curvaceous parts of the bone, where two of the rotator cuff muscles originate, specifically *the subscapularis* and *the infraspinatus*. If you look back at the acromion process, the *deltoid* attaches here. If you look at *the medial border*, the rhomboids attach here. A last landmark that is super important is *the choroid process* (it looks like a bird's beak). This is where important muscles attach anteriorly to your scapulae, such as *the pectoralis minor*, *the coracobrachialis* and *the biceps brachii.*

I often invite participants into an intimate relationship with the bony landmarks of their scapulae, using gravity and the floor as a fulcrum. Here, participants can push, press, pivot, release, roll, yield, melt, and slide and glide over the bones. I have offered an example in Figure 3.34. As you rest in gravity and sense–perceive the scapulae, you are meeting bone and soft tissues. You can differentiate bone and tissue in your sense–perception through directed awareness. Both bone and soft tissue enjoy connection and relationship, particularly the deep fascia surrounding bone. Becoming familiar with the bony landmarks of the scapulae and transmitting this knowledge is wonderfully enlivening and educational for participants. The more participants can sense the bony landscape of their scapulae, the more these wonderful supports arise into awareness.

Examples of practice: Sense–perceiving the bony landmarks of the scapulae

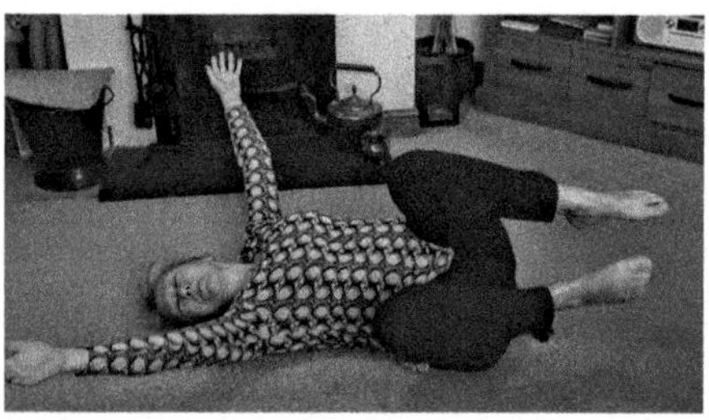

(a)

Invite participants to enjoy landing in their scapulae, noticing all their fulcrums supporting them.

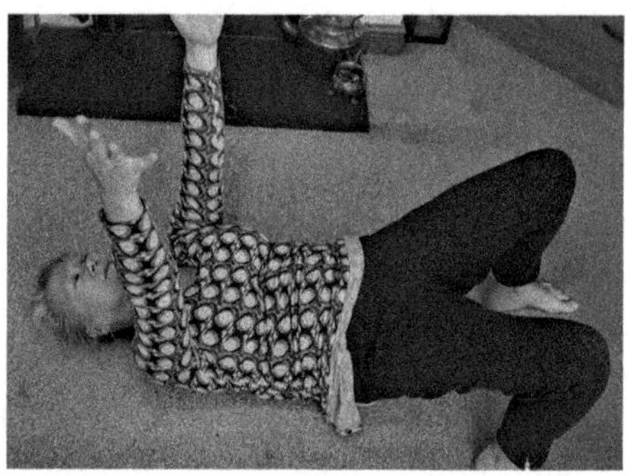

(b)

Invite participants to sense–perceive their bony scapulae through gentle compressions and decompressions, exploring ridges, crests and smooth surfaces.

FIGURE 3:34A–B: Karin Rugman. Photographer: Anika Rugman.

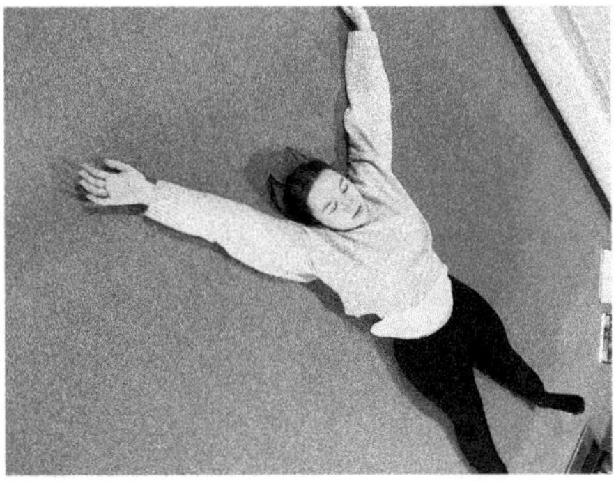

(a)

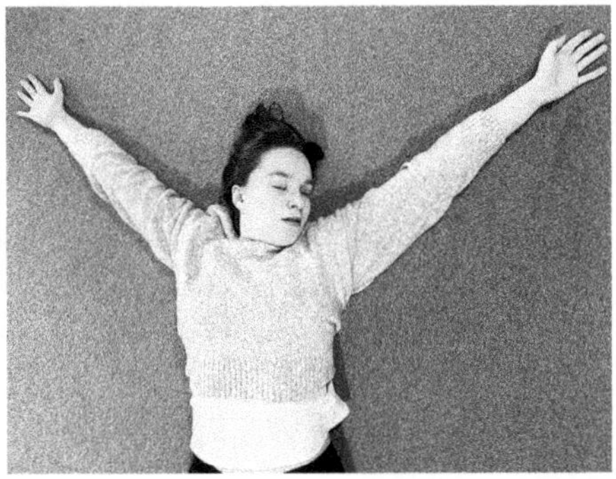

(b)

Breathe into the fluid space in the glenoid fossa, open and explore bi-lateral width.

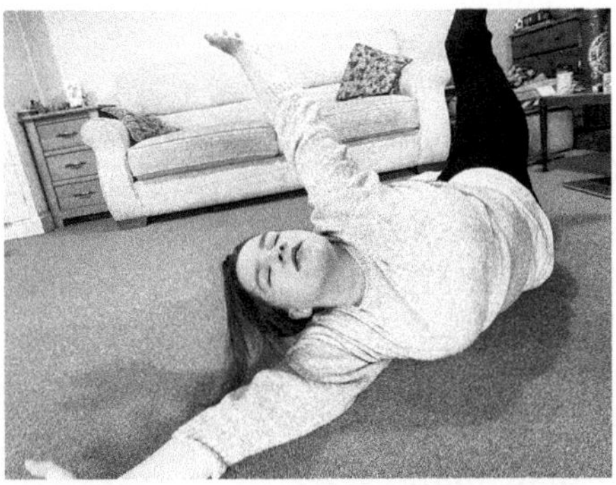

(c)

Invite participants to sense–perceive the lateral and medial border, and the spine of their scapula.

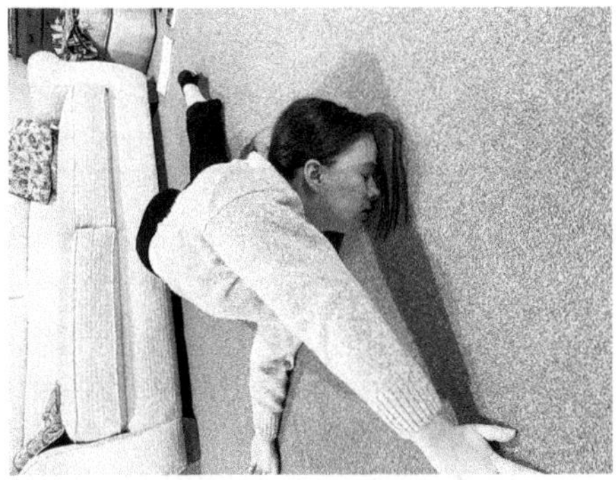

(d)

Invite participants to hang-out on the edges of the scapulae, sensing-perceiving how the bones enjoy a little pressure, compression and decompression. The fascia around these bones enjoys different pressures and sliding and gliding.

FIGURE 3.35A–E: Natasha Martin: exploring the bony landmarks of the scapulae. Photographer: Amanda Williamson.

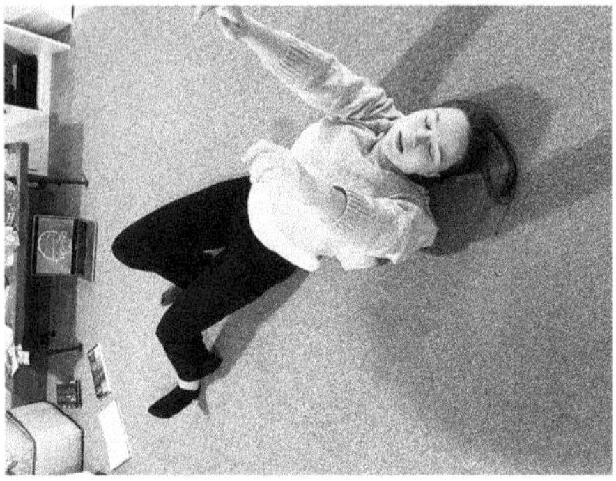

(e)

Invite participants to meet and connect with their scapulae: resting, stilling, listening, massaging, rubbing, rolling, pivoting, pushing and releasing. Listen into these bones, sensing the self-regulatory intelligence of soft myofascial tissue, and the powerful fulcrums they provide.

FIGURE 3.35A–E: Natasha Martin. Photographer: Amanda Williamson. (*Continued*)

The glenohumeral, sternoclavicular, acromioclavicular and scapulothoracic joints

Participants who are new to practice often think that shoulder mobility starts in the glenohumeral joint. On the contrary, shoulder mobility is created through a

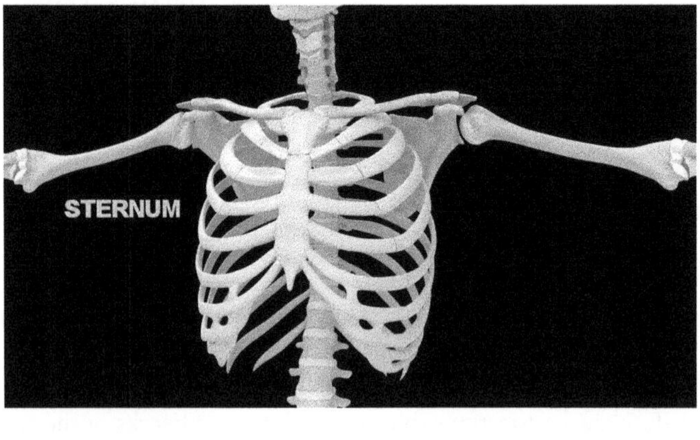

FIGURE 3.36: The shoulder girdle.

fluid relationality and articulation between the following joints: the glenohumeral, sternoclavicular, acromioclavicular and scapulothoracic joints. If you glance at Figure 3.36, you will notice the scapulae are connected to the clavicles anteriorly at *the acromioclavicular joints*. This is where the acromion process of each scapular meet and articulate with each clavicle. It is also crucial to share that the clavicles connect with the sternum at *the sternoclavicular joints*. Note, these are synovial joints – so fluent. The scapulothoracic joint, is a wonderful fluent joint. It is not a true joint, but rather a gliding fascial surface between the anterior surface of each scapula and the thoracic ribcage. The scapulothoracic joint suffers terribly when we don't move our shoulder girdle or circle our arms; often its fascial fluid nature becomes dry and crystallized. While playing in gravity, gentle sensory articulations in the glenohumeral, acromioclavicular, sternoclavicular and scapulothoracic joints helps to free tension throughout the shoulder girdle and also raises awareness of the inter-relational fluency between these joints. Additionally, circling the arm as you tip, pour and play around each scapula brings fluency to the scapulothoracic and glenohumeral joints. It is vitally important to always bring awareness to the inferior and anterior nature of the shoulder girdle. Participants new to practice are usually unaware the shoulder girdle has connective synovial articulations with the clavicles and sternum.

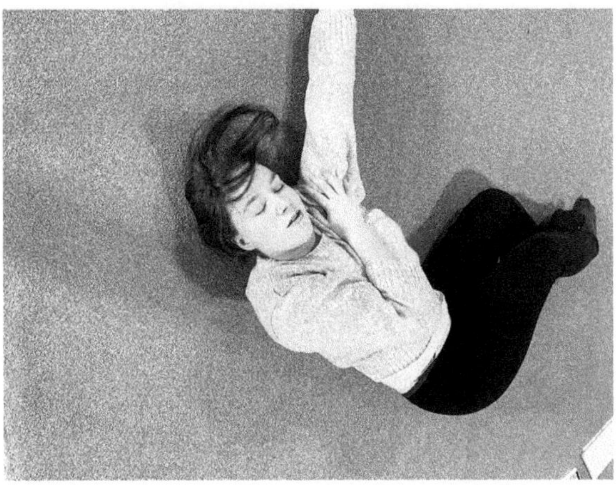

FIGURE 3.37: Natasha Martin: sensing her joints through self-touch and movement. Photographer: Amanda Williamson.

Invite participants to sense–perceive their clavicles. These are very profound bones. Note, they articulate with the sternum medially through two synovial joints and laterally at each acromion process through two more synovial joints.

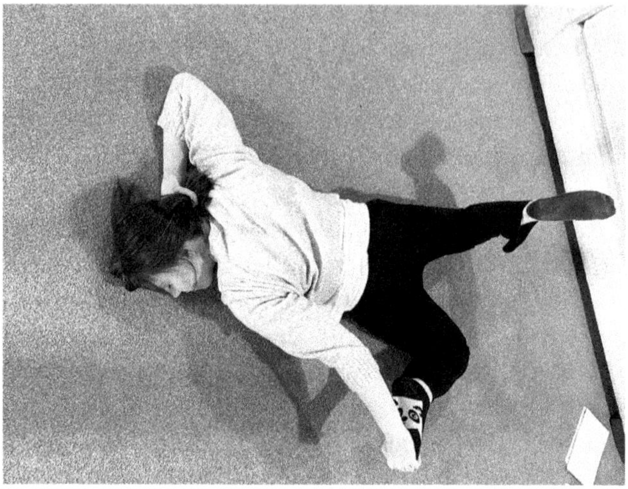

FIGURE 3.38: Natasha Martin: resting in her clavicals. Photographer: Amanda Williamson.

Invite participants to sense–perceive and initiate gentle movement in the sternoclavicular and acromioclavicular joints.

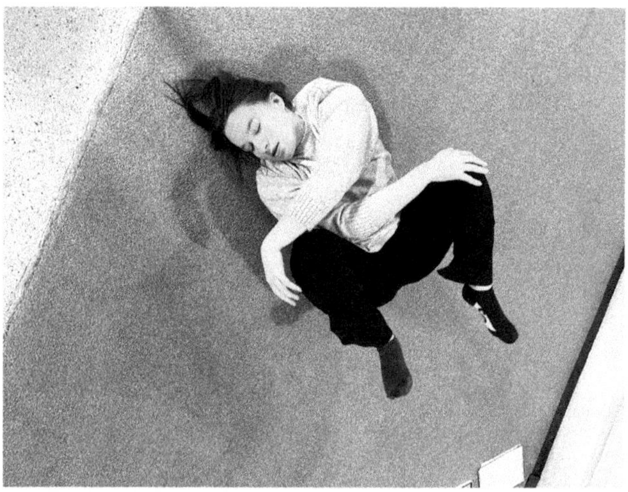

FIGURE 3.39: Natasha Martin: initiating movement from her sternoclavicular and acromioclavicular joints Photographer: Amanda Williamson.

When participants soften, explore and soft tissue roll around their scapulae they are often invited to circle and spiral their arms, easing out, and sensing space in the glenohumeral joint, as well as bringing fascial fluency to the scapulothoracic joint. The glenohumeral joint is vitally important to explore, but notably with awareness of how the sternoclavicular, acromioclavicular and scapulothoracic joints also move in fluid relation. Joints love to move together, sensing their connective fluency. As you circle your arms you can bring awareness to the scapulothoracic joint, the fascial landscape living under the scapulae that allows the scapular to move smoothly in relation to the thoracic cage (it supports elevation, depression, protraction, retraction, and medial and lateral rotation). This joint is beautifully integrative, connecting the movement of the scapula across the thorax, with movements of the arms. The glenohumeral joint is also a synovial joint, offering the mobile articulation between the head of the humerus in the glenoid fossa. It is a ball-and-socket joint and has an incredible range of movement, such as flexion, extension, abduction, internal and external rotation. It allows the lovely wide circumduction of the arm, but it is important to share with participants that the acromioclavicular, sternoclavicular joints and scapulothoracic joints are all involved when you circle your arm in an integrative fluent way. The glenohumeral joint is the most mobile joint in the human body. When you circle your arm, following your own movement, you are likely to be engaging flexion, extension, abduction, adduction, medial and external rotation. All these movements help to release many of the tissues that cross from the scapulae to the humerus and increase awareness of the fluid mobility within the shoulder joints. Of course, in somatic movement work, we are not using linear functional movement, but rather inviting the arms to open and play expressively. Unusual movement pathways

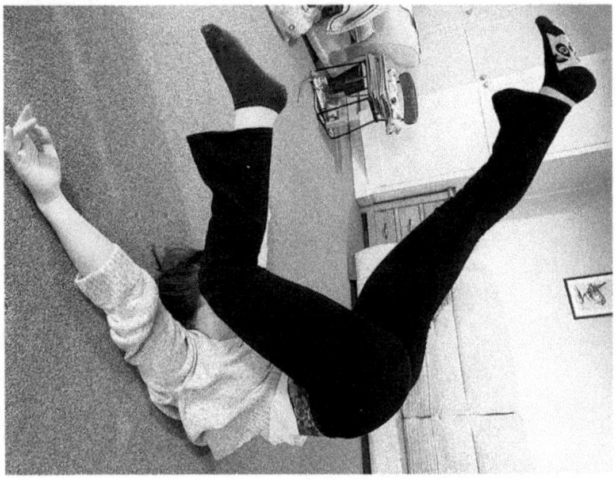

FIGURE 3.40: Natasha Martin: rolling onto her scapulae. Hanging-out with her scapulae. Photographer: Amanda Williamson.

that awaken and enliven the fascial tissues are extremely important because the fascia surrounding the scapulae needs new pathways to re-pattern habituated movement and soften stiff myofascial tissues. In short, when we follow and unwind the arms, we invite incredible fluency in the muscles and fascial tissues surrounding the scapulae and the forementioned joints. Exploring the incredible range of movement in the glenohumeral joint while simultaneously sense–perceiving the sternoclavicular, acromioclavicular and scapulothoracic joints is a key to deep release and tissue fluency.

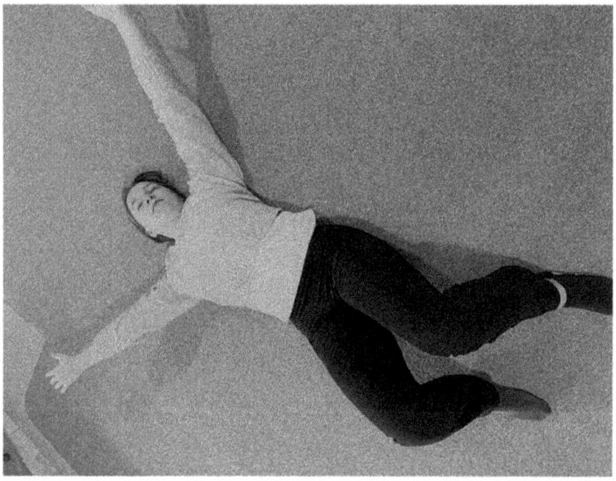

FIGURE 3.41: Natasha Martin: landing in the grace of her scapulae. Photographer: Amanda Williamson.

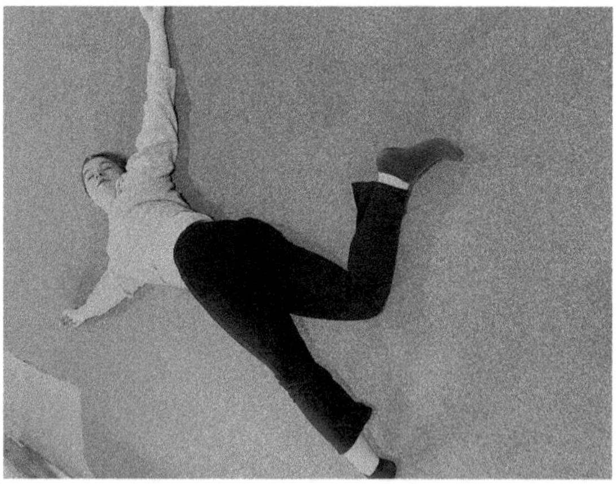

FIGURE 3.42: Natasha Martin: noticing her synovial joints and surrendering. Photographer: Amanda Williamson.

The four rotator cuff muscles

Nestled deeply into the scapulae we find the rotator cuff muscles snuggly originating in the fossae of the scapulae. These four deep muscles all originate on the scapulae and attach to the humerus. Markedly, these four muscles all cross the glenohumeral joint, connecting the scapulae with the arms. These four muscles stabilize the shoulder joint, keeping the head of the humerus in the glenoid fossa. Thus, when you move the head of your humerus, your shoulder blades also move. Tension and holding in these muscles affects the fluency and mobility of the glenohumeral joint, as well as the health of the entire scapulae. Moving with attuned awareness of these muscles and their lovely fascial extensions over the glenohumeral joint may also support a strengthening of the tendons. Often clients literally 'hold' their arms in, pulling in their scapulae medially, which compresses the rhomboids, trapezius, the rotator cuff and the glenohumeral joint. Here people are retracting their bilateral width – their expanse and 'presence' from the world. Sensing, rolling, tipping, yielding, compressing and decompressing the soft tissues of the rotator cuff muscles releases tension deeply held in the scapulae. Specifically, the rotator cuff muscles are:

- *the supraspinatus muscle*, which originates in the supraspinous fossa and attaches onto the superior facet of the greater tubercle of the humerus;
- *the infraspinatus muscle*, which originates in the infraspinous fossa and attaches onto the middle facet of the greater tubercle;

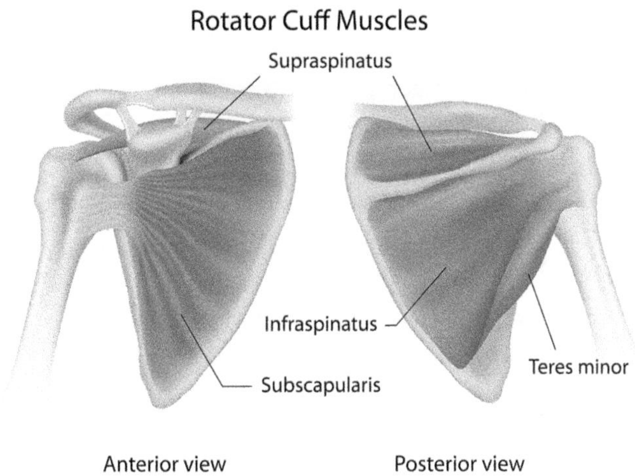

FIGURE 3.43: Rotator cuff muscles.

- *the teres minor muscle*, which originates on the middle half of the lateral border of the scapula and attaches onto the inferior facet of the greater tubercle;
- *the subscapularis muscle*, which originates in the subscapular fossa and attaches onto the lesser tubercle.

Example of practice: Sense–perceiving the rotator cuff muscles

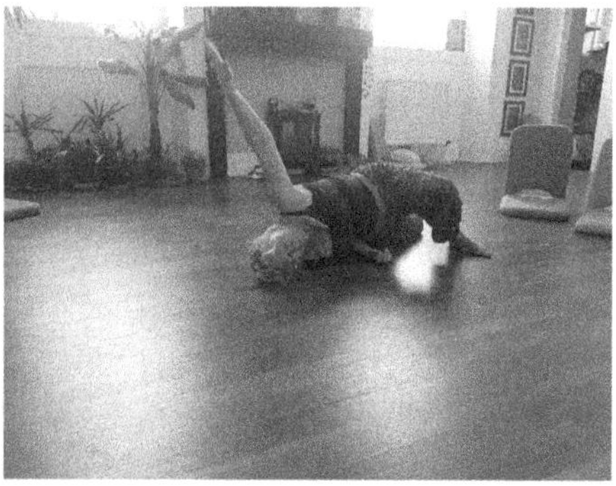

(a)

Bring awareness to the soft tissue of the rotator cuff muscles, snuggling and enfolding your scapulae bones and extending out into your humerus.

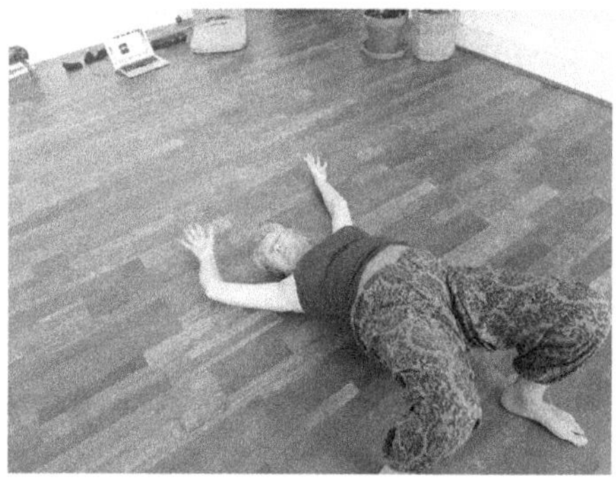

(b)

Direct movement through your arms, noticing the rotator cuff tissues crossing the glenohumeral joint and attaching to the humerus.

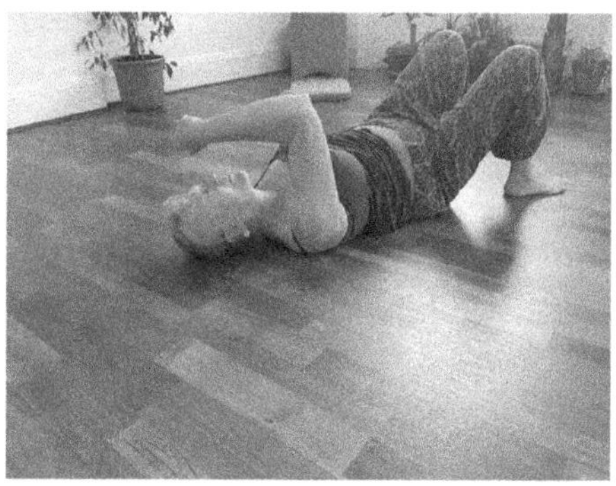

(c)

Sense the rotator cuff muscles that snuggly live in the fossa through gentle compressions, decompressions and releases.

FIGURE 3.44A–C: Karin Rugman. Photographer: Scott Closson.

The sternocleidomastoid and trapezius (supporting social engagement)

> The eleventh cranial nerve, or 'accessory nerve', is one of the keys to the well-being of the entire musculoskeletal system. Because it innervates the trapezius and sternocleidomastoid muscles (SCM), which enable the movement of the head and neck, tension on one side of these muscles pulls the shoulder, spine, and entire body out of alignment [...] together they make the outer ring of muscles in the neck, shoulders and upper back.
>
> (Rosenberg 2017: 20)

When participants soften into gravity, bringing sensory awareness to their occiput and scapulae, they have a wonderful opportunity to sense–perceive, explore and soften their trapezius. Additionally, they have the opportunity to release their sternocleidomastoid as they pour their head from side-to-side. In Chapter 2, we touched on how when both these muscles are released and softened it helps to bring us into a balanced state of health. In short, both muscles play key role in our ability to be socially engage because they are innervated by the accessory nerve, one of the four cranial nerves that engage the ventral branch of the vagus nerve. Soft tissue rolling the cranium with the cervical spine and scapulae following will ease out tension in both these muscles, inviting the accessory nerve into a state of health.

The trapezius loves to rest and soften in gravity. This is because it is often asymmetrically held, may have multiple trigger points, and many patterns of tension held in the upper, middle and lower fibres. Note, each person will have a different pattern of asymmetry and tension in their trapezius. Because of this, offering functional exercises with 'a one size fits all mentality' may not reach and resolve those holdings unique to an individual. Participants can sense where they feel stiff, where they feel pain and where they need to release. It is important to support self-regulatory agency, noted in Chapter 1. The participant who is attuned to their own sensory-motor feedback loop and their own pain receptors knows far more about the state of their trapezius than the therapist.

Observe in Figure 3.29 (the trapezius) just how large *it is*. This community of living tissues have multiple origination and insertion points. The tissues originate from the external occipital protuberance and the nuchal ligament all the way to the spinous process of C7. They then carry-on originating from C7 all the way to T12 – thus the tissues of the trapezius originate a fair way down your midline. It is thus important to invite participants to sense–perceive and explore self-regulatory movement along their midline – all the way from their occiput to T12 in their thoracic vertebrae.

Notice in the images above how the trapezius then moves laterally and anteriorly reaching out (curving around you), inserting on the spine of the scapulae, the acromion process and on the lateral part of the clavicle. In order to feel socially engaged and enter a ventral state, the trapezius needs to soften and balance into a state of fluency (only the upper fibres of the trapezius are innervated by the spinal accessory nerve). Bringing sensory-perceptual awareness to the trapezius through slow-time self-regulatory movement invites the accessory nerve into healthy expression, allowing its nature and role to take expanse within you. In anatomical language, the trapezius elevates, depresses, rotates and retracts the scapulae. While these terms feel rather functional, they are incredibly useful words to offer in improvisational processes underpinned by somatic awareness, guiding participants to explore elevation, depression, rotation and retraction through attuned self-regulatory improvisational play. The trapezius is a beautifully integrative muscle, connecting the occiput, cervical and thoracic spine, scapulae and clavicle.

Most participants are unaware the trapezius originates on their occipital bone, moving all the way to T12. In short, most people are unaware that tension in their shoulders is often caused by a dysfunctional relationship between their occiput, cervical and thoracic vertebra, the spine of the scapulae, the acromion process and the clavicle. Finding these incredible connections and somatically playing all along the midline, and then out laterally in relation to the spine of the scapulae, the acromion and clavicle is an incredibly integrative experience. This invites participants to become aware of lateralization.

Rosenburg points out, asymmetry is a real problem in the trapezius. He notes, asymmetry can compress the spinal nerves and also affect the heart and the lungs (2017: 112). Thus, the trapezius, when twisted and held in a state of holding, causes problems. Because the tissues of the trapezius are so accessible, lying just beneath the skin, this expanse of tissue is a fantastic place to start to unwind and repattern. In order to resolve dysfunction in the trapezius it is helpful to invite participants to explore asymmetry, rather than force symmetry and balance. Asymmetrical play, attending to one side of trapezius (through softening, yielding, stretching, expanding, compression, decompression and release), and then attending the other side, is one of the best ways to resolve asymmetrical holding. In my work, I offer that asymmetrical play is the precursor to symmetry, dissolving hypertonicity. This starts to stimulate the accessory nerve, enlivening the tissues and inviting balance.

The trapezius has many origins and insertions. For our purposes here, it is important to remember it originates on the occipital bone, the ligamentum nuchae and the spinous processes of T1–T12. The trapezius wraps around you anteriorly and inserts on the spine of your scapula, acromion and clavicle. The important thing to note here is the relationship between the occiput, cervical and thoracic spine, the spine of the scapulae, the acromion process and clavicle. As you unwind, remember from earlier, the trapezius is innervated by the accessory nerve that moves out of the jugular foramina between the temporal and the occipital bone and down into the tissues of the trapezius. Thus, moving the occipital bone and temporal bones in relation to the cervical and thoracic spine and out into the shoulder girdle invites all the tissues into integrative awareness and regulatory balance. It is incredibly important to develop an intimate relationship with the trapezius, especially if you struggle with feeling safe and socially engaged. This muscle

> is one of the very first muscles that we humans use as babies. When a baby lies on its stomach, its first movement is to arch its back and lift its head using the trapezius muscles. Then, with its head up, the baby can turn its head and look around using the sternocleidomastoid muscles.
>
> (Rosenburg 2017: 108)

The sternocleidomastoid (Figure 3.28), like the trapezius, is also innervated by the eleventh cranial nerve (the accessory nerve). Thus, the sternocleidomastoid also plays an integral role in supporting our social engagement. As Roseburg clearly shares

> Because these two muscles are innervated by a cranial nerve, they are different from the other 660 skeletal muscles in the rest of the body, which are all innervated by spinal nerves. Tension in any of these muscles can cause pain, reduced range of movement, and stiffness. Dysfunction in the sternocleidomastoid and trapezius muscles, by contrast, is related to a host of serious health issues that we usually do not associate with muscular problems.
>
> (Rosenberg 2017: 105)

Glance back to the image of the sternocleidomastoid (Figure 3.28) and notice how it originates on the manubrium of the sternum and the clavicle. It inserts on the mastoid process of the temporal bone. Dysfunction in this muscle is common and will affect the entire shoulder girdle. Sometimes these muscles shorten on one side. Sometimes one side is stiff. The sternocleidomastoid has easily accessible origination and insertion points. It is another fantastic example of how our cranial bones and shoulder girdle are so deeply connected. If you place your fingers on your sternum (manubrium) and the medial part of the clavicle, you can feel where this muscle is originating. If you then place your other hand and fingertips on the mastoid process on your temporal bone, you can feel where this muscle is attaching. It is a lovely clear connection, or curvaceous climb of living tissues from the sternum to the mastoid process.

The trapezius and sternocleidomastoid are only two of the twenty muscles that move the neck, but they are vital to our well-being and self-regulatory agency. Both these muscles, as Rosenberg notes, are 'determining factors in the shape and health of the spine' (Rosenberg 2017: 103). 'If the eleven cranial nerve is dysfunctional, it results in a lack of proper tonus in these muscles, stiff neck, migraines and difficulties rotating the head from side to side' (Rosenberg 2017: 20).

One of the defining features of my work is the very obvious expressive play with asymmetry, and the sheer delight of moving into asymmetry and distortion. Asymmetrical play during self-regulatory movement is a precursor to balance and symmetry. For example, one side of the trapezius may be emotionally held, and this misalignment, in turn, has caused restrictions and pain. The other side may be soft and dropped, with little proprioceptive awareness arising into consciousness. Quite naturally during a self-regulatory movement process, participants will move towards and sense–dwell in their trigger points, easing out pain, or indeed, enliven, stretch, push and weight bare on the side that is hypotonic.

Example of practice: Sense–perceiving where the trapezius originates

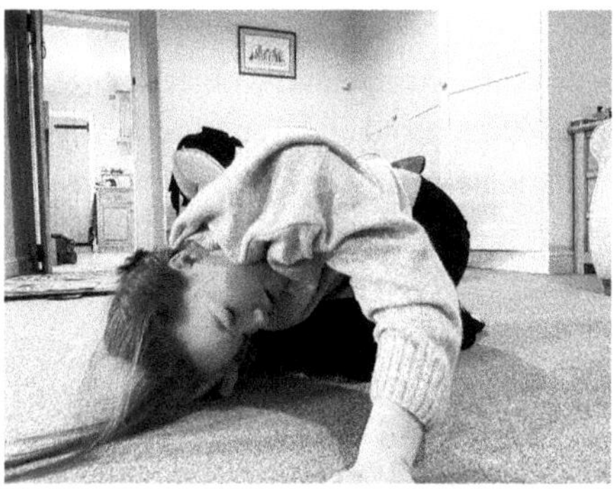

(a)

Invite participants to initiate movement from their occipital bone, with the vertebral column following and responding. Sense–perceive the originating points of the trapezius between the occiput through to T12.

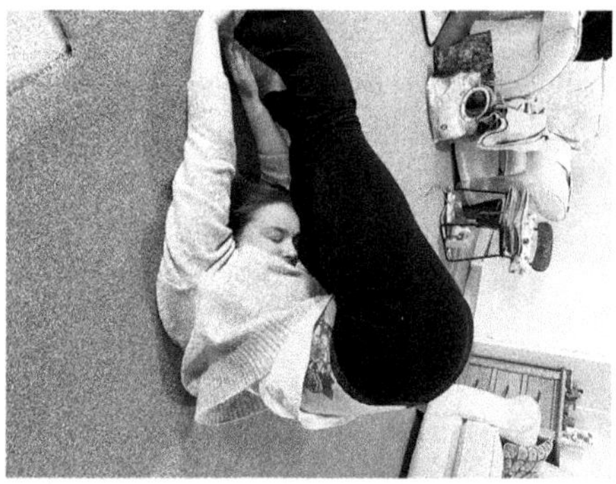

(b)

Invite participants to sense–perceive the originating points of the trapezius, from the occipital protuberance all the way down the midline to T12.

FIGURE 3.45A–C: Natasha Martin. Photographer: Amanda Williamson.

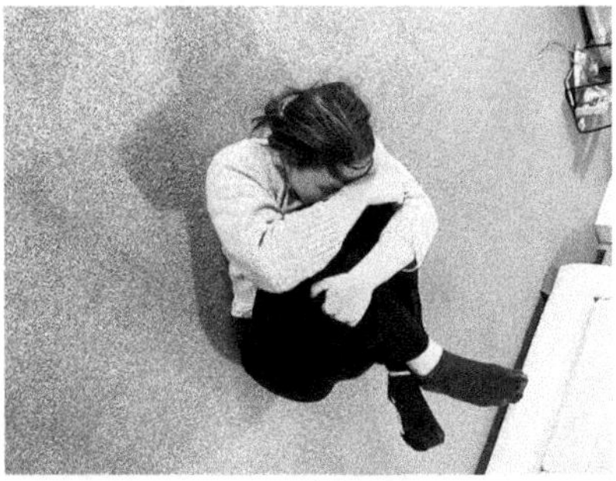

(c)
Sense and play along the midline, inviting the occiput, cervical and thoracic spine into integrative awareness.

FIGURE 3.45A–C: Natasha Martin. Photographer: Amanda Williamson. (*Continued*)

Example of practice: Sense–perceiving the insertion points of the trapezius

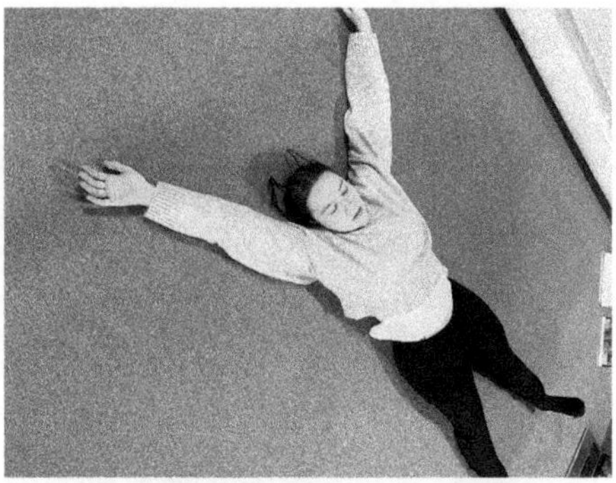

(a)

Begin by sense–perceiving the trapezius symmetrically, resting the soft tissues in gravity. Invite breath awareness. Bring your awareness to the soft tissues of the trapezius, noticing how they grow down and out along the midline (from the occiput to T12). Notice how they envelop you anteriorly attaching to the spine of the scapulae, the acromion and clavicle. Move your awareness around the origination and insertion points. Sense–perceive the mass and expanse of soft tissue lying just beneath your skin.

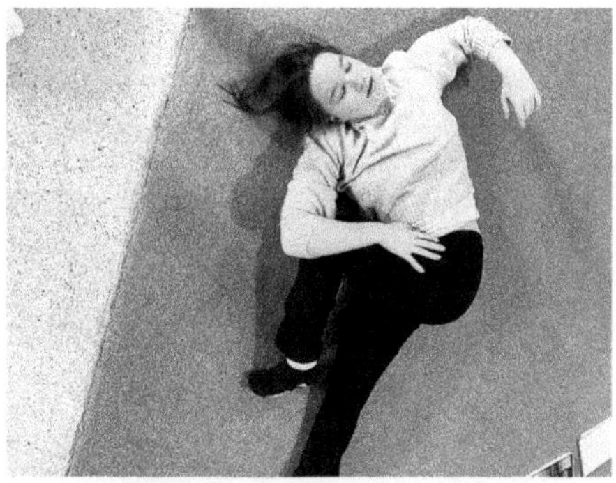

(b)

Sense–perceive the gentle clavicles with breath awareness. Bring awareness to how the trapezius wraps around you and attaches to your acromion process and clavicles. Sense the soft tissues enfolding around your shoulder girdle.

FIGURE 3.46A–D: Natasha Martin. Photographer: Amanda Williamson.

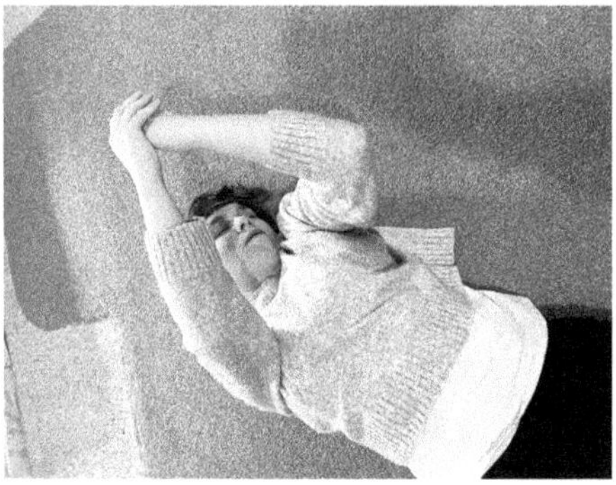

(c)

Sense–perceive the spine of the scapula. Bring awareness to the trapezius connecting onto this lovely ridge. Invite gentle compressions, decompressions and releases.

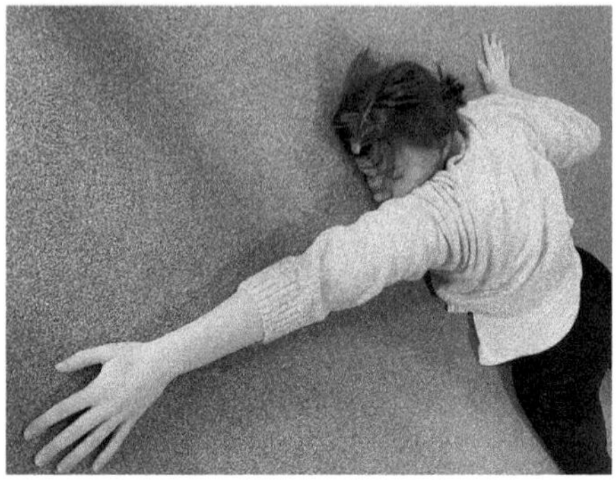

(d)

Sense–perceive the acromion process. Sense how the trapezius connects to this strong part of your scapulae.

FIGURE 3.46A–D: Natasha Martin. Photographer: Amanda Williamson. (*Continued*)

Asymmetrical play: A precursor to symmetry and balance in the tissues

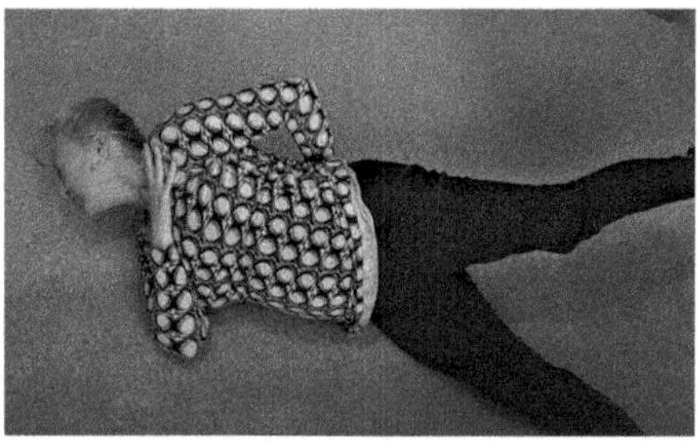

(a)

Invite participants to sense–perceive their trapezius and move with self-regulatory awareness, easing and stretching the tissues. Sense from the occiput to T12, out to the spine of the scapulae, acromion process and clavicle.

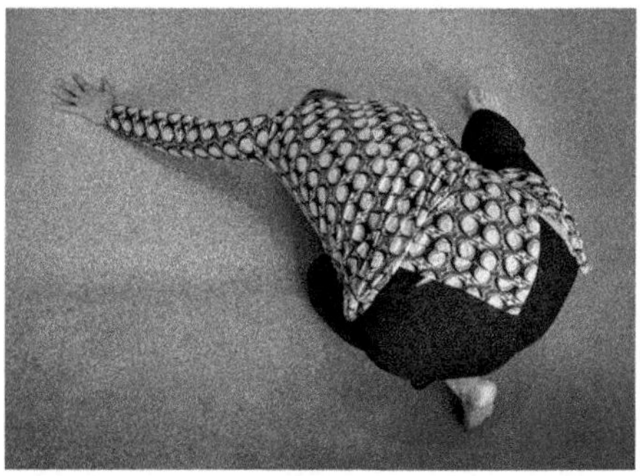

(b)

Invite participants to notice where they feel tension or pain in the trapezius, and listen to how the tissues want to express and ease pain.

FIGURE 3.47A–B: Karin Rugman. Photographer: Anika Rugman.

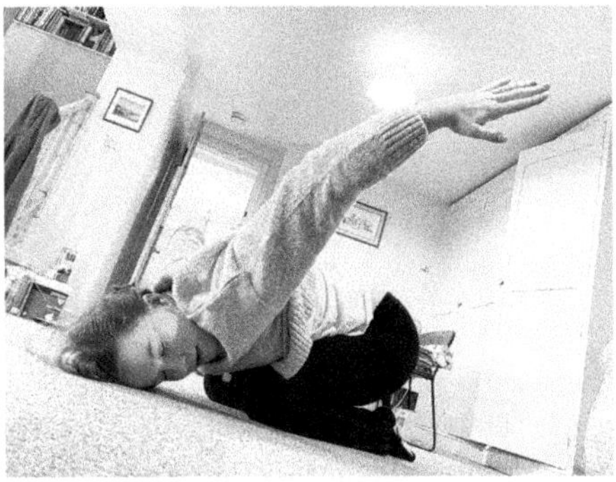

(a)

Invite participants to move in response to where tensions are calling for stretch, lengthening, expanding and stretching.

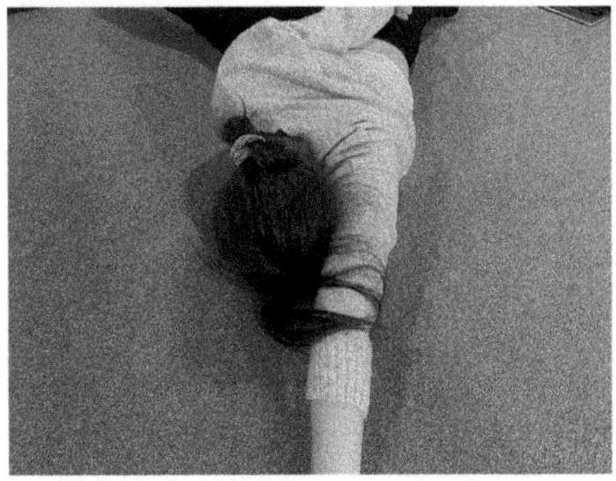

(b)

Invite participants to explore one side of their trapezius, listening into mechanoreceptors. What do these tissues need?

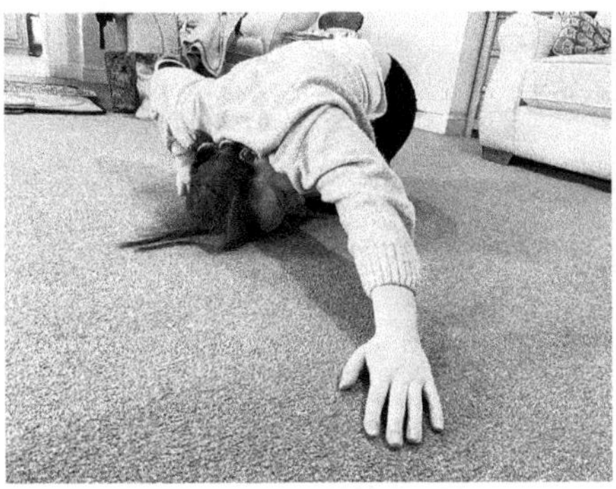

(c)

Do they need lengthening through reach on one side?

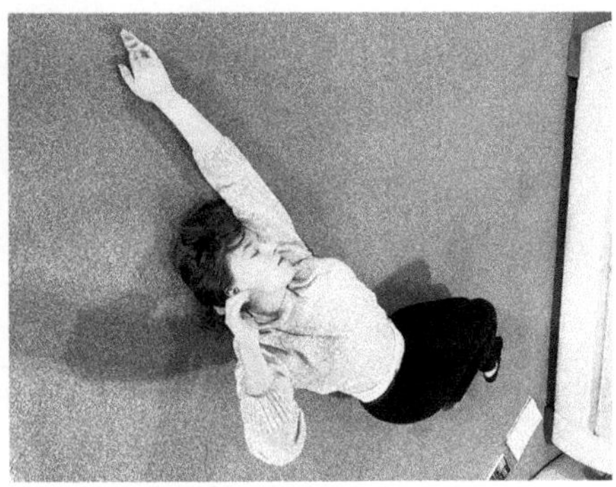

(d)

Do they need compression and pressure?

FIGURE 3.48A–D: Natasha Martin. Photographer: Amanda Williamson.

Practice: Sternocleidomastoid release

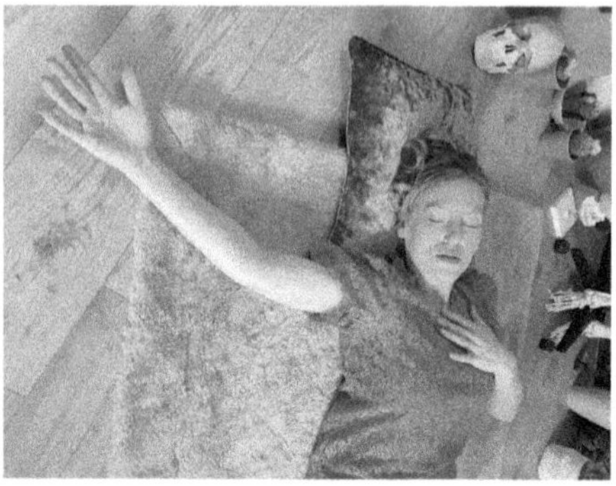

(a)

Invite participants to sense–perceive and softly touch the originating fibres of the sternocleidomastoid, the manubrium and clavicals. Rest awareness in breath.

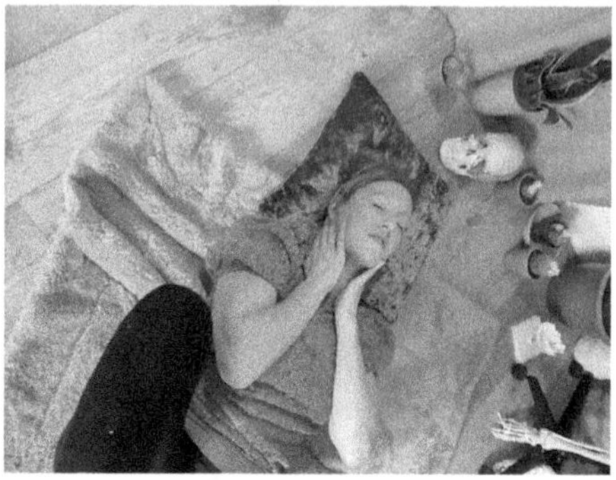

(b)

Invite participants to sense–perceive and tenderly touch the insertion fibres of the sternocleidomastoid, the mastoid process of the temporal bones. Rest in breath.

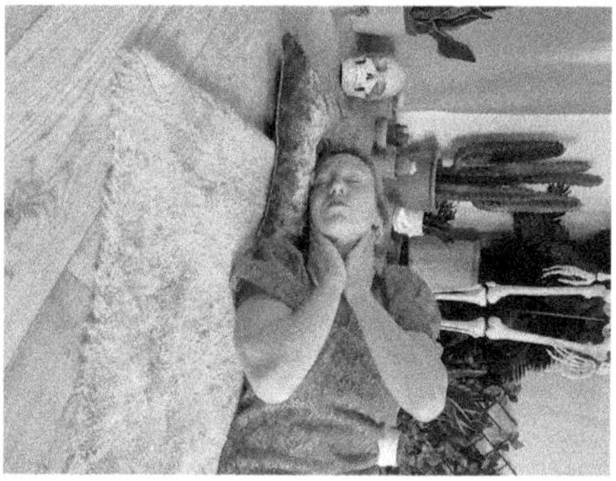

(c)

Somatically play between the organization and insertion points, with breath awareness, releasing the weight of the cranium and tipping and pouring the head from side-to-side.

FIGURE 3.49A–C: Amanda Williamson. Photographer: Scott Closson.

Key offerings and learnings

Sense–perceiving the scapulae is offered to:

- Sense structural support, attending to the shape and landscape of the scapulae.
- Sense the myofascial tissues surrounding, attaching or orginating from the scapulae.
- Sense the fluid articulations and relationality among the glenohumeral, sterno-clavicular, acromioclavicular and scapulothoracic joints. This brings awareness to the fluid nature of the shoulder girdle and the anterior and posterior joints that create the shoulder girdle.
- To open the glenohumeral joint, easing the soft tissues of the rotator cuff that pass from the scapulae and attach onto the humerus.
- To release and bring awareness to the trapezius and sternocleidomastoid.
- To lengthen, strengthen and stimulate the rotator cuff muscles, supporting a sense–perceived connection between the scapulae and the arms.
- Note, different somatic practitioners might bring awareness to different tissues that attach or originate or pass over the scapulae, such as the latissimus dorsi, for example.

The sacrum as a fulcrum of support and tissue re-organization

The sacrum provides the most tremendous fulcrum of support and soft-tissue re-organization when you lie in gravity at the beginning of class. When we release into gravity in a supine position the sacrum is easily sensed–perceived. The sacrum is the large upside-down triangular bone at the base of your spine. It intersects with the hip bones to form the pelvis, through the sacroiliac joints. The beautiful shape of the sacrum supports the weight of the upper body; this bone spreads and distributes the weight across the pelvis and down into the legs. It is sometimes referred to as *the keystone* of the pelvis because it provides incredible support for the spinal column. The sacrum, from the Latin 'holy bone', is an essential fulcrum to experience in gravity. As with the bony scapulae, it meets the ground easily when lying in a supine position and is, therefore, another natural fulcrum. The sacrum is made of five fused vertebrae – these are S1–S5. Of note, the sacrum connects and articulates with the final lumbar vertebra L5 superiorly, and with the coccyx (tailbone) inferiorly. This is also the location of the nerves of *the cauda equina.* Distilling your consciousness in this beautiful holy area and inviting tender, sensitive and attuned movement to arise from the lumbosacral region is extremely important because the nerves that pass through these tiny foramina form the sacral plexus.

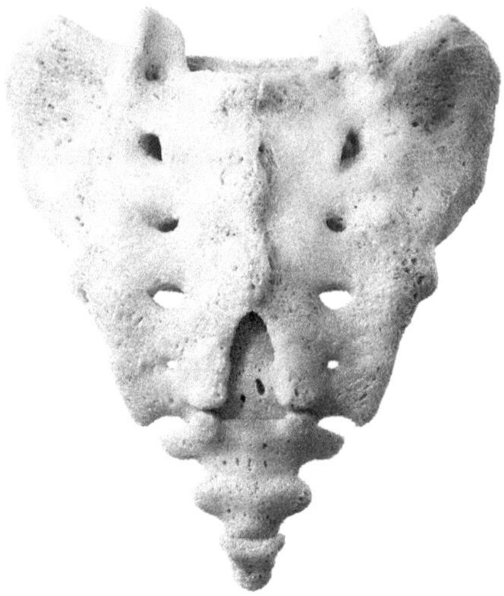

FIGURE 3.50: The sacrum.

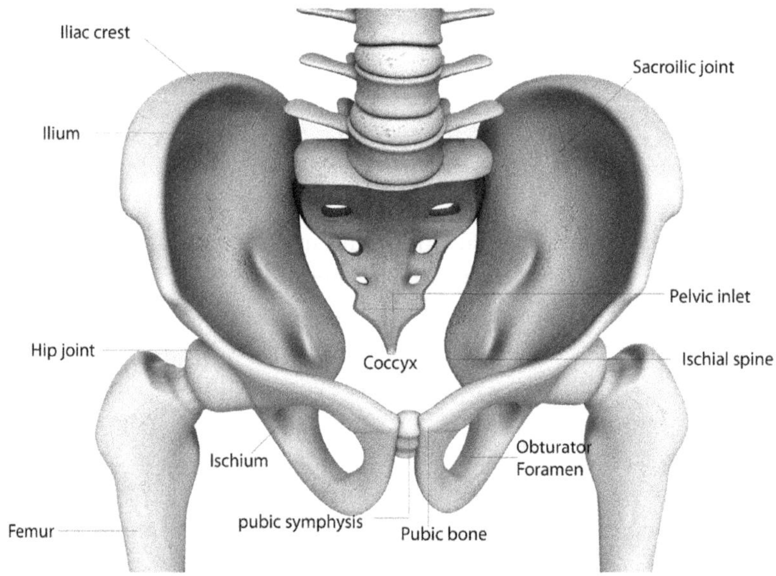

FIGURE 3.51: The pelvis.

There are many reasons why sense–perceiving and enjoying self-regulatory movement arising from the sacral region is important – there are too many to list here. However, self-regulatory movement around the following four areas feels particularly healing.

The sacral plexus.
The sacroiliac joints and lumbar–sacral joint.
The thoracic–lumbar fascia.
The parasympathetic nerves and the pudendal nerve.

The sacroiliac joints and lumbar–sacral joint

It is not the sacrum alone that is a natural fulcrum, but rather the entire pelvis (the pelvic bowl), as well as the lumbar–sacral region. The pelvis is created from the three following intersecting bones:

- *the ilia*: these are the largest bones in the pelvis, and you can make contact with each ilium easily by feeling along the posterior, superior and anterior parts of the iliac crest – the iliac crests enjoy gentle touch, compression and decompression
- *the pubis*: this is the bone that connects to the ilium through a joint called *the pubis symphysis*
- *the ischium*: these bones are often referred to as 'the sits bones' – again these bones are easy to contact.

It is absolutely delicious to soft tissue roll around all the bones in the pelvis, but notably, always inviting the rest of the body to tenderly follow, unwind and respond. As you breathe, sensing and following pathways of regulatory ease, it is very likely you are inviting healthy mobility in your *sacroiliac joints* and *lumbo-sacral joint*. When we sense into the sacrum, the *sacroiliac joints* often feel tight and restricted; people often perceive little mobility at their sacroiliac joints. Conventional anatomy reports, 'there is little movement at the sacroiliac joints'. There is movement, and this movement, however small, is absolutely vital to health and well-being. The lumbo-sacral joint is often under considerable strain, and this joint just loves to rest and unwind in gravity. There are two joints that are important to sense–perceive. Specifically,

- *the lumbo-sacral joint*: this is where L5 meets and articulates with S1 (the lumbar–sacral junction)
- *the sacroiliac joints*: this is where the wings of the sacrum (the alae) meet and articulate with the ilium

Using all the bones that form the pelvis as mini fulcrums inter-relationally is a lovely way to bring health and well-being to the lumbo-sacral joint and sacroiliac

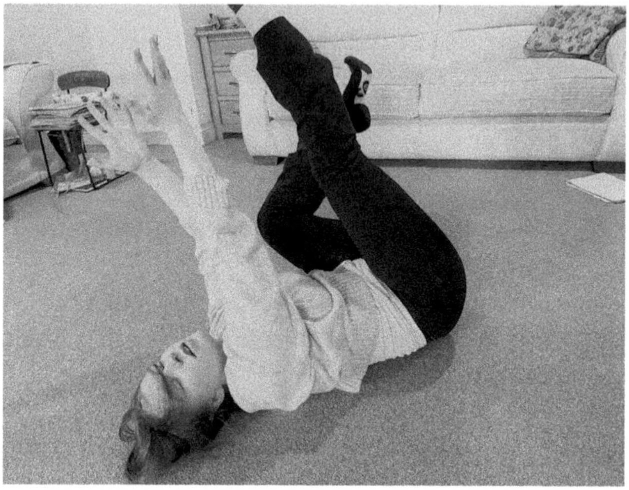

FIGURE 3.52: Natasha Martin: sensing her lumbar–sacral region. Photographer: Amanda Williamson.

joints. Below we are tipping, pouring, rolling and yielding around our pelvic bones, with particular awareness of the sacrum. As we initiate movement from our sacrum and pelvis, we invite the rest of my body to follow and unwind.

The lumbo-sacral joint is often under considerable strain when we are vertical because this joint is baring the weight of the vertebral column above it. This joint lives between L5 and S1 (the bottom of the lumbar vertebrae and the top of the sacral vertebrae). When we settle, rest and move in gravity we can ease this joint,

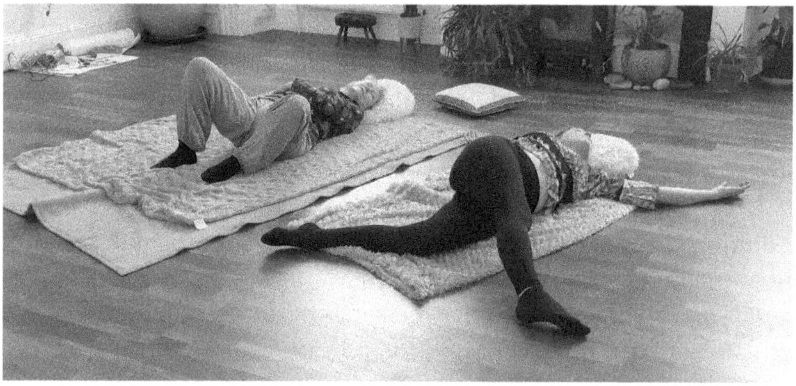

FIGURE 3.53: Karin Rugman and Amanda Williamson: Easing their lumbar vertebrae: Photographer: Scott Closson.

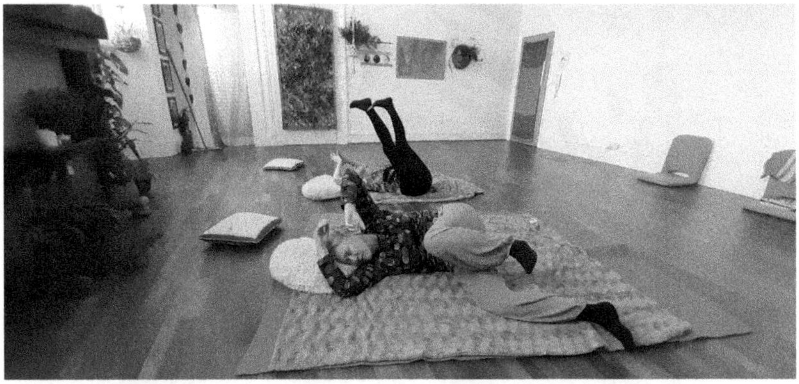

FIGURE 3.54: Amanda Williamson and Karin Rugman: bringing awareness to their sacrums. Photographer: Scott Closson.

releasing tension and stress held in this area. The sacroiliac joints, formed between the wings of the sacrum and the ilium, are also invited into health when you soft-tissue roll around pelvis. Softening in the lumbar–sacral region and listening for a gentle movement response to arise, invites these joints into expression.

The sacral plexus

When participants sense–perceive their sacrum and pelvis, movement usually emerges from their lumbar–sacral region out through their legs. This is very integrative, and as you facilitate you often witness a very fluid connection between the lumbar–sacral

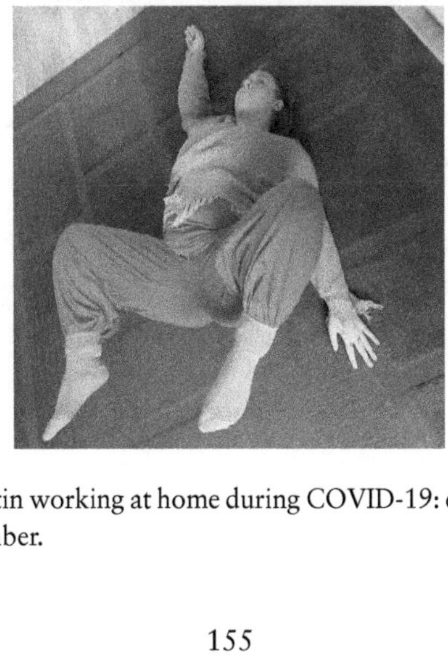

FIGURE 3.55: Natalie Austin working at home during COVID-19: enjoying sensing her sacrum. Photographer: family member.

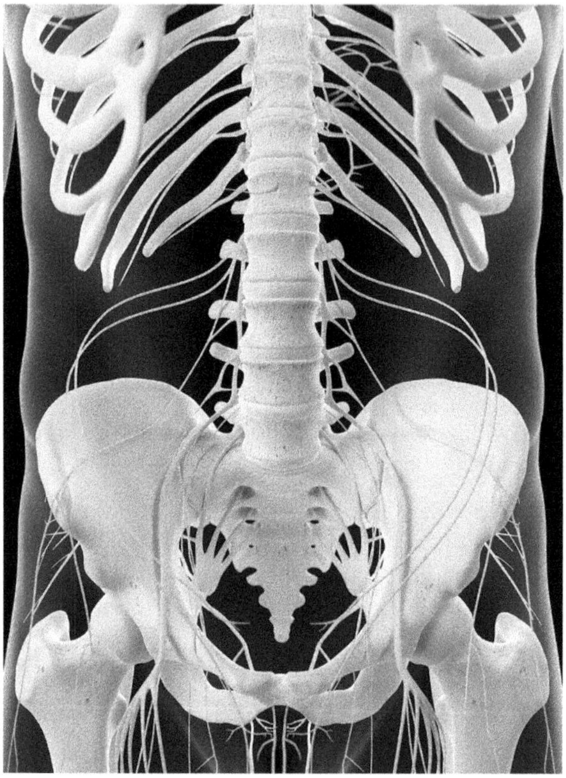

FIGURE 3.56: The sacral plexus.

vertebra and the legs. Participants are intuitively sense–perceiving their sacral plexus. The sacral plexus is located in both the lumbar and sacral vertebrae. Specifically, this plexus of nerves is formed by the spinal nerves in the lumbar region, L4 and L5, as well as the sacral nerves S1 to S4. The sacral plexus extends out of the lumbar–sacral region and down into the legs. As participants explore the relationship between their sacrum and legs, they are engaging the sacral plexus.

Notably, the sciatic nerve, which is a very long nerve, emerges from this area (specifically from L4, L5, S1, S2 and S3). Attuning to the lovely connection between our lumbo-sacral region and our legs flosses our sciatic nerve.

The thoraco-lumbar fascia

When participants soften in the lumbar–sacral region, they also have opportunity to soften, ease and change the viscosity of the thoraco-lumbar fascia. This is

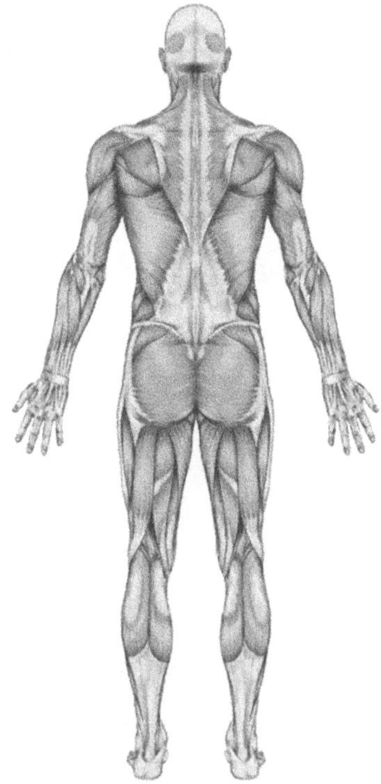

FIGURE 3.57: The thoraco-lumbar fascia.

a large area of fascial connective tissue that connects with many muscles, such as the latissimus dorsi, the quadratus lumborum and gluteus maximus. It is often referred to as a nodal area and moving with awareness of this fascial tissue and its expanse and connectivity can reduce back pain.

The parasympathetic nerves and the pudendal nerve

We noted in Chapters 1 and 2 that the parasympathetic nerves emerge from the sacral region at S2, S3 and S4. Thus sensing and perceiving the sacrum is often very relaxing and peaceful, especially when combined with initiating movement from the cranial bones – and playing consciously with the head–tail connection. Of note here, *the pudendal nerve* (formed by S2, S3 and S4) innervates your sexual organs and often participants report an incredible flow of energy when sense-perceiving their sacrum. This is a very important experience, connecting participants with a transpersonal life-force. This process transcends how sexuality has

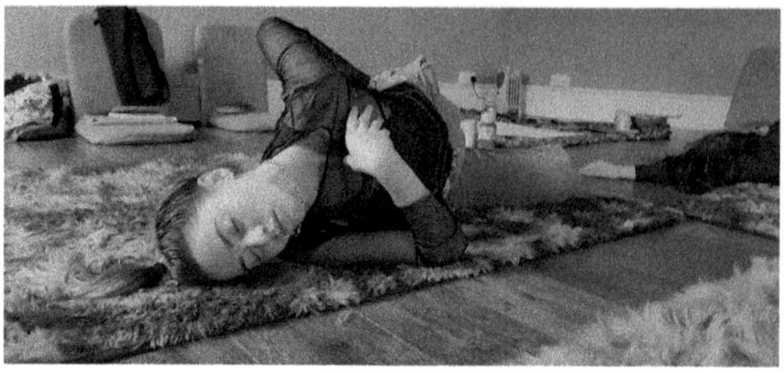

FIGURE 3.58: Sylvia Gregory: sensing the life-energy from sacrum to occiput. Photographer: Amanda Williamson.

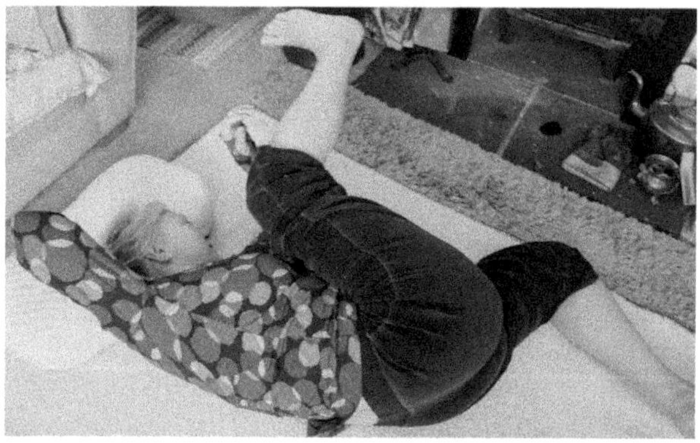

FIGURE 3.59: Karin Rugman: sensing the connection from her sacrum to her legs: Photographer: Amanda Williamson.

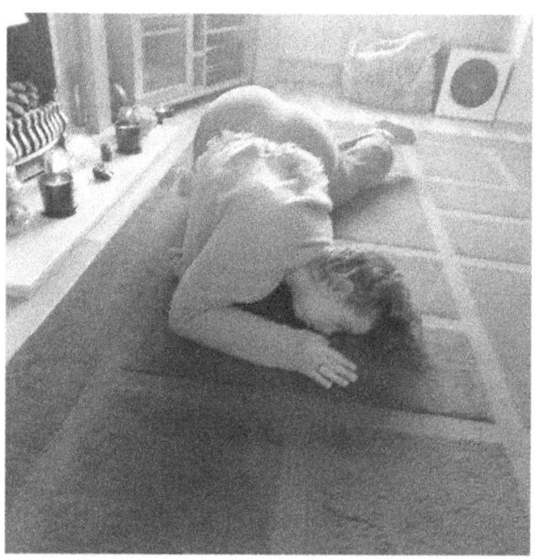

FIGURE 3.60: Natalie Austin working at home during COVID 19: life-force sensing: Photographer: family member.

been enculturated and constructed. There is an incredible opening to life-energy sense–perceived in the sacrum and pelvis, moving all the way to the cranium. A very deep contact with the life-force from the sacrum and pelvis is arising, both through attuning to the parasympathetic nerves, as well as through the craniosacral system (the free flow of cerebrospinal fluid within the dural tube). This is a primal life-force that begins in the third week of embryonic development with the appearance of the primitive streak (this is further defined in Chapter 6). Suffice to say, sense–perceiving the sacrum innervates the parasympathetic nerves and opens movers to an energy in the sacral region which is deeply illuminating and healing.

Key offerings and learnings

Participants are invited to develop a sense–perceptual relationship with their sacrum and pelvis to:

- To release strain in the lumbar–sacral region.
- To explore and invite fluency (however micro) in the sacroiliac joints.
- To explore the relationship between the sacral plexus and the legs, flossing the nerves.
- To soften the thoraco-lumbar fascia.
- To sense the parasympathetic nerves, aiding rest and sensing the life-force opening in the pelvis.

Conclusion

When we explore fulcrum support and tissue reorganization for long periods of time in gravity through self-regulatory movement, we are not simply rolling around with no rhythm or reason. We are attending to the release of especially important tissues throughout the body. In this chapter, I have presented some of the key tissues we can reorganize in the studio by resting in our fulcrums and following our own sensory movement pathways. For every tissue, I have pinpointed, there are thousands more interrelated tissues. All these unmentioned tissues will also be reorganizing and finding ease as you gently, tenderly and creatively play in gravity, with breath awareness. Different practitioners may pinpoint different tissues in the studio. In this chapter, I focused on tissues and structures that are relevant in terms of finding support in your own body, aiding parasympathetic release and social engagement.

To an outsider, it often looks as if participants are simply rolling around the studio floor. In contrast there is a rationale underlying why I do what I do. Because we do not approach health in a mechanistic way, it is hard for outsiders to understand how health can be rooted in sensing, feeling, perceiving and following self-regulatory movement. This chapter has provided an example of the physiological and anatomical complexity underlining the apparent simplicity of somatic movement dance practice. Let us move to the next chapter, where I attend to the co-regulatory presence of the heart-centered witness.

4

Co-regulation, Cardio-ception and the Transpersonal Witness

Your words,
seeped into my bones,
dropped my awareness into breath and heart,
landed me in ground.
Invited me to soften and release.
Wrapped me in silk
and enfolded me in warmth and safety.
I imagined a bird being
held gently, carefully being
set free to fly again.
A child being held by her mother's
gentle touch.

(Reflective writing by Karin Rugman after dyadic witnessing and moving)

Part 1: Co-regulation and cardio-ception

> The heart's electromagnetic field is by far the most powerful produced in the body; it is approximately five thousand times greater in strength than the field produced by the brain, for example. The heart's field not only permeates every cell in the body but also radiates outside of us; it can be measured up to eight to ten feet away with sensitive detectors called magnetometers.
>
> (Childre and Martin 1999: 33)

The processes shared throughout this book are rooted in self-regulation, but they are always held in the presence of a compassionate non-judgemental witness, who holds either group processes, or one-on-one sessions. Therefore, these processes are co-regulatory, where the health of the therapist is equally important, if not vital, in the efficacy of practice. The concept of co-regulation within my work is rooted in the pioneering research of Steven Porges (2017), Doc Childre and Howard Martin (1999), as well as my own empirical investigation with students and clients over what is now, decades. These open minded scientists demonstrated that when people's nervous systems interact, they can either regulate or deregulate each other. Thus, the state of our nervous system affects those around us and vice versa (Porges 2017). A deregulated nervous system is disturbed by fear, anxiety and thus sympathetic arousal. A regulated nervous system is inspired by peace, safety and sociality. Applied to somatic movement dance therapy, I offer it is extremely important that the therapist regulates their own nervous system prior to working with a client or group. I always train students to release stress, strain and anxiety, which causes sympathetic arousal in their own tissues, in preparation for working with participants and clients. Most significantly, I offer that heart-centred sensing and moment-by-moment breath awareness is the foundation (the heart) of co-regulation.

Self-regulatory movement is possible on your own, especially if you have been practising for years, have learned to shift your nervous system into parasympathetic release, have developed attuned sensory-perceptual–imaginal movement awareness, and have a strong sense of *the inner-witness*. In fact, one of the aims of somatic movement is that participants take their experiential learning beyond the studio walls so they can self-regulate in other contexts, remaining calm and with an integrated sense of Self. Self-regulation is however, far more effective in the presence of a non-judgemental compassionate witness. I thus train students to become heart-centred witnesses through a number of subtle embodied skills, some of which I share below. These embodied skills help them to balance their own tissues, in turn creating a peaceful heart-space, full of breath and ease, for Other.

I noted in Chapters 1 and 2 that breath awareness and particularly conscious diaphragmatic breathing reduces the heart rate, lowers blood pressure and innervates the vagus nerve. Breath awareness is the most efficacious and necessary inroad into the parasympathetic. Less commonly known is that sense–perceiving the heart also supports a shift into the parasympathetic and supports a ventral vagus state. Thus, sense–perceiving the heart and breath is the first stage of self-regulation and the entraining of the co-regulatory compassionate witnesses. Developing a sensed relationship with the organ of the heart, its position, weight, rhythm and quality, is highly effective for students training, staff leading and participants attending. Heart-sensing may sound spiritual or hippie, or perhaps mystical, symbolic or metaphorical. Heart-sensing can certainly feel deeply spiritual and mystical; however, as I will share in this chapter, the health benefits of heart-sensing are also now scientifically grounded.

Because the heart lies at the centre of many spiritual traditions, heart-sensing could easily be dismissed as rather romantic, wishful thinking, simply poetic and

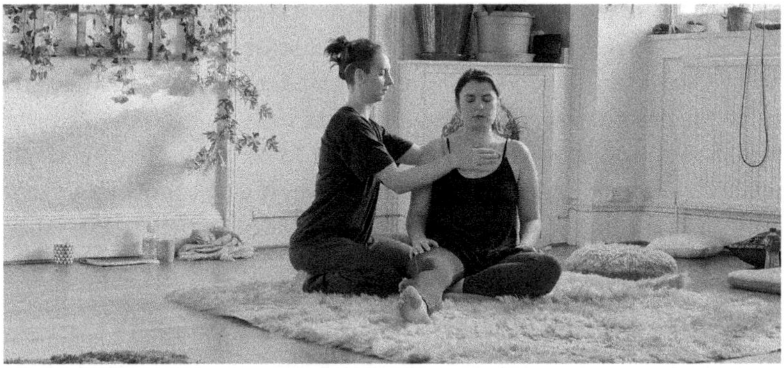

FIGURE 4.1: Jessica Cotton and Ella West: heart-sensing and moment-by-moment breath awareness. Photographer: Amanda Williamson.

certainly not grounded in science. There has, however, been a wonderful meeting of spirituality and science since the 1970s, extensively developed through research untaken at the HeartMath Institute (1999). Many of the HeartMath scientific findings explain why sensing the heart is so vital to our well-being. Sensing the heart not only reduces sympathetic activity and innervates the parasympathetic but also releases stress-reducing hormones and thus helps to self-regulate emotions. For those who practise heart-centred meditations on a daily basis, it will come as no great surprise that science has now validated the importance of heart-sensing – something many meditative traditions already knew. The ongoing research at the HeartMath Institute is rather beautifully inspired by asking why so many ancient mystical and religious traditions focus on the organ of the *heart*? Their research has shown that heart-sensing contributes to the health of the entire organism.

> Core heart feelings affect both branches of the autonomic nervous system. They reduce the activity of the sympathetic nervous system (that branch of the system that seeds heart rate, constricts blood vessels, and stimulates the release of stress hormones) and increase the activity of the parasympathetic nervous system (the branch of the system that slows the heart rate and relaxes the body's inner systems), thereby increasing its effectiveness. In addition, the balance between these two branches of the nervous system is enhanced so that they work together with increased efficiency. The collaboration results in diminished friction and wear and tear on the nerves and internal organs.
> (Childre and Martin 1999: 15)

Many ancient spiritual and religious are *cardio-centric* (heart-centred), while the western secular world is largely *cephalon-centric* (brain-centred). In some spiritual traditions, the heart is perceived as the centre of our being, emotion, sensation, morality and often an organ where one can sense or converse with the mystical presence of God. Cardio-centric philosophy and poetry can be observed from antiquity to the present day. Egyptian, Sufi and Christian mystical traditions have prayer rituals that centre on the heart. Plato and Aristotle wrote extensively about the heart. For example, Aristotle identified the heart as the most important organ in the body, and the first to develop in the embryo (Alberti 2010: 7). And he was correct, as Childre shares:

> The heart starts beating in the unborn fetus before the brain has developed. Scientists still don't know exactly what triggers the beating, but they use the word 'autorhythmic' to indicate that the heartbeat is self-initiated from within the heart. As the brain develops, it grows from the bottom up. Starting from the most primitive part of the brain (the brainstem), the emotional centers (the amygdala and the hippocampus) begin to emerge. It is well known to brain researchers that the thinking brain then grows out of the emotional regions. That speaks volumes about the relationship of thought to feeling.
> (Childre and Martin 1999: 9)

In traditional Chinese medicine, 'the heart is seen as the seat of connection between the mind and the body, forming a bridge between the two. It's said that the heart-blood houses the *shen*, which can be translated as both "mind" and "spirit"' (Childre and Martin 1999: 8). 'In the Kabbalah the heart is the Central Sphere, the only one of ten to touch all the others, and it's reputed to hold the key to the mysteries of radiant health, joy, and well-being' (Childre and Martin 1999: 8). Scientists now know when the heart is honoured as a site of consciousness and felt fully in our sense–perception and awareness, our well-being greatly improves. HeartMath scientists soon realized that ancient cultures and spiritual traditions had developed their own sophisticated knowledge of the heart. 'All these conceptions have a common view of the heart as harbouring an "intelligence" that operates independent of the brain yet in communication with it' (Childre and Martin 1999: 8).

The intense focus on the brain as the centre of consciousness (and emotional and cortical processing) reflects Cartesian dualism at its most extreme, where heart and head are separated, and the heart is divested of its neurological, hormonal and electromagnetic consciousness. Rechtschaffen notes below, there is quite a gap in how the heart is perceived within the medical paradigm and how the heart has been, and is still, talked about symbolically and metaphorically in multiple languages. He notes:

> Western conventional medicine speaks of the heart solely in terms of its physiological function. In that medical definition, the heart is a multichambered muscular organ

> crisscrossed with electrical circuitry. The heart is often described as a pump and the arteries as pipes – essentially the biological equivalent of the well pump and plumbing in your house. This description is in such marked contrast to our emotional sense of the heart that one is left wondering if there's any connection whatsoever between the literal and figurative, the physical and the mystical.
>
> (Rechtschaffen 1999: x)

Further,

> [t]he difference between the physical and emotional definitions of 'heart' is rooted in the body/mind split so pervasive in medicine today. We've separated the role of our thoughts and daily stresses from the effects that they produce in the physical body. Throughout their medical training, physicians are told of bacterial, metabolic, toxic, and other causes of physical illness, yet the relationship of our thoughts and emotions to effecting physical change is for the most part ignored. This has in large measure led to a medical model that can be dehumanizing, focusing solely on the specific physical manifestations of disease, thus losing sight of the whole person.
>
> (Rechtschaffen 1999: x)

With

> the emergence of scientific medicine (and the separation of mind and body, head and heart), theoretical ideas about the mind and body transplanted emotions to the mind. And the heart became an organ of the body: mechanized, predicable, subject to decay and the barometer (rather than the instrument) of emotional experiences.
>
> (Alberti 2010: 17)

The transition from a cardio-centric to a cephalon-centric world

> took place under the influence of processes that we might broadly associate with modernity. The construction of the subject as a thinking being, the cognitive processes located in the brain rather than in the soul, and not in the body, meant that it was the brain that would be prioritized in discussions of emotions and the self. Since the nineteenth century and the segregation of the body and the mind into a series of parts, it has become commonplace for the brain to be the organ most associated with life (indeed brain health has succeeded heart health as the number one criteria for determining life).
>
> (Alberti 2010: 7)

Pre-modern medicine and indeed many forms of non-western indigenous medicine new something of the heart that science is catching up with. Seismically disrupting the head/heart split, scientists discovered the heart has a brain containing at least 40,000 neurons, and this intelligent organ is not only involved in emotional processing (as one might intuit) but also cortical decision making. Childre shares:

> In recent years, neuroscientists have made an exciting discovery. They've found that the heart has its own independent nervous system – a complex system referred to as 'the brain in the heart'. There are at least forty thousand neurons (nerve cells) in the heart – as many as found in various subcortical centres in the brain. The heart's intrinsic brain and nervous system relay information back to the brain in the cranium, creating a two-way communication system between heart and brain. The signals sent from the heart to the brain affect many areas and functions in the amygdala, the thalamus, and the cortex.
>
> (1999: 10)

HeartMath's research demonstrated how the heart directly affects emotions and reasoning, because the amygdala, thalamus and the cortex respond to the heart's signals – thus our heart is involved not just with emotional processing (often assumed) but cortical reasoning as well. Historically scientists had 'presumed that the brain made all the discissions', but research since the 1970s has demonstrated that the heart sends a wealth of information back to the brain and thus is highly involved in perceptions, decision-making and reasoning (Childre and Martin 1999: 10). It has been shown that the heart responds with 'its own distinctive logic' and does not necessarily obey all the orders sent by the brain (Childre and Martin 1999: 10). Research also demonstrated that 'the heart appeared to be sending messages back to the brain that the brain not only understood but obeyed' (Childre and Martin 1999: 10). They discovered that negative emotions throw 'the nervous system out of balance' creating heart rhythms that are 'jagged and disordered' (Childre and Martin 1999: 13–14). In contrast, they found positive emotions 'increase order and balance in the nervous system and produce smooth, harmonious heart rhythms' (Childre and Martin 1999: 13–14). Cultivating heart intelligence has been scientifically shown to:

facilitate brain function
adjust balance in the autonomic nervous system
lower blood pressure
increase stress-relieving hormones
increase immune responses

> and, positive emotions such as happiness, appreciation, compassion, care, and love not only change patterns of activity in the nervous system, they also reduce the production of the stress hormone cortisol.
>
> (adapted from Childre and Martin 1999)

Childre shares that the heart communicates with the brain and the rest of the body in four ways 'for which there is solid scientific evidence: neurologically (through the transmission of nerve impulses), biochemically (through hormones and neurotransmitters), and biophysically (through pressure waves)' – and in addition, 'energetically (through electromagnetic interactions)' (Childre and Martin 1999: 28–29). 'Through these four communication systems, the heart has a significant influence on the function of our brains and all our body systems' (Childre and Martin 1999: 29). In terms of neurological communication, 'the signals the heart sends to the brain have a regulatory influence on many of the autonomic nervous signals that flow out of the brain to the heart, to the blood vessels, and to other glands and organs' (Childre and Martin 1999: 30). However, 'the signals that the heart sends back to the brain also cascade up into the higher centres of the brain' and thus the heart affects 'the activity of the cortex – that part of the brain that governs our higher thought and reasoning capacities' (Childre and Martin 1999: 30). These 'pathways linking the heart with our higher brain centres' serves to explain how 'information from the heart can modify' our 'mental states and feeling states' (Childre and Martin 1999: 30).

Biophysically, with every beat of the heart pressure waves are produced that send arterial blood to the organs and glands, and every cell in the body. These pressure waves have been shown to increase the electromagnet activity in the brain; thus, our beat or pulse not only delivers fresh oxygenated blood to our capillaries and every cell in the body, but additionally, these waves affect the electromagnetic field produced in the brain (see Childre and Martin 32).

> As many doctors know, the pattern and quality of the energy emitted by the heart is transmitted throughout the body via the heart's electromagnetic field. Just as cell phones and radio stations transmit information via an electromagnetic field, recent research has led some scientists to propose that a similar information transfer process occurs via the electromagnetic field produced by the heart. The heart's electromagnetic field is by far the most powerful produced in the body; it is approximately five thousand times greater in strength than the field produced by the brain, for example. The heart's field not only permeates every cell in the body but also radiates outside of us; it can be measured up to eight to ten feet away with sensitive detectors called magnetometers.
>
> (Childre and Martin 1999: 33)

'The neural, biochemical, biophysical and electromagnetic messages that the heart sends to the brain have a profound influence on our physiological, mental, emotional processes' (Childre and Martin 1999: 34). As Childre shares, the interaction between the heart and brain is most readily witnessed through heart rate variability. Heart rate variability patterns, or heart rhythms, 'have consistently emerged as the most dynamic and reflective of inner emotional states' (Childre and Martin 1999: 35). He notes, 'in negative emotional states such as anger and frustration, the HRV pattern is incoherent, random and jerky' whereas in 'positive emotional states such as appreciation, love and care, the HRV pattern in coherent and ordered' (Childre and Martin 1999: 35). Interestingly, and rather wonderfully, and reflecting the ancient heart-centred spiritual traditions of the world, these scientists found that when we focus on our hearts, the heart and brain come into synchronicity, and the health benefits of this balance affect not only the person, but those around them. Adapting Childre's remarks, this has incredible social implications, where balance and awareness of our own heart can support the health of those around us, and enhance community and social well-being (Childre and Martin 1999: 35).

> HeartMath demonstrate that when we focus our attention on our hearts, the synchronization between the heart and brain increases. Experiments suggest that the energetic interaction between the heart and brain plays a part in this process. Furthermore, research evidence indicates that the energetic information contained in the heart's field isn't detected only by one's own brain and body but can also be registered by the people around us.
>
> (Childre and Martin 1999: 34)

Further, he iterates, the heart's electromagnetic field is dramatically affected by emotional states.

> Frustration produces an incoherent signal, while appreciation creates a harmonious, coherent one. Core heart feelings – care among them – generate coherence in the heart's field, while stressful feelings produce incoherence. The resulting energy is transmitted throughout our bodies, and the fact that it radiates outside of the body has tremendous social implications.
>
> (Childre and Martin 1999: 160)

The somatic movement dance field has been highly influenced by eastern traditions. Sensory movement processes often focus on sensing the living presence of different organs. Thus, much practice in the field invites participants to direct their awareness to specific organs – not simply to think about these organs or talk about them symbolically or figuratively. Somatic movement dance practice has never been cortico-centric, or merely symbolic or metaphorical where the heart is concerned. It is through slow-time experiential sensing that one is invited to listen to the messages and sense–feeling of the heart, and most importantly, balance awareness of the brain and the heart. Childre makes an important distinction in his research and it something that many somatic movement therapists are well versed in. He notes, one has to move one's attention and awareness to the heart itself, in order to balance the nervous system; and one has to learn to differentiate between two intelligences – the heart and the head.

> The head – that is, the brain or mind – operates in a linear, logical manner that serves us well in many situations but limits us in others. Sometimes we need more than analysis and logic to solve a problem or unravel a complex emotional issue. Heart intelligence provides an intuitive, direct knowingness that's an essential aspect of our overall intelligence. When heart intelligence is engaged, our awareness is expanded beyond linear, logical thinking.
>
> (Childre and Martin 1999: 105)

Further,

> experiencing heart intelligence with continuity requires building a reliable partnership between the heart and the head – a partnership that starts when you learn how to distinguish between these two interactive but very different sources of intelligence and can tell when your thoughts and feelings are being directed by the heart and when they are not.
>
> (Childre and Martin 1999: 17)

It is interesting that the HeartMath institute make a very clear distinction between talking and thinking about the heart and actually feeling the presence of the heart. This shift from cortical thinking to sensing is the foundation of all somatic movement practices; moving your awareness away from thinking (living in your head so to speak) and redirecting your awareness into the living intelligence (the mind of) various organs and body systems is foundational in the field. Bonnie Bainbridge Cohen's work initiated many dancers and practitioners into this tradition; hence, somatic movement processes are deeply rooted in sensing-perceiving the living presence of various organs. My own practice is rooted in breath and heart-sensing – slowing down enough to receive afferent information streaming back into the central nervous from the respiratory and cardio-vascular system. Therefore, heart-sensing is a very real, but subtle sensory-perceptual activity and skill, underpinned by directing your sensory awareness into your heart itself – noticing your autorhythmic beat – your pulse – the intelligence arising from your living heart tissues, beating at the centre of your being – the centre of your mandala.

Research from the Institute of HeartMath also discovered

> that *intelligence* and *intuition* are heightened when we learn to listen more deeply to our own hearts. It's through learning how to decipher the messages we receive from our heart that we gain the keen perception needed to effectively manage our emotions in the midst of life's situations and challenges. The more we learn to listen to and follow our heart intelligence, the more educated, balanced, and coherent our emotions become [...] Without the guiding influence of the heart, we easily fall prey to reactive emotions such as insecurity, anger, fear, and blame, as well as other energy draining reactions and behaviours.
>
> (Childre and Martin 1999: 13)

Further,

> Since the act of evoking heart intelligence has been shown to facilitate brain function, adjust balance in the autonomic nervous system, lower blood pressure, increase stress-relieving hormones, and increase immune responses, it shouldn't surprise us that our bodies experience a sensation of well-being clear down to the cellular level – a sensation that we ourselves can induce. We feel better mentally and emotionally as a result of heart intelligence. And in the long run, that sensation translates into physical health.
>
> (Childre and Martin 1999: 15–16)

Noted earlier, it is common to know that good diaphragmatic breathing supports oxygenation, slows the heart beat and lowers blood pressure. It is less common to know that sensing the heart also slows the heart rate, lowers blood pressure and reduces stress hormones. Thus, sensing the heart and breath simultaneously, or moving one's awareness between the two, is an advanced empirical investigation I offer students when they are learning to become compassionate non-judgemental witnesses. I share with students and clients that anger and frustration, for example, creates increased disorder and incoherence in the heart's rhythms and in the autonomic nervous system, thereby affecting the rest of the body. When this happens,

> the sympathetic and parasympathetic branches of the autonomic nervous system are out of sync with each other, battling for control over the heart-rate – the sympathetic trying to speed it up and the parasympathetic trying to slow it down. In contrast positive emotions such as love, care, and appreciation create increased harmony, order and coherence in the heart' s rhythms and improve balance of the nervous system.
>
> (Childre and Martin 1999: 36)

Because out dominant culture has taught us think rather than feel, it is sometimes very difficult for facilitators and trainee students to access their heart. Sensing breath and easing the tissues around the heart, the scapulae, the diaphragm and thorax, when held in an environment of safety and non-judgment, can support a participant to slowly and safely sense their heart-space. Through the silent sensing of breath and heart an authentic sense of love or compassion can emerge. The simple act of caring for your heart is an act of self-love. Additionally, witnessing another person while in the presence of your heart, entrained as a compassionate witness, can generate feelings of self-worth for self and Other. When training somatic movement dance therapists, I share and offer processes that investigate the following, through empirical embodied practice-as-research. Further below, I offer a few examples of the students researching their own heart and how their heart affects others:

1. The heart has a brain that is involved with both emotional processing and cortical processing.
2. The heart has the strongest electromagnetic field in the human body and this field extends beyond Self and affects others.
3. If our heart is disconnected from our head and we are stressed, our HRV will be incoherent, and this incoherence will affect Self and Other.
4. Feelings of anger and frustration, stress and anxiety create an incoherent HRV.
5. Feelings of compassion, care, love and kindness create a coherent HRV.
6. That focusing on the heart and sensing the presence of the heart balances the nervous system, lowers heart rate, blood pressure and reduces stress releasing hormones and enhances the immune response.
7. That touch is electric. When we touch, we send an electromagnetic signal into the body of other: if our heart-rhythms are coherent, our touch will have a positive effect on Other. If our heart rhythms are incoherent, our touch is likely to deregulate Other.
8. Moving into a peaceful sense–perceived relationship with heart and breath, will support positive emotions and coherent rhythms between therapist and client.
9. We live in a culture that prioritizes awareness of mind over heart; thus, we bring the heart's intelligence into conscious awareness, balancing the head and heart.
10. The heart's electromagnetic field is dramatically affected by emotional states.
11. The electromagnetic field generated by the heart envelops the entire body and extends out in all directions into the space around us. The heart's electromagnetic – is by far the most powerful produced by the body – it can be measured many feet away [...] (Childre and Martin 1999: 34).

(all the above adapted and paraphrased from Childre and Martin's research 1999)

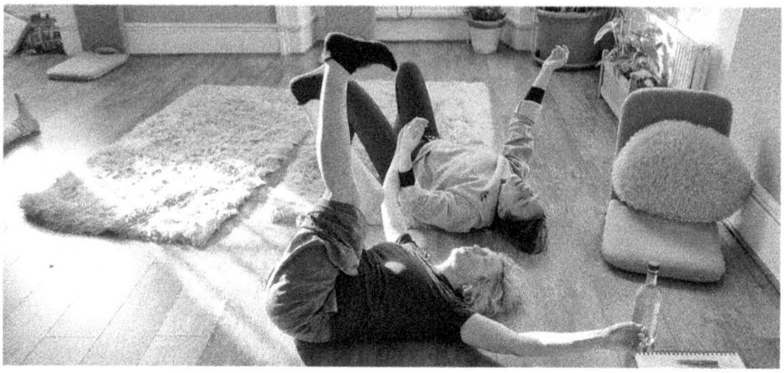

FIGURE 4.2: Emma Thompson and Melanie Brierley: sensing my heart and sensing my electromagnetic field – extending my heart field to you. Photographer: Amanda Williamson.

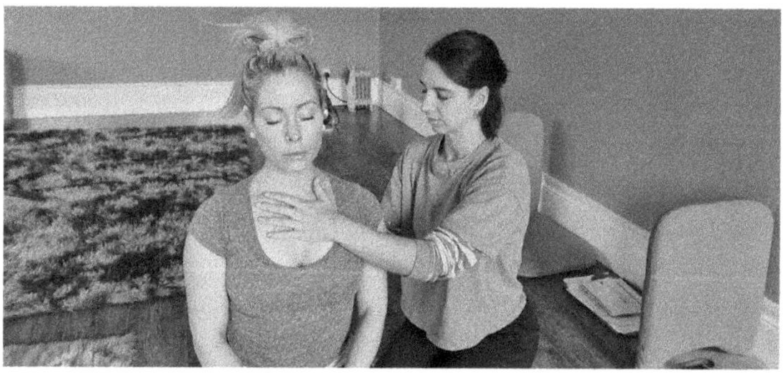

FIGURE 4.3: Sarah Pinch and Jessica Cotton: before supporting a person's heart, I regulate my own through breath awareness and cardio-ception. Therefore, my touch and presence is likely to have positive effects on Other. Photographer: Amanda Williamson.

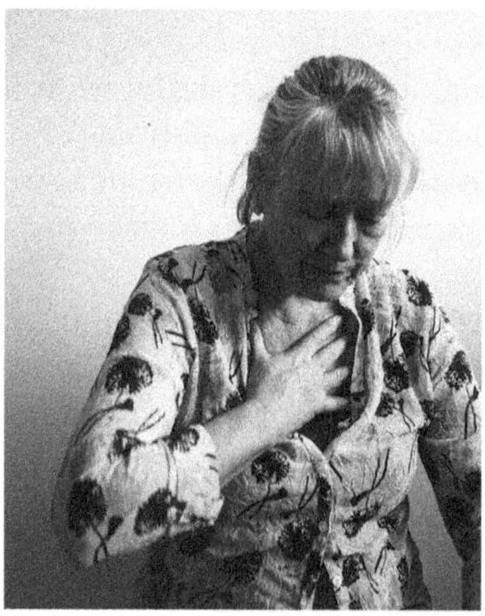

FIGURE 4.4: Karin Rugman: Moving with awareness of her heart. Photographer: Anika Rugman.

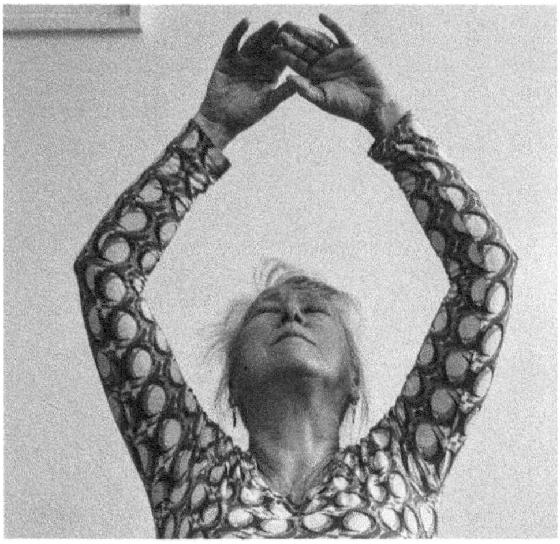

FIGURE 4.5: Karin Rugman: Moving with awareness of her heart. Photographer: Anika Rugman.

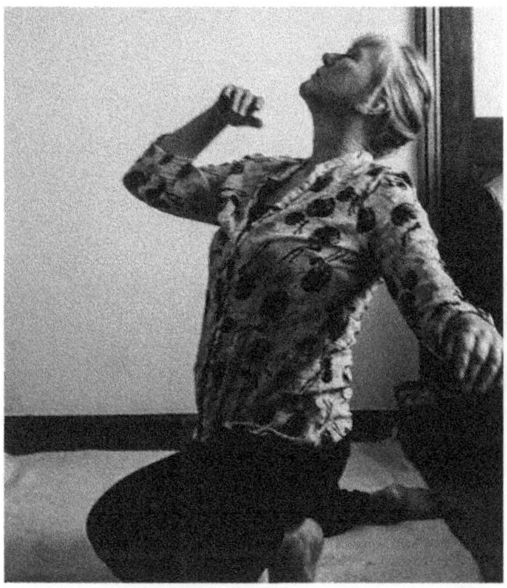

FIGURE 4.6: Karin Rugman: Moving with awareness of her heart. Photographer: Anika Rugman.

At first, I found it hard to sense my heart, I couldn't find it. Now my hand is always on my heart! In the studio and even with my family. I also placed my hand on my heart at work. It helped me feel less worried or fearful. I work in a situation that is quite bullying, it feels like that. Now as soon as I get to the studio, I place my hand on my heart and breathe. I have to lie down first and ease my neck and shoulders, then after this I sense my heart. I am a slightly different person in my heart. Here I feel rest and almost love for myself. That comes and goes. When I work with someone, I always place my hand on my heart. It keeps my focus, like a deep point within me that is very grounded and intelligent. I am shifted and changed by this way of working – a new consciousness within the body is arising.

(Stacey Nelson)

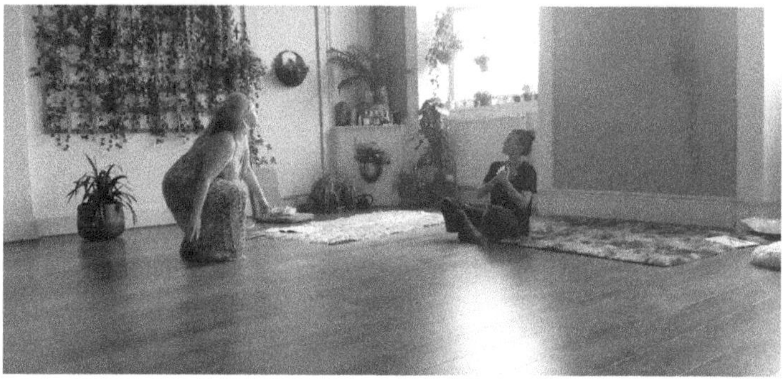

FIGURE 4.7: Vanessa Tucker and Miranda Henderson: witnessing you through my heart and breath. Photographer: Amanda Williamson.

> I have learned so much about my heart and my head. I go instantly back into my head when I leave the studio. I often don't even realize. At night I lie in bed with my hand on my heart and breathe. It makes me both sad and strong. Sad because this knowledge is kept away from the public and I find general life difficult. Strong because I realize my heart has a lot to say, and it makes me a better person. I realize that living in your heart or being able to recognize a difference between heart and head takes time. In the studio I have time, so much time. I love it. But at work there is no time for my heart. When I practise somatic movement dance my heart is allowed to be there, alive with another person. It is a different soft knowing, an ancient feeling. Here I feel connected to the stream of deep life again, I guess I mean my soul. Yes heart-sensing connects me to my soul, those more expansive energetic feelings that tend to know there is more to life, and life beyond this life.
>
> (Sarina May)

Dyadic heart-sensing

The dyad is one of the most common structures used in somatic movement dance modalities that use improvisation underpinned by somatic awareness to support self-regulation. The dyad underpins one-on-one work and involves the therapist witnessing the participant moving in front of her. Below is a basic description of the dyad, written from my own practice. I note other practitioners might use a different language or a slightly different process, but many practitioners are likely to be using self-regulatory processes underpinned by the witness and mover.

> The therapist sits quietly, sensing gravity, the ground underneath her, and her breath-flow. She moves her awareness away from exteroception (the external world) into her internal

world of sensing and feeling. She senses her living tissues moving and the presence of her own heart. She is contacting her autonomic nervous system. She notices and sense–perceives motility (bio-flows pulsating, altering, waving, and rippling within her own body). She brings her awareness to movement within her thorax and diaphragm – the rise and fall of breath. She invites her autonomic nervous system to move from sympathetic charge into parasympathetic ease, attending to breath and heart moment-by-moment. The participant lies in gravity in front her. The therapist invites the participant to move her awareness from extroception (shutting her eyes) to interoception (sensing breath and heart). She shuts her eyes, senses her breath, releases her weight into gravity and senses the ground supporting her tissues. She is invited to sense the physical presence of her heart and the rise and fall of breath. The participant is being invited to regulate her own autonomic nervous system. The therapist witnesses the participant sensing her interoceptive awareness. Both therapist and participant attune to gravity, breath and heart. Together they are moving from sympathetic arousal into parasympathetic awareness. The therapist does not look at the participant through her eyes, but rather de-focuses, and receives the participant's presence through her own living tissues and interoceptive awareness. The therapist invites the participant to sense–dwell in afferent information, noticing how their tissues need to ease, loosen and dissolve through slow-time movement. The participant follows movement pathways of loosening, easing and releasing. The participant is invited to tip, pour and roll, curl and uncurl, yield and push, reach and pull, stretch, lengthen and soften along the floor, using the ground as a fulcrum – a pivotal support. The therapist does not judge, analyse, evaluate or criticize the participant's movement. She does not decide if they can move well or judge their body type. The therapist welcomes the smallest shyest movement expression, to the largest reach, sweep or curve (and any movement range in between). The participant follows her own self-regulatory movement desires and pleasures. She is encouraged to find pathways that feel delicious, pleasurable and comfortable. Breath awareness and interoception underlie the process. After around 20–30 mins, the therapist invites the participant to come to stillness, staying in touch with breath and the resonance of her moving time. The participant is invited to rest in self, and after 5 more minutes opens her eyes, receiving the external world, while staying in touch with her breath and heart.

They come together, staying in contact with breath and heart. The participant is invited to reflect on her moving experience through language or through symbolic mark-making. The therapist does not speak. She listens. She listens, engaging all her senses.

From the outside, this looks an amazingly simple structure. The participant moves and the therapist witnesses. However, underlying this apparent simplicity is moment-by-moment breath awareness, cardio-centric sensing and other embodied skills I share below. Without these embodied skills, it would be hard to support and maintain co-regulation; the therapist would be disengaged and distracted. Additionally, before the participant has entered the studio, I always share with trainee students that the therapist should prepare and self-regulate her own body. Let's take a look.

Preparing to work with someone

If the therapist is stressed and edging towards sympathetic arousal (or fight-or-flight), she will deregulate her client. All participants, including therapists, are likely to be deregulated before they enter the studio. None of us, even therapists, who often appear balanced and calm, can escape the multiple stresses and strains of life. We can however learn to manage them through bottom-up somatic processes that invite the nervous system into homeostasis. I offer four inter-related embodied processes. These processes support therapists to bring balance to their own nervous system, in preparation for working with participants. The fourth process, that I attend to further, integrates the opposites, inviting the archetype of wholeness to hold the process. I refer to these four processes as: *parasympathetic ease-and-release (immobilization without fear), open-hearted social engagement (the ventral vagus), stimulating the spinal nerves (mobilization without fear), and the mystical integration of the opposites*. All involve sensing the heart, breath and engaging the vagus nerve, but have slightly different orientations. Parasympathetic ease-and-release is deep liberation from sympathetic arousal and involves innervating the parasympathetic division of the autonomic nervous system. In the first state, immobilization without fear, the therapist is sense–dwelling in her inner world, augmenting deep tissue release, unravelling sympathetic holding in gravity, with breath and cardio-ception. The second state, the ventral vagus (opened hearted social engagement) still involves engaging the parasympathetic division but pays more attention to the group of cranial nerves that innervate the ventral branch of the vagus nerve, shared previously in Chapter 2. The third process attends to a hybrid state termed mobilization without fear (stimulating activity combined with safety). The fourth gently senses and integrates the opposites within Self. Below, I offer these four interrelated processes that prepare therapists to work with others peacefully and spaciously.

Immobilization without fear

When participants enter the studio, they need to feel safe, and continue to feel safety throughout the session. Co-regulation is a process of attunement, 'in which the nervous and cardiovascular systems of the practitioner and client maintain and build a therapeutic container based on trust and safety' (Shea 2016: 60). Feeling safe is the most vital aspect of self-regulation. The therapist is part of the environment, and therefore her nervous system must also be safe. Therapists also feel fear, stress, tiredness and imbalance. Because of this, it is important that the therapist finds safety in her own nervous system before the session begins and maintains balance and homeostasis throughout the session. In order to bring the nervous system into a state of balance the vagus nerve must be in a state health. Noted in Chapter 2, the vagus nerve is the longest nerve in the parasympathetic nervous system, regulating nearly every organ in the body. The vagus nerve arises into a state of health through breath awareness and cardio-ception, in particular. When I train therapists, I invite them to experientially explore and empirically investigate the five areas below. I invite them to sense–perceive these elemental processes before they work with a client, and practice maintaining sense–perception of these elements while they facilitate and witness. The therapist is invited to release into gravity and sense–perceive

- the movement and aliveness of breath, and in particular her diaphragm; in physiological terms this is *referred to as diaphragmatic breathing*
- the living presence of her own heart; in physiological terms this is to referred to as *cardio-ception*
- the internal state of her autonomic nervous system; this is called *interoception.*
- *gravi-ception:* releasing her tissues into ground and surrendering her weight and mass into earth
- *sensory-motor perception:* afferent sensing and conscious awareness of efferent motor expression.

The ventral vagus

Dropping peacefully into a deep parasympathetic state is essential so the therapist can bring balance to her nervous system. This heals and balances the therapist

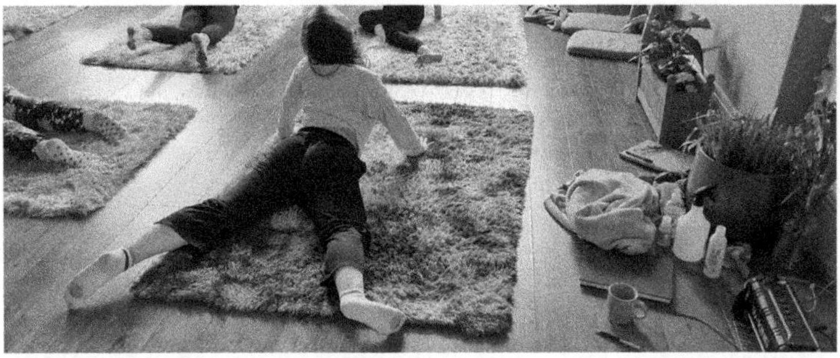

FIGURE 4.8: Natasha Martin: unwinding and releasing energy (holdings) in her sympathetic chain. Photographer: Amanda Williamson.

and in turn will support the client's nervous system to calm, soothe and soften. However, the therapist also needs to socially be engaged, with a soft open face, and a welcoming heartful presence. All these details, no matter how small, influence the efficacy of practice. Therefore, I offer that after entering a deep parasympathetic state, the therapist needs to open out into a state of social engagement. Noted in Chapter 2, social engagement still involves maintaining good vagal tone (innervating the parasympathetic and staying in contact with breath and heart), but also involves releasing tension in the face, jaw, neck and shoulders. If your facial tissues are holding anger and fear, your shoulders are tense and your jaw is tight it will deregulate not just you, but your client. Therefore, opening out into social engagement involves releasing tension in the face, jaw and shoulders. Worth reminding us again, there are five cranial nerves involved in social engagement: *the trigeminal nerve (V)*, *the facial nerve (V11)*, *the glossopharyngeal nerve (CN 1X)*, *the vagus nerve (X)* and the *spinal accessory nerve (X1)*. Together these nerves innervate the ventral branch of the vagus nerve. I invite you to notice again that all these nerves involve ease and balance in your face, jaw, neck and shoulders. Thus the therapist is invited to continue preparing her body, moving with attentive awareness of the living tissues below.

- Soften into gravity, releasing the sternocleidomastoid and trapezius. Sense–perceiving and releasing these muscles invites the accessory nerve into health. The spinal accessory nerve is one of the five cranial nerves involved in social engagement and the innervation of the ventral branch of the vagus nerve.
- Contact breath-flow in the tissues: the thorax and the diaphragm. The ventral branch of the vagus nerve is innervated by good diaphragmatic breathing.
- Sense–perceive the living presence of your heart. Bringing awareness to your heart is particularly important in innervating the ventral vagus.
- Soft-tissue-roll contacting the caudal–cranial axis, inviting the parasympathetic nerves into expression. Notice the gentle nature of these nerves.
- Open your eyes (moving between eyes shut and eyes closed), and start to release tension, or ease out, the muscles around the eyes.
- Release tension in the sympathetic chain between T1 and L2. Releasing tension in this area invites the parasympathetic to override the sympathetic.
- Unwind tension in the jaw: The trigeminal nerve innervates the muscles of mastication and is one of the nerves involved in social engagement.
- Soften, unwind and stimulate the facial muscles. The facial nerve controls tensing and relaxation and is one of the nerves involved in social engagement.
- Soften in the mouth: invite toning and sounding and sighs. This starts to bring the glossopharyngeal nerve into health.

Mobilization without fear

- Start to open your eyes, sometimes moving with eyes shut, eyes open.
- Start to reach and stretch through the limbs, stimulating the peripheral nerves.
- Start to push away from the earth, stimulating your bones.
- Explore weight baring, stimulating bones and joints.
- Explore moving through different planes of action, with different speeds, forces and directions.
- Shake, hum, tone, open the eyes wide, stretching and relaxing the jaw.
- Start to push away from the floor and reach out through your limbs, changing rhythm, speed and force, stimulating the sympathetic branch of ANS. Here you are stimulating the spinal nerves but in relaxed state; thus the ventral circuit is activated.
- Play and spiral between horizontal to the vertical.
- Stand up, breath shake and sound.
- Noted in Chapter 2, this is referred to as stimulating activity combined with safety.

The heart-centred transpersonal witness and the mystical integration of the opposites

We live in a world where we are constantly judged. Our intellectual capabilities are judged, what we have or have not achieved is judged and indeed how we look is judged. We are also enculturated into judging ourselves. Most of us have a loud overpowering inner critic, which puts us under enormous pressure. We rarely enjoy

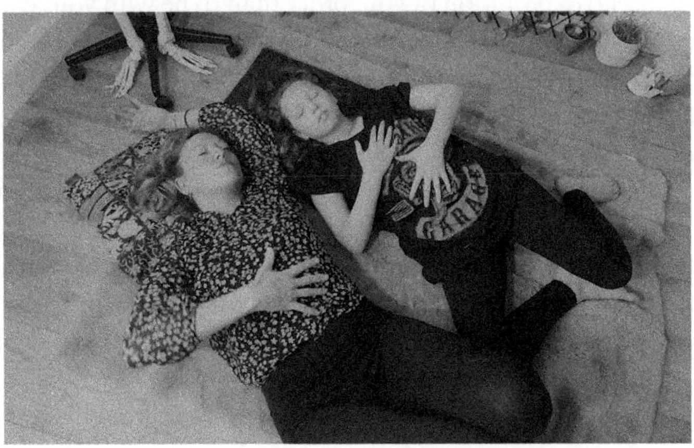

FIGURE 4.9: Amanda and Tala: sensing each other's heart field. Photographer: Scott Closson.

situations where we not judged. We rarely enjoy situations where we are witnessed and listened to with compassion and empathy. The somatic studio is one place where people are not judged, criticized, analyzed and evaluated. Thus, the term non-judgemental witness is used frequently to entrain somatic movement dance practitioners into a non-judgemental way of being. This takes time and is often a life-long process – an empirical embodied investigation and reflection. Not being judged, but rather being witnessed with compassion is integral to self-regulation. Being invited into a process where your movement, body, emotionality and soul's life-journey is valued and witnessed through the living heart of the therapist is a great relief for many participants. The roots of non-judgemental witnessing are Jungian in origin and the term is commonly associated with a strand of somatic practice called Authentic Movement. Jung developed the idea that the therapist is an archetypal guide (an energy of wholeness), not a critic who analyses, judges or hierarchically uses their education to make a diagnosis rooted in pathology. The term non-judgemental witness is used in many somatic movement trainings. I prefer to use the term *heart-centred transpersonal witness*, denoting, (1) the therapist is staying in touch with her own body experience, receiving and witnessing the participant's movement through her interoceptive sensations (especially her heart and breath); and (2) there is something larger than the personal supporting the therapeutic process. The therapist becomes, as I share, a heart-centred witness, attuning to a transpersonal life-force, which is a qualitatively different experience to watching and observing someone from a place of ego-consciousness and persona. Our familial situation may not have brought us the witnessing and holding we needed as children. Our workplaces are, more often than not, places of competition and production, with little time to listen and support others with compassion. Moving in the presence of a heart-centred transpersonal witness, who empathizes with your suffering, and has no expectation of you, other than to be with you, witnessing you untangle the suffering in your tissues, or finding your creativity and connection to life again, is incredibly healing. Without this presence, it is extremely hard to heal from trauma, anxiety and depression. Learning to be a heart-centered transpersonal witness has both physiological and spiritual elements that are not separate, but rather, in Jungian terms, embrace the vast spectrum of our psyche, and particularly our ability to access and sense the transpersonal.

The etymological roots of 'compassion' come from the Latin, meaning 'co-suffering'. Thus, compassion involves feeling for others. Empathy is from the Greek roots empatheia, meaning pathos, 'feeling as another', and denotes we can feel and be with another person's suffering. The etymological roots of these terms are rooted in feeling and sensing – they are not purely intellectual constructs. When students are training as therapists, compassion and empathy are feeling-full empirical embodied investigations, rooted in cardio-ception, breath awareness and sensory awareness. Hence compassion and empathy are physiologically entrained in the studio. Noted above, sensing the heart and breath entrains and supports a field of compassion.

Sense–perceiving your heart balances your nervous system and brings your heart rhythms (heart rate variability) into coherence and balance. Most interestingly, we also know that the electromagnetic field of your heart affects those around you (Childre and Martin 1999). If your heart rhythms are coherent, your electromagnetic heart field will support the participant to regulate. If your heart rhythms are incoherent, you will deregulate your participant. Thus, heart-sensing is one of the most important aspects of witnessing and develops compassion from within every cell of your body, extending and nurturing the person you are working with. This way of training notably attunes therapist and clients to the 40,000 neurons in their heart (their heartbrain).

The therapist moves into her cardio-ceptive and breath awareness as she witnesses. She attunes to her own body, accessing what I refer to as the transpersonal realms of breath and heart. Everyone breathes or is breathed by the life-force, and everyone came into being through the autorhythmic beat of their heart. I use the word transpersonal here to denote that through sensing breath and heart people can access a transpersonal consciousness, qualitatively different from ego-consciousness. When we settle into breath and heart and move into the parasympathetic, we open out into a receptive state of consciousness, beyond the limits of our personality and ego. By entering the transpersonal realm of breath and heart, the therapist is inviting the field of her heart to hold and support the process. She invites her ego with all its imposing thoughts and constructs to take a break. She does not judge, analyze, transfer or impose her narrative onto the mover; rather she remains present through moment-by-moment breath awareness and cardio-ceptive sensitivity, welcoming and holding the participant's movement journey with compassion. If the therapist is disembodied and in ego-consciousness, she will remain a distant observer and is likely to move into analysis, judgement, projection and evaluation. Hence, I use the term heart-centered transpersonal witness to signify there is something larger than the personal witnessing and holding the process. Underpinning the concept of the heart-centred witness is the therapist's ability to sense, feel and care about her own heart, which enables her to stay balanced for the participant, in turn creating a field of electromagnetic coherence (Childre and Martin 1999). Thus, therapist and client are of equal importance in the process.

Just as we have spirals in our 'fingertips', so too, we have 'clockwise and counter-clockwise spirals in our hearts' (Buckberg 2002: 142). The heart is in fact a double helix, just like the flowers, galaxies, snails and seashells that surround us. Sensing the heart, especially with knowledge that our autorhythmic beat and blood flow is supported and sustained within a double helix enables therapists and participants to experience and sense a dimension of Self that is spun by nature, just as mother spider spins her web. Transpersonal Self knows she is nurtured by a life-force, beyond her individuality and ego – perhaps beyond words, but more easily felt in a parasympathetic state of consciousness. Our growth and becoming, just like a seashell, is of Fibonacci's logarithmic spirals. Spirals are a primal part of our being. This knowledge also supports the development of the transpersonal witness – she who is attuned to the transpersonal life-force.

When therapists settle into gravity, contacting their breath and deepening into cardio-ception, a different sense of Self thus emerges (or a different state of experiential consciousness). This is also the transpersonal Self Eckhart Tolle writes so exquisitely about – a state of awareness that arises with breath awareness and by directing awareness to internal bodily sensations (1999). It is a transpersonal awareness, rooted in life-force or source sensing, that quietly exists underneath the loud overpowering and judgemental egoic mind. We know breath awareness and interoception slows the heart rate and regulates breathing – notably all the ingredients that invite participants into a parasympathetic state of consciousness (Williamson 2020c). Therefore, I share with students that the transpersonal Self can only be sensed and animated through breath awareness, cardio-ception and interoception. The transpersonal witness, thus, prefers a particular physiological state, for she cannot arrive when we are riddled with stress, sympathetically charged, egoically driven or identifying solely with disembodied mind. Transpersonal Self arrives when we have turned away from the exterior world and our ego-consciousness loses its control. It is important to develop a strong ego to survive and grow in the world and therefore ego-consciousness is crucial and has its place (especially in your early life). However, if ego-consciousness is running our lives, expanded states of consciousness (of non-duality, of surrendering into sensory-perceptual awareness of the life-force) are constrained and buried, and thus often unattainable. A deeper authentic Self, located right at the centre of our being, can only be accessed when we move away from the one-dimensional consciousness of ego into the expansive worlds of sensing breath and heart, bringing mind and body together in a state of non-duality. The transpersonal heart-centred witness is not a fixed state, but rather a state of experiential awareness. This is the shift from ego-consciousness into a transpersonal state, usually hidden by ego-consciousness.

The mystical integration of the opposites: Holding a space of wholeness and integration

Carl Jung also wrote about a transpersonal Self, often concealed by egoic self. Freud, considered Ego, from the Latin 'I' the centre of our consciousness, identity and personality. However, Jung proposed the centre of our authentic identity or personality was not located in the ego, but rather in the true 'Self', a transpersonal fulcrum at the centre of our being. Self with a capital S, was for Jung, our true transpersonal centre. Equally, for Jung, Self can only arise when the ego's control is loosened.

> Capital Self is used to distinguish 'between the "self" of everyday usage (which refers to ego or persona) and Jung's "Self" which transcends the ego and adheres the age-old capacities of the species' (Stevens 1994: 61). Through a Jungian lens, 'the term Self is used for a totality or for a mainly "not me" force in, or at the centre of, the psyche which is usually not experienced as the conscious "I"' (Papadopoulos 1992: 49). Capital Self is expansive and extensive – the daemonic centre of all psychic life – the archetype of wholeness.
>
> (Williamson 2020e: 152)

Interestingly for Carl Jung, the daemonic Self is both immanent and transcendental by nature – or more accurately, the transpersonal Self has integrated, synthesized and balanced the opposites. Thus, for Jung, Self's expansive nature can only truly manifest when the opposites have been integrated, such as body/mind, mind/heart and mater/spirit. Self, for Jung, was considered an archetype of wholeness that mediates between all the opposites. She is teleological, actively supporting people to move towards wholeness. Thus, when I train students to become therapists, I propose we always invite the archetype of wholeness (the true centre of our being which is the 'I-I' – a mystical connection to the life-force) to hold and witness the process. Jung was at pains to point out that people live (on mass) from their ego-consciousness, at a great cost to their authentic being. For Jung there were many more dimensions and experiences of consciousness. Ego is only one – and a limited one at that. Jung also located Self in spirit (breath) that lies at the centre of the mandala (Hayes 2013).

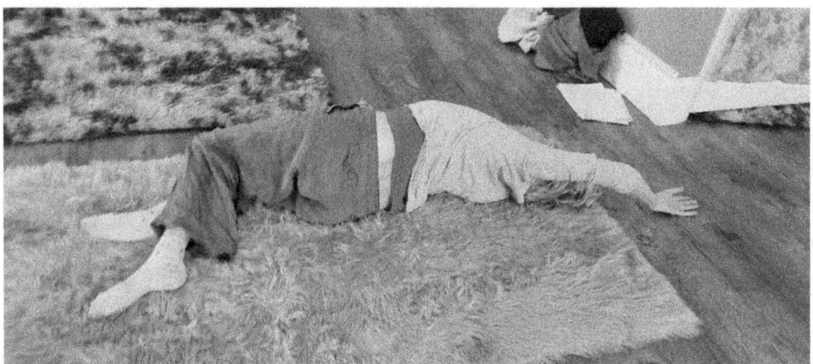

FIGURE 4.10: Hazel Rose: Moving with awareness of her heart. Movingsoma group. Photographer: Amanda Williamson.

Further, Jung believed Self arises, or may become visible, through imaginative play, where people can integrate the opposites as they arise from the unconscious into awareness: mind/body, body/spirit, heaven/earth, inner/outer, male/female, for example. Much healing takes place in the somatic studio through integrating and exploring the continuum between the opposites, which in turn supports experiences of non-duality. For example, studio practice may offer processes that explore the continuum between gravity/space, inner/outer, unconscious/consciousness, high/low, front/back, sympathetic/parasympathetic, left/right, structure/fluidity, spirals/linear, inner/outer and inhalation/exhalation. Opposites are an inherent part of our humanness. Jung believed the opposites have a regulating function in the psyche. 'If for example, your life is analytical, controlled and ego driven, a powerful regulating energy will arise, where you find yourself desiring freedom and creativity' (Snowden 2020: 192). Many people arrive in the somatic studio because they are not satisfied with the mechanistic paradigm that makes no room for theocentric soulful dimensions. In contrast to the mechanistic paradigm, somatic movement dance makes space for a whole spectrum of experiences, from the deeply material to the transcendental. In Jungian discourse, this might mean, for example, balancing the animus (male) and anima (female) aspects of your personality, or bringing to consciousness and integrating the shadow aspects of self (Snowdon 2020). In studio practice, integrating the opposites is not simply a mental activity, but rather an embodied activity where we invite participants to explore the continuum between mind/body, gravity/space, inner/outer and the caudal–cranial, for example. When I am training therapists, I offer there are subtle physiological–spiritual dimensions to self-regulation and co-regulation. When the therapist witnesses, she is not an inert lump with a slumped over body, peering through two eyes, disengaged and disinterested. Rather, she has cultivated an awareness of Self that resides in the transpersonal realms of breath (spirit) and heart, and in the metaphysical integration of the opposites. Self, in Jungian thought, is the meditator of individuation – from her pivotal centre, she meditates the opposites, eventing us towards wholeness and a state of non-duality.

Experiencing an expanded state of consciousness is common for participants in the somatic studio. In contrast to pursuing higher states of consciousness, dependent on transcendental realms, separating from *materia* (the terrain of transcendental meditation and monotheistic religions severed from their mystical roots), expanded states of consciousness are, in contrast, dependent on integrating and synthesizing the opposites. Hence our *materia* (breath, heart, sensory receptors and motor neurons, for example) are always involved in the expansion of consciousness. As therapists integrate mind and body, heart and head, spirit and earth, a sense of non-duality often pervades their experience. This aliveness and sense of non-duality can be entrained by learning to hold and synthesize the opposites in the studio. Hence, I offer that when the therapist sits down and prepares her body to receive another person's living body, she also holds and integrates the following opposites in her sensory-perceptual awareness. The therapist

- directs her awareness to breath and heart. She is mind and body
- sense–perceives gravity (the earth calling her) and the space around her. She is gravity and space
- sense–perceives her caudal–cranial axis (she is high and low)
- sense–perceives her lateralization (she is left and right)
- sense–perceives her inhalation and exhalation (she is outer/inner)
- sense–perceives her structure (her skeletal system) and her fluid body (her bio-tensile three-dimensionality). She is structure and fluidity
- senses the proximal space around her body, and the space in front, behind, above and below, and to the left and right of her
- sense–perceives distal space (the space between her and the studio walls, and beyond to the sky and stars) (she is spacial and non-spatial).

Most of the processes listed above are rooted in integrating the opposites. Some are rooted in enlivening sensory receptors and listening to, sensing and softening into space. All attune the body to the senate. All invite the body to inhabit gravity and space with aliveness and integrity. While these are subtle offerings, they attune the therapist to the existence and integration of the opposites, creating a holding environment of assimilation and wholeness. As participant's move into the archetypal and instinctual realms of the unconscious negotiating many opposites during their moving time, the therapist contacts the archetype of wholeness – the daemonic centre of their psyche, which transcends duality. She is no longer 'me' or even 'we', but rather 'I–I'. She holds the great spiral and continuum between mater and spirit. This is a lifelong process of empirical investigation and a process of entrainment. One rarely feels they have reached this state in totality, or one may reach this state momentarily.

Part 2: Self-regulation and the imagination

Throughout this book, you can see images where participants are dropping their awareness deeply into their sensate (through anatomical and physiological focus points and pathways) and simultaneously engaging their imagination, as they unwind and release. Noted in Chapter 1, a distinctive difference between somatic movement dance therapy and mechanistic health is how the imagination plays an essential role in health and healing. On a physiological level, movement underpinned by the imagination supports the discovery of novel and playful neuromuscular pathways, inviting habitual movement patterns to melt and fall away. Imaginative movement also augments the dexterity and fluidity of the skeletal–muscular system, supporting fascial health, in particular. However, the imagination is also considered a guide, and often lensed through a Jungian frame. Thus, the imagination is considered the playful bridge between consciousness and the unconscious. When we dance with the imagination, it is believed unconscious contents are expressed in symbolic form and can then be integrated into consciousness. This starts to open participants to a path that Jung called *individuation*. Individuation is, in a sense, the holy grail – a life-long process in which the psyche (including conscious and unconscious parts seeks integration, unification, balance and wholeness). We have many dimensions of our being that need attention, care and encouragement to self-regulate, such as our inner world of emotions, and our existential dimensions. We feel a great schism when we are trapped in our persona and ego-consciousness. Our heart longs for development and expression beyond our jobs, our persona and economic pressures. Jung referred to this as a process where the archetype of wholeness, the authentic Self, confronts the ego – a stage where we can longer live in one-dimension, and a point in our lives where unconscious aspects of Self are calling for integration.

While somatic movement is a bottom-up feeling therapy attending to the stress living tissues hold, self-regulation often moves beyond the physiological into imaginal realms, or more accurately, practice seeks to integrate the physiological with the imaginal. Thus, self-regulating the complexity of our multidimensionality often attends to our body, mind, spirit and soul (differing experiences of consciousness and expressions of our vast pysche). Postpositivist arts therapies, such as the somatic movement/dance paradigm, do not reduce mental health to mechanistic approaches found in psychiatry that tend to limit the human psyche to the organ of the brain, or root health in physiology alone (see Snowden 2020: 192). In contrast, the psyche is perceived as inherently sacred, occupying a vast spectrum from the physiological to the transcendental. The imagination, spirituality and the numinous are thus perceived as essential to our growth, and our mental well-being (Jung [1969] 2003).

When dancers and somatic practitioners, such as Mary Starks Whitehouse, Janet Adler (Haze and Stomstead 1999; Whitehouse 1999a, 1999b, 1999c, 1999c, 1999d), Anna Halprin (2015) and Daria Halprin (2002) applied Carl Jung's theories to movement, a whole new aspect of somatic movement/dance opened out into our collective awareness, commonly termed *active-imagination-in-movement*. Active-imagination-in-movement is thus another defining feature of the somatic dance movement field. Active-imagination is deeply rooted in Carl Jung's theories, particularly the following:

- The imagination is the bridge between the unconscious and consciousness.
- The imagination is teleological, seeking wholeness, unification and integration.
- The imagination is the bridge to the soul–soul bridges source (spirit) with ego and the world of family, culture and society.

- Imaginative play invites unconscious aspects of the psyche to arise into consciousness through symbolic form.
- Imaginative play can access the personal and collective unconscious.
- The collective unconsciousness is simultaneously archetypal (transcendental) and instinctual (earth bound).
- The self with a capital S, is considered the true Self, often hidden and suppressed by the ego and persona.

Carl's Jung's theories underpin many of the processes and values in field of somatic movement and dance. The non-judgemental witness, the inner witness, shadow work and symbolic moving and mark-making are all rooted in Jungian theory. The integration of his ideas into movement shapes many of the therapeutic principles we use in the studio. For example, the idea the therapist is an archetypal guide who witnesses without judgment has its roots in Carl Jung's work (Snowden 2006: 89). Sometimes the influence of Jung is unambiguous; the somatic movement therapist will make clear references to Jung. However, the influence of Jung is often implicitly felt, rather than explicitly vocalized. In such cases, Jungian ideas have become *naturalized.* His ideas have been integrated so completely, and with such a passion, over many decades, the original source is sometimes forgotten. Each time a practitioner uses active-imagination-in-movement, or applies ideas such as the non-judgemental witness, myth, archetype, dream and symbol, for example, they are applying and animating theories and concepts researched and popularized by Carl Jung. The integration of Jungian and post-Jungian psychology and spirituality is vividly witnessed in Anna Halprin's and Daria Halprin's somatic movement modality (2002, 2015). Both practitioners pioneered the imagination-in-movement as a therapeutic tool and catalyst for healing. Authentic movement is another movement practice where you can vividly witness the integration of Jungian spirituality and psychology into movement (Pallaro 1999).

All the arts therapies, including somatic movement and dance, have been profoundly influenced by Carl Jung's model of the psyche. Through his legacy the imagination is commonly viewed as the subtle bridge between the unconscious and consciousness. Further, the imagination is viewed as teleological, meaning the imagination holds an innate regulatory drive towards integrative wholeness. Jung viewed the psyche as dynamic and constantly changing, but ultimately moving us towards wholeness, even when we feel we are regressing, or having an awfully hard time (Jung [1969] 2003, [1953] 2003, 1993). Hence, the imagination-in-movement is not a thing, easily quantified, but rather a living breathing process eventing us towards wholeness, through all life's ups and downs. The imagination is the bridge to the soul – perhaps the most subtle delicate realm of our being that often feels great pain when the exterior world tears and pulls us away from our heart, and our transpersonal connection with breath, spirit and source.

For Jung, the imagination was not an irrational part of our being, but rather a deeply intelligent guiding force. This care and belief in the imagination as an intelligent force has instrumentally shaped the somatic movement dance field. Imaginative movement and dance is thus highly valued in the studio. When the imagination enters our moving time, she shows us areas of our life that need tilling, attending and healing. For example, a mover might encounter a trickly landscape full of black thorns, or sense a bleak figure, dourly shadowing their skin. In such cases, the imagination is sharing (breaking into consciousness through symbolic movement) areas of life that need attending and tilling. Animals often arrive when we attune to the sensory-imaginal, bringing us courage and acuity when we feel frail, broken and damaged. She soulfully underlies the places participants travel to, the trails of sensation they follow and the imaginal landscapes they dance in. She is a catalyst for healing. The imagination thus offers us an expansive fulcrum – a pivotal dimension, around which the psyche revolves, offering us landscapes, images, symbols and metaphors, that help to integrate unconscious aspects of self, and synthesize the opposites.

She

The embodied imagination is never far away when we start sensing, feeling, perceiving and moving. She softly starts to whisper through our breath or cries through our hearts as our arms reach out into space longing for connection. Sometimes she surrenders our suffering to the earth. The imagination is the most complex facet of our work for she does not like to be captured and rarefied within the positivist paradigm. She is timeless, endless, ongoing, continuous and infinite – sounding, sighing, murmuring, mouthing, rustling and hissing through our movement. Sometimes she strikes out boldly in our mark-making and moving – sometimes she is too shy to come into symbolic form. She may arise as a snake winding through our vertebral column, or as an owl resting with large eyes in our sphenoid bone. She may spiral us into a pool of water on the studio floor, where we lie, surrounded by verdant grass, with a ladybird kissing our skin. When she arrives, within a Jungian frame, she has purpose and meaning and forms a key part of the self-regulatory process in the studio. The imaginal aspects of practice are much harder to quantify and qualify, especially within the pervasiveness of the positivist paradigm. The imagination and Jung's theories provide a self-regulatory framework for unconscious contents to express in symbolic form.

I call the imagination *she* because her arrival invites the deep feminine aspects of our being into expression (Hayes 2013, 2014; Hartley 2014, 2020; Williamson 2020e, 2018). For Jung, work with the unconscious is to be in soul (*esse in anima*) – to be with the depth of the injured feminine (Hannah 2013) – to be in a creative process in which the conscious point of view is in continual dialogue with the unconscious psychic matrix out of which it springs' (Nagy 1991: 77). We are ensconced by dehumanizing institutions where the human body and its beautiful sensory and imaginal capacities are diminished in service of the economy. The feminine aspects of practice are also of polytheistic imagining, devalued and feared by patriarchal religions. Our lives are discoursed within many institutions that cause dissociation from our sensory-perceptual imaginal capabilities. Such institutions favour mind or spirit and propagate rarefied religious symbols (with a one size fits all mentality). When the imagination moves in the somatic movement field, she is polytheistic (Williamson 2018). She does not produce symbols belonging to one religious' group. Rather she produces images and symbols relevant to one's personal life in all its complexity, highs, lows and suffering, as well as transpersonal symbols emerging from the deep well of the collective unconscious. She is a vital source of self-knowledge in our field, supporting participants to feel and reflect on how their soul wants to heal, and how their life-journey wants to unfold (Williamson 2018).

The imagination often arises with a vitality when we sense our breath and the living tissues of our heart. Thus, moving with awareness of our living physiology prepares the receptive ground for the imagination to speak. If a participant is sympathetically aroused and invited into somatic movement improvisation, they are likely to express agitated anxious movement and little growth will occur. In contrast, if the participant has released into a parasympathetic state, they are ready to receive images, symbols and impressions from aspects of their being, usually imperceptible when stressed. Thus, I note, the parasympathetic is particularly important when sensing and accessing the imaginal. If the body is overwhelmed and stressed, it is extremely difficult to sense–perceive the subtle transformative power of the imagination. If the body is relaxed, receptive and open, growth and change is possible. The imagination is always there, but often buried under sympathetic stress. She arrives more fully when we are quiet, stilling and resting in our tissues. She arrives when we have enlivened our body with attentive awareness. If we are dissociated from our body and deregulated with stress (which is often the case), the subtle realms of the embodied imagination remain hidden.

The imagination, feeling and sensation are all right brain hemisphere activities. Sensing, feeling and perceiving, especially with deeply entrained sensory awareness of your breath and heart (interoceptive awareness), are processed by your right hemisphere, while thinking is processed by your left hemisphere (Shea 2016: 59). Thus, we must note, the field is categorically a right hemisphere activity. The field is firmly rooted in sensing, feeling, perceiving, moving and imagining, which are all predominantly right brain activities. This does not mean the left hemisphere is not involved, or that we attribute creativity, imagination or indeed healing to the right hemisphere alone, but rather we invite the left hemisphere with its emphasis on language, reasoning, critique and logic to take a good long break in the studio. This is an essential part of self-regulation; inviting people into a safe space where they can access other aspects and dimensions of their consciousness. Much of our work supports people to access parts of their being that stir through right brain hemisphere activities, where intuition, feeling, image, impression, rhythm, dreaming and emotions are processed. We spend most of lives living in our left hemisphere, thinking, analyzing and criticizing, rather than sensing, feeling and accessing our imaginal capacities. Western culture with its emphasis on the cerebral cortex perceived as the zenith of human achievement has and continues to enculture the mass populous into left hemisphere beings. Carl Jung wrote extensively on how western culture has created left hemisphere beings, who worship logic, reason and linear thinking. Neurologically speaking, the field of somatic movement and dance has grown to provide spaces of balance, where the right hemisphere, with its emphasis on creativity, intuition, sensing and feeling can take its rightful place as an integral and purposeful part of our lives. As soon as we sense and feel, the right hemisphere starts processing, and thus the imagination often arrives, whispering and expressing through our tissues. It is difficult, if not impossible, to offer somatic movement and dance without the imagination contemplatively calling us and whispering through our tissues.

Jung developed Freud's *free-association* method, calling it *active-imagination*, positioning the imagination as the subtle bridge between consciousness, the personal unconscious and the collective unconscious. When participants are sensing, perceiving and moving, held within a Jungian frame, both layers of the unconscious may appear in symbolic form. However, in reality, a vast range of movement material often emerges in one session. Participants may initially let go of accumulations of daily stress in their tissues, then perhaps move into and through layers of their personal unconscious, often expressing their soul's struggle within familial or societal problems – and sometimes they might then move into angelic/transcendental or animalistic/instinctual realms emerging from the collective unconscious. As participants follow their sensory improvisatory imaginal trails, movement may emerge from consciousness, the personal unconscious or the collective unconscious. Jung developed a model of the unconscious where the imagination and its symbols are perceived as essential to our growth. His model has profoundly influenced the western psyche, especially in relation to the art therapies, and somatic movement dance education is not an exception. Below, I outline both Freud's and Jung's model of the unconscious. Note Jung's more expansive model because it is highly relevant to studio practice.

Freud's model

1. Consciousness/ego (the centre of our identity and personality).
2. Pre-conscious (unconscious contents from the personal unconscious teetering on the edge of consciousness – pushing through).

3. The personal unconscious (repressed sexual desires, repressed traumatic memories, impressions, memories and forgotten memories – uncomfortable experiences in waking life that become repressed).

Jung's model

1. Ego-consciousness (persona – we think it is the centre of our personality).
2. Personal unconscious (repressed personal experiences, including childhood memories/traumas, subliminal images/impressions from the past – everyday life experiences that feel uncomfortable and thus become repressed).
3. The collective consciousness (a deeper and ancient layer of the unconscious shared by every human being across cultures – this is the level of dreams, mythology, symbology, the medicine man, lucid dreaming, instinct and archetype).
4. Self with a capital S, is the true self behind the ego and persona (Freud and Jung's basic model adapted from Snowden 2006).

When participants attune to the sensory-imaginal, a vast range of movement material emerges from both conscious and unconscious aspects of the psyche. All material is welcome. Sometimes movement emerges that expresses from the ego, personality and persona. This is often the case with people who are new to somatic movement practice. They feel comfortable sharing movement that is culturally recognizable and acceptable. You may notice Tia Chi like movement, classical lines or yoga stretches emerging as they start to improvise. You may witness common gestures, such as reaching high, or bending low. *Persona*, from the Latin, meaning 'actor' and related to 'mask' refers our public face, and the parts of ourselves we are happy to share, deemed socially acceptable. It is necessary for individuals to build a strong persona to survive in the world. However, as Jung noted, this dominant mask hides other aspects of our rich and vast psyche, such as our shadows, and the numinous/spiritual dimensions of Self. As participants become familiar with attuning to, and following their own sensory-perceptual pathways, held in a space of non-judgement, they start to let go of culturally acceptable movement and begin to let go of controlling their movement.Sometimes movement emerges from the personal unconscious where repressed personal experiences, childhood memories, or subliminal images and impressions arise through movement. At this stage, you may notice movement that expresses sadness, shame, depression and grief. Sorrow, longing, somatic collapse, fear, frustration and anger might symbolically express. This type of movement is especially important, indicating the participant has many aspects of their life-journey that need witnessing, attending and tilling in the studio. At other times, symbolic movement may emerge from the collective unconscious, or the transpersonal unconscious. Movement that emerges from this deeper layer usually has a numinous or instinctual quality and is of great significance, indicating the participant is moving in archetypal or instinctual realms. Often symbols such as the spiral, the circle or the zigzag emerge. Animals, such as a snake or bird, might appear. The collective unconscious contains both instinct and archetype – thus this level of awareness holds the vast continuum between instinct (infra-red) and spirit (ultraviolate). Often participants start to shape-shift into reptiles and mammals, listening to their quality, energy, temporality and spatiality. At other times people might meet angels, or spirit guides, inviting the quality of these archetypes to express through their movement. Archetype, from the Greek arche, means imprint or pattern. Archetypal patterns appear cross-culturally, expressing through symbols and myths. Transpersonally shared struggles express through symbolism and dream-like form in the studio. The archetype may arise in our movement when we sense–dwell and dream-in-sensory-awareness, or when we enact myth through movement, or when we welcome embodied symbols to arise through our movement. Jung believed the collective unconscious is 'infinitely mysterious', full of ideas and 'seeds of the future' – in this way, it has visionary dimension (Snowdon 2020: 198). We recognize each other's symbols, such as the circle or the spiral, that move us into wholeness. We recognize the wise women or medicine man who visits our moving time, letting us know we belong to the great circle of birth and decay. We recognize the angel who visits, surrounding us with love. We recognize the spiral that moves us forwards and often backwards as we journey together through life's ups and downs in the studio. We recognize the power of the crocodile waiting for prey, homolaterally lurching forward, belly close to earth, in water and mud.

Moving into practice

Emotion, feeling and sensation are inextricably linked and therefore hard to define or extrapolate from one another. However, directing awareness into sensation, below the threshold of emotion is one of the defining features my practice, and a skill I teach. Before I offer somatic movement processes rooted in the imaginal, I always invite participants into the peaceful and expansive realm of the parasympathetic first. When we have reduced the emotional stress and suffering held in our tissues, we are softer and thus more receptive and open to imaginal dimensions. If we are riddled with hyper-tension and sympathetic stress, the delicate energies of the imagination and soul become buried. It is thus essential to support participants to initially self-regulate their autonomic nervous system, so they can find peace, restitution and ease in their tissues. The emotional–glandular–sympathetic anguish held our tissues can become extreme, and if we become locked in habitual hyper-arousal, it is extremely hard to contact other dimensions of consciousness that are essential to our growth. The parasympathetic offers a very special landscape to prepare your tissues, where you are not emotionally overwhelmed. Safe emotional processing and transformation is thus heavily reliant on dropping into sensation first. Through introceptive and proprioceptive sensing, over time, one can begin to trace imprints, impacts and patterns of holding. Dropping into sensation is a level of awareness where (1) you can begin to feel the impacts of familial, cultural and societal trauma in your body, (2) you can begin to feel how your mental and emotional state is affecting your living tissues and (3) you can begin to release these impacts slowly, crafting and transforming them through the moving-imagination and creativity. This is why sensation is so very important and integral to somatic movement dance therapy.

Notably, we do not drop participants into the sensate to seek out suffering and di-ease explicitly. On the contrary, we move into the sensate and parasympathetic to move towards life – to balance the nervous system and oxygenate the tissues. It is from this calm space we invite the imagination to arise and show us areas that need tilling and attending. It is from these preparatory processes that emotions, shadows, complexes and difficult experiences can artfully take form and arise in the tissues slowly, supported by breath, crafting their energies through symbolic form. Dropping into sensation first lays the receptive ground for a deep listening to the imagination.

Example of practice with Karin Rugman: Self-regulating through the embodied imagination

The mover lies on the floor and closes her eyes. She is invited to sense her breath, gravity and ground. She attunes to her autonomic nervous system, sense–dwelling in interoceptive awareness. Her nervous system starts to calm. She is invited to notice

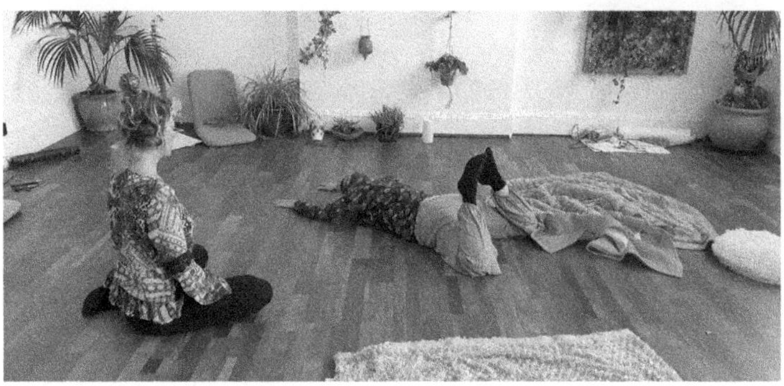

FIGURE 4.11: Karin Rugman: easing her tissues in gravity. Photographer: Scott Closson.

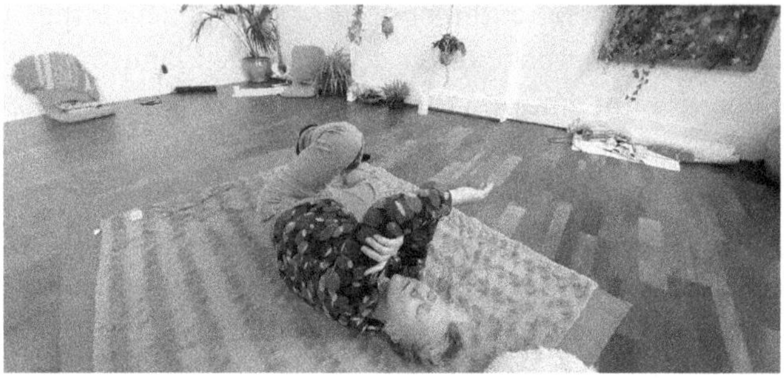

FIGURE 4.12: Karin Rugman: easing pain in her arms. Sensing, listening and following pathways of unwinding. Photographer: Scott Closson.

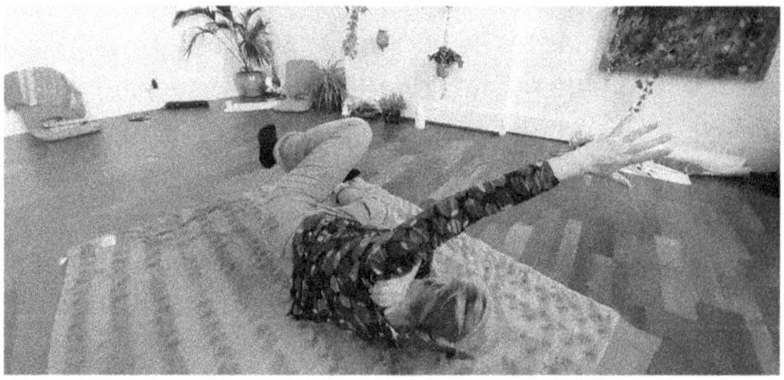

FIGURE 4.13: Karin Rugman: easing her scapulae. Photographer: Scott Closson.

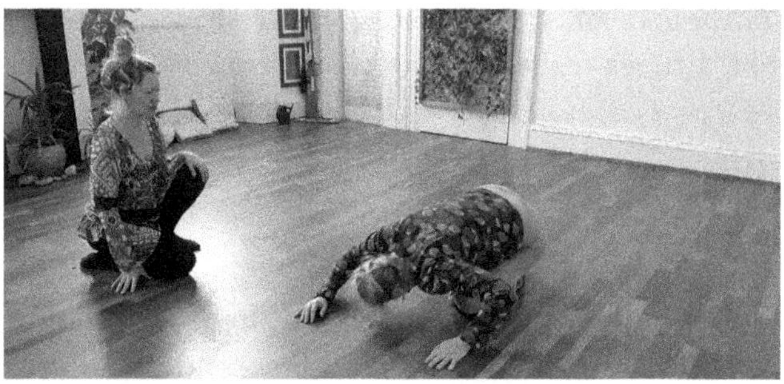

FIGURE 4.14: Karin Rugman: following sensation. Photographer: Scott Closson.

movement (motility) within her: she brings awareness to her breath rising and falling, her thorax expanding and softening. She drops her awareness into her diaphragm, inviting breath to take space within her. She senses her living tissues and releases sympathetic holding, attending to areas of restriction through small micro movements.

She is invited to sense where her tissues are calling for ease. She follows pathways of fluency and release. She unwinds tensions, torsions and sympathetic holding using gravity as a fulcrum: she pushes and releases gently. She listens to her sensory receptors and enjoys traveling consciously with her motor neurons.

She is loosening, unraveling – sensing, feeling, perceiving and moving. She is invited to soften, tip, pour, roll, release and yield in gravity, easing out places of pain and tension.

She is invited to notice images or impressions arising from within. Images and landscapes start to arise. She follows these landscapes and impressions curiously, noticing their colours, textures, shapes, symbols and energy. She does not analyze them, but allows their energies and textures and tones to arise into awareness.

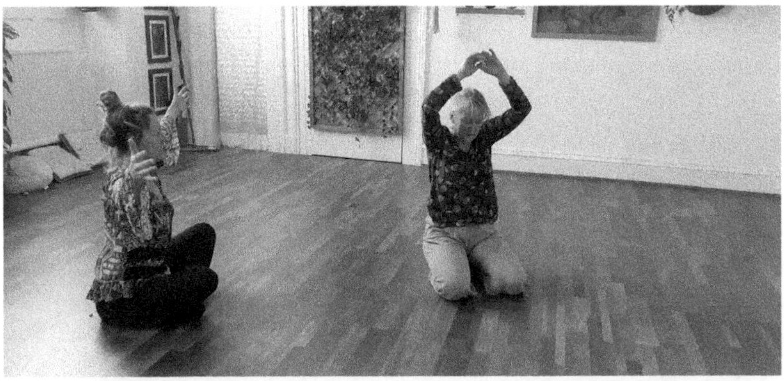

FIGURE 4.15: Karin Rugman: noticing images arising within her psyche (body/mind). Photographer: Scott Closson.

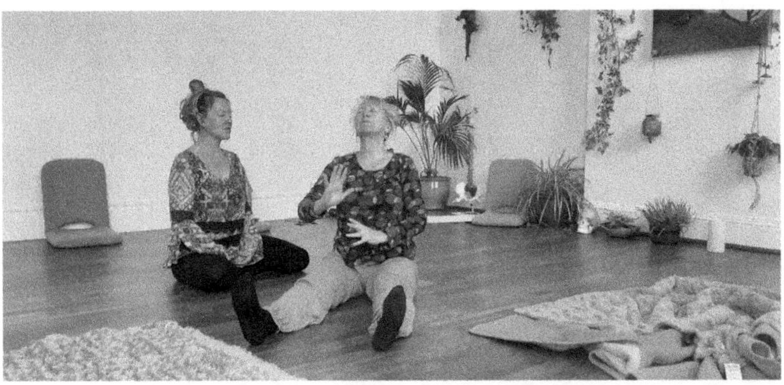

FIGURE 4.16: Karin Rugman: sensing an image arising along her midline. Photographer: Scott Closson.

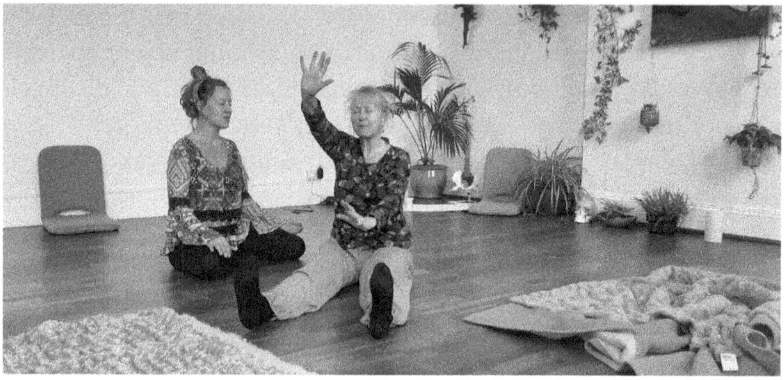

FIGURE 4.17: Karin Rugman: touching jewels on a cavern wall. Photographer: Scott Closson.

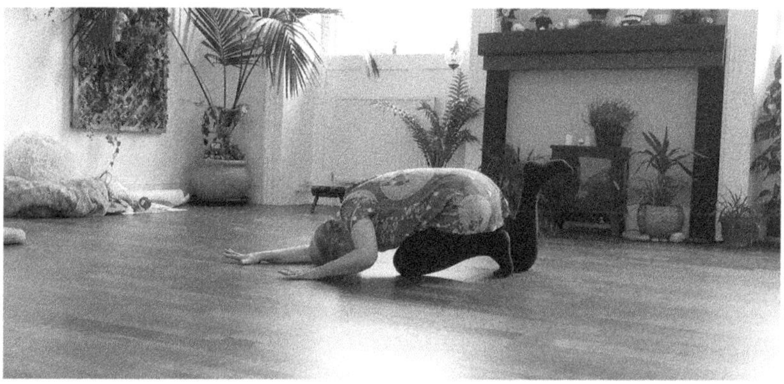

FIGURE 4.18: Karen Rugman: sense–perceiving heaviness. Photographer: Scott Closson.

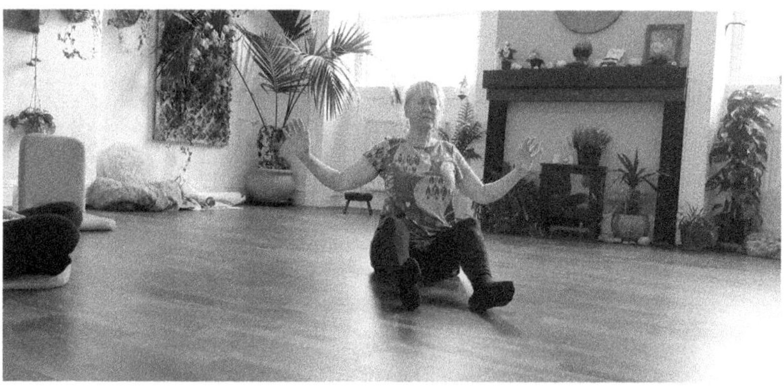

FIGURE 4.19: Karin Rugman: sense–perceiving heart. Photographer: Scott Closson.

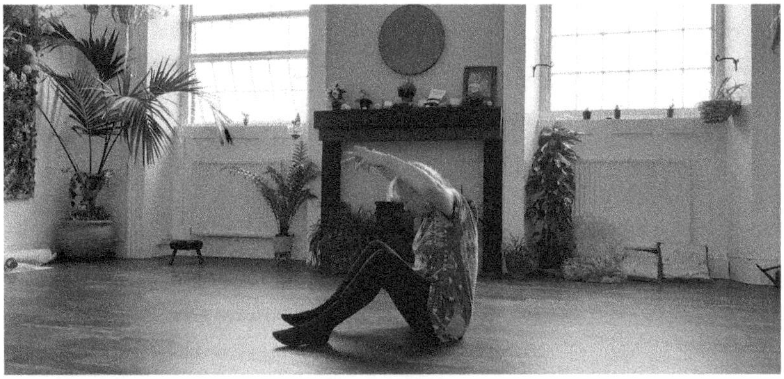

FIGURE 4.20: Karin Rugman: embodied waves washing over her. Photographer: Scott Closson.

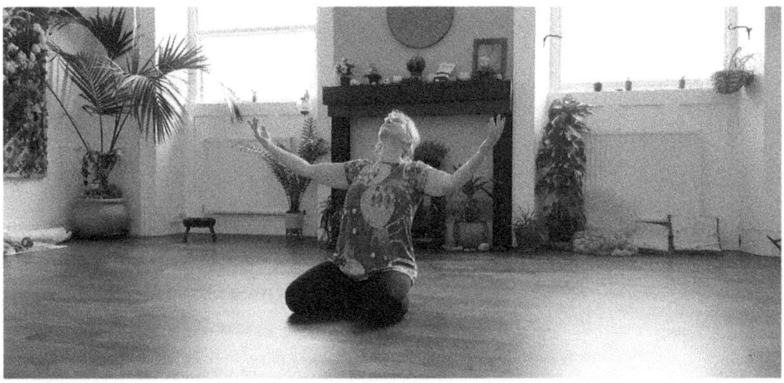

FIGURE 4.21: Karin Rugman: attuning to the vast sky above. Photographer: Scott Closson.

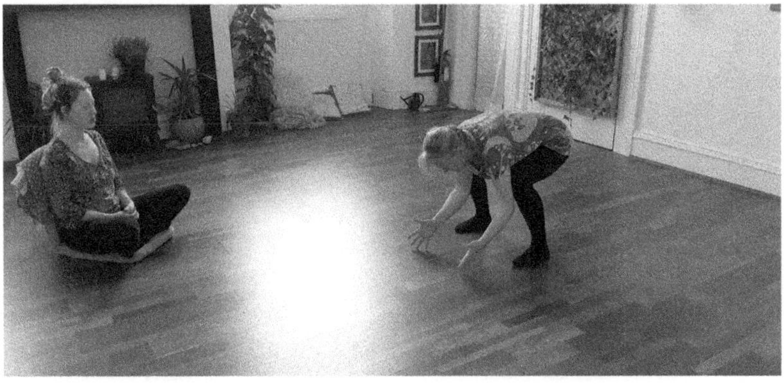

FIGURE 4.22: Karin Rugman: tilling sand. Photographer: Scott Closson.

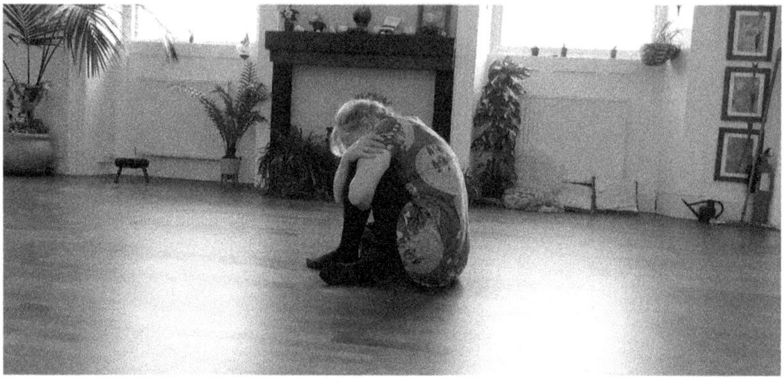

FIGURE 4.23: Karin Rugman: disappearing into rock. Photographer: Scott Closson.

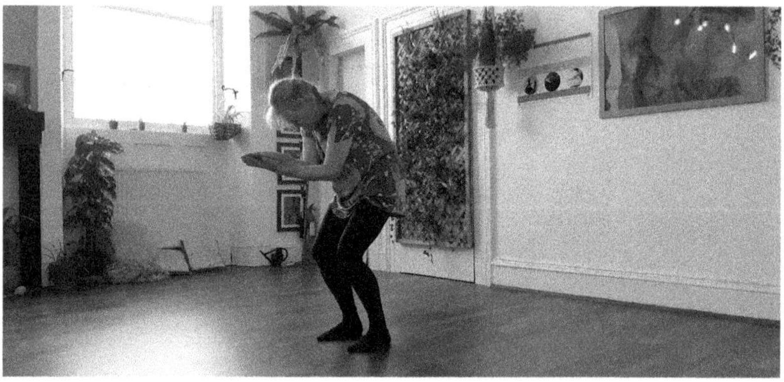

FIGURE 4.24: Karin Rugman: holding a sacred stone. Photographer: Scott Closson.

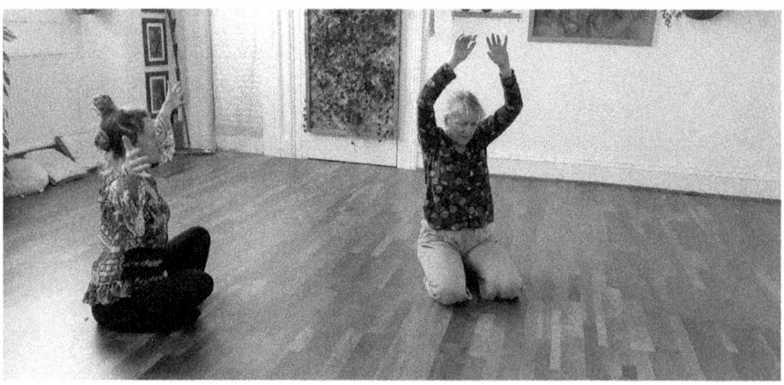

FIGURE 4.25: Karin Rugman: cool cleansing sacred water. Photographer: Scott Closson.

She is invited to come to stillness. She rests in breath and the energetic resonance of her moving time. She picks up her pencils and begins to mark-make and write.

Somatic movement dance therapists always invite participants to reflect on, and integrate their moving experience into conscious awareness. Reflection after moving is a vitally important aspect of practice that supports participants to make meaning from their often-profound sensory experience. Participants are encouraged to write, speak or mark-make from their felt-sense after moving. A felt sense 'refers to a way of knowing that is not just logical, but is responsive, that is awake to the bodily evocative dimensions that make words personally relevant' and meaningful (Todres 2007: 31). In short, language or mark-making is encouraged to tenderly unfold from kinaesthetic, sensory, emotional and imaginal feeling. This is often referred to as *the somaticization of language and symbol* in the field (Williamson and Eddy 2014: 186). This is a unique process where words are encouraged to arise from an authentic connection to the moving experience (sometimes called phenomenological or embodied writing). Such processes invite participants into the intimacy of phenomenological language – 'a method where participants are invited to stay in contact with sensory-perceptual imaginal flows that continue to stir and feel meaningful' after moving (Williamson 2018: 183). This method stands in stark contrast to the everyday usage of 'objectified language' that can often be 'disengaged, dissociated, and abstracted from the individual heart and living experience of the participant' (Williamson 2018: 80). Embodied language seeks authentic words that grow out of real feelings and sensations, rather than perpetuating the use of objectified words – 'words that betray our deeper experience [...] banal words, ready-made words, truisms, slogans, etherealized generalized words' (Johnson 2014: xiv). There are many ways to support reflection and integration post moving. Below, I outline some important approaches that support the participant to reflect and integrate their experience.

> The therapist always invites the participant to speak first and to stay in contact with their breath and heart (and the resonance of their moving time), as they share their moving experience verbally. The therapist refrains from projecting or transferring their own narrative onto the participant. They refrain from analysis, judgment, and critique. They listen, staying in contact with gravity, ground, space, breath and heart. The embodied presence and quality of the therapist's listening are vitally important, providing a heart-felt grounded presence where the participant is witnessed and heard without judgment.

I often invite the participant to speak in first-person and present tense as they share their moving experience.

Figurative, symbolic and metaphorical reflection

For example, I am moving. I am feeling the sea washing over my hands. I am raising my arms in darkness, touching jewels – little lights are falling over my fingers and hands. I am feeling warmth in my heart as I curl and uncurl in sand. I am sinking, breathing, softening into sand – waves are lightly washing over me. I am rippling and waving. I am embedding in sea. I am seabedding. Sun is landing kissing my face and I am opening my arms – reaching wide. Gemstones are falling on my heart – tending, whispering, loving – I am opening, receiving, collecting love. I am full of gratitude.

Making meaning and integrating

I am learning to be in the world with me by my side. I bring my felt-sense into my head, or my mind into my body – I will grow strong with the sea washing over my troubles.

Inviting participants to share in first-person and present tense supports them to stay in touch with their body experience, to remain present with the resonance and symbols of their moving time, and to listen for words that are authentic and meaningful. This also helps people to remain present in their body experience while talking, healing the rift between objectified language, and language that has heart and authenticity.

Participants are often invited to mark-make after they have moved. This is sometimes referred to as 'somaticization' in symbolic drawing (Williamson and Eddy 2014: 186). Mark-marking enables participants to bring their inner life and moving experience onto the page – sensations, emotions and images are further crafted into symbolic form. When lensed through a Jungian frame, the symbols that arrive on the page are considered teleological, supporting growth. Participants are invited to reflect on their mark-making and symbols, and through this process they can begin to integrate unconscious contents into conscious awareness.

Noted above, participants may be invited to write from the imaginal resonance of their moving time. They allow words to fall onto the page that arise out of the moving experience itself. Writing from sensation and the imagination often brings forth poetic writing full of imagery and symbols, such as the poetry shared by Karin Rugman below. Through a Jungian frame, this type of writing is also considered to bring unconscious contents into conscious awareness, enabling the participant to attend to areas of life that need healing and attention.

Karin Rugman writes after moving:

> Emerging from the darkness of a cavernous place, damp and heavy with the fruits of the sea, I come from the earth.
> The swelling tide washes over me, cleansing and refreshing. Light floods into my eyes, my veins.
> Heaviness draws hands down toward sand.
> They till the seabed, filtering the grains through fingers. Scattered pieces.
> I dig deeper and find a precious stone.
> Cupping it between hands I feel a sacred energy filling me with warmth.

This was a particularly significant session for Karin. Nature is often a strong source of imagery for participants – a place of inspiration and hope. The images that arose from her moving time were all of nature – each symbol was full of meaning, offering healing, cleansing and enfolding her. Within her process she came across a sacred stone. She pulled the stone out of the earth (materia) and up through her midline, resting it in her chest and eventually pushing it up above her head, raising it to the heavens (transcendental). The stone that rose up from the depths of the earth, through her tissues, was particularly important to her. By moving with, and symbolically drawing the stone, she gathered strength and reflective knowledge about her place in the world and the issues that were binding her freedom. Notably, her process was both personal and transpersonal. The transpersonal symbols offered healing to her personal struggles. This play between personal struggles and transpersonal imagery creates a great relief for many participants. It is in the somatic movement studio that one can turn to the transpersonal for support, offering strength to continue one's path that is

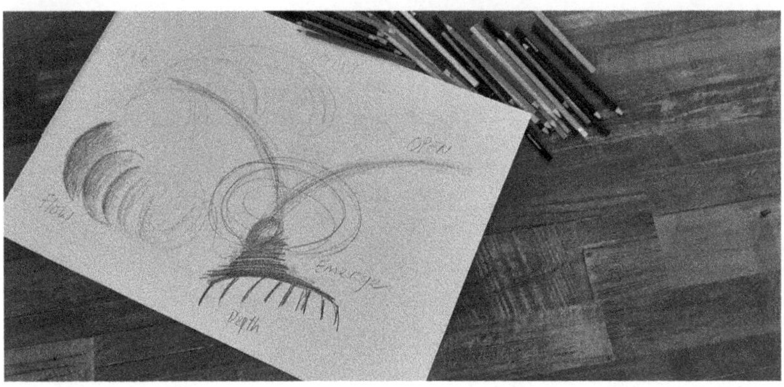

FIGURE 4.26: Photographer: Amanda Williamson. Image by Karin Rugman.

not always easy. The transpersonal plays a very important role in the efficacy of self-regulation.

Of note, her process also moved between the instinctual earth-bound and archetypal sky-bound aspects of the transpersonal. She was enfolded by stone, washed by salty sea and touched jewels on a cavern wall, eventing her towards illumination and wholeness. This play between deep immanence (nature/instinct) and transcendence (spirit/archetype) is another extremely important aspect of of self-regulating the psyche. Participants are negotiating and synthesizing the opposites. It is here, in the realms of the transpersonal that our earthy suffering and existential worries can be shared and explored creatively.

Key offerings

Because somatic movement integrates and attends to so many levels of our being, I propose it is a highly advanced self-regulatory moving bodywork modality. As we draw this chapter to a close, let us build on the list offered earlier in Chapter 1, surveying the key elements of self-regulation in the field. Self-regulation in the field is additionally explored and offered through the following:

- Sensory-imaginal processes that integrate physiological, emotional, spiritual and soulful levels of our being.
- Sensory-perceptual imaginal processes that invite unconscious contents to arise into consciousness through symbolic form.
- The co-regulatory presence of the heart-centered witness who holds the possibility of integration and wholeness for the client.

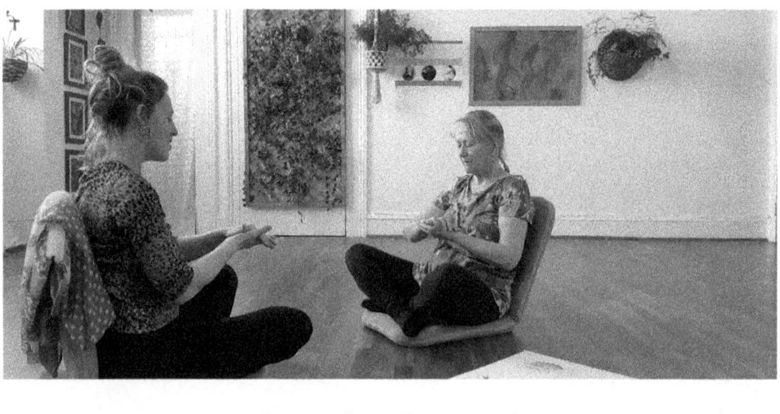

FIGURE 4.27: Karin Rugman and Amanda Williamson: closing our session. Photographer: Scott Closson.

- Self-regulation is supported by the heart-centered transpersonal witness, sensed and cultivated through moment-by-moment breath awareness and cardio-ception.
- The therapist prepares their body before practice, calming their nervous system down and moving into a parasympathetic state, resonate with nature.
- Self-regulation and co-regulation are underpinned by feeling safe: safety is invited by releasing sympathetic holding and moving into parasympathetic release. This state invites receptivity, ease, restitution, calmness.
- The imagination is expansive and perceived as a teleological guide, moving participants towards wholeness.
- Carl Jung's theories are a bedrock of knowledge in the somatic movement dance paradigm, and his concept of the personal and collective unconscious plays a significant role in many somatic movement modalities.
- Non-judgemental witnessing plays an essential role in self-regulating.
- Somatic movement dance therapists do not diagnose and seek out pathology; rather they support participants to move towards life through peaceful processes that re-balance the nervous system, releasing impacts, assaults and imprints slowly and over time.
- Embodied language is offered as a method that heals the rift between objectified banal words and the deeply feeling-full body.
- Symbolic mark-making is offered as a method that further visualises unconscious contents, supporting participants to integrate unconscious contents into awareness.
- The imagination supports the dexterity and fluidity of fascia and the skeletal muscular system, supporting participants to find new movement pathways.

5

Co-regulatory Touch and Myofasical Softening

Touch is used across a variety of bodywork health professions. Just as cranio-osteopaths, chiropractors and massage therapists use touch, somatic movement and dance therapists/specialists also use touch. In fact, the skilled use of touch is one of the defining features of the field. Qualified practitioners are often trained in somatic touch and bodywork processes underpinned by experiential anatomy and physiology. Bodywork and hands-on may be offered prior to moving, or during moving. Often bodywork is followed by a movement response, increasing self-regulation. Touch may be offered to guide and support improvisational movement. Gentle hands-on work soothes the nervous system and softens sympathetic arousal in the tissues and is one of the most effective ways to support self-regulation and parasympathetic release. The production of cortisol is reduced when safe healthy touch is applied, cascading healthy chemicals through the tissues, such as oxytocin, dopamine and serotonin. Practitioners may offer touch in one-on-one practice and in community groups. In the wake of COVID-19, defining why we use touch has

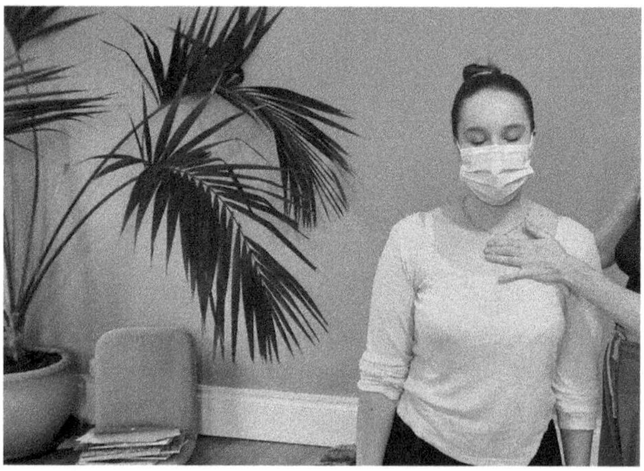

FIGURE 5.1: Movingsoma students training in touch. Photographer: Amanda Williamson.

become even more important. Additionally, still using PPE and safeguarding both practitioner and client is at the forefront of the profession.

Of note, somatic movement dance practitioners do not manipulate or correct a person's body, while they lie on the bodywork table, passively receiving touch. In contrast, touch is offered to support a person to self-regulate through their own movement expression and sense–feeling, and through their internal somatosensory system. Thus, participants are invited to actively respond to touch, perhaps softening into the therapist's hand, and using their hand as a fulcrum, or moving improvisationally with and from touch. The intention of touch is further offered to support easeful movement, creativity and the imagination. Touch is offered for the following reasons, greatly enhancing a client's ability to self-regulate. For example, practitioners might offer a touch to:

- reconnect participants to their sensory-motor feedback loop
- enhance afferent sensing and conscious efferent motor expression
- support expressivity, creativity and the imagination-in-movement
- bring consciousness to living tissues and body systems that are often beneath consciousness
- support fascial release through soft-tissue rolling and easeful motor pathways
- support skeletal–muscular alignment
- support anatomical differentiation and movement integration
- calm and balance the nervous system (reduce sympathetic arousal and support parasympathetic ease)
- locate specific body tissues and systems, objectively and subjectively
- teach anatomy and physiology through subjective experience and objective knowledge
- release habituated patterns of neuromuscular holding, soften hypertonicity and re-balance tissues
- enhance the imagination-in-movement, supporting skeletal-muscular dexterity and movement fluidity
- connect with Self, others and the community group through the non-verbal language of touch, dance and movement
- enhance moment-by-moment breath awareness and cardio-ception, reducing sympathetic arousal, and integrating mind and body
- offer touch-based processes that explore presence in Self and with other.

While you can effectively self-regulate through your own attuned improvisation, especially using the floor as a fulcrum, co-regulatory somatic touch is one of the most effective ways to support myofascial release, resolve knots and trigger points and ease the nervous system. The quality of touch, energy, support and presence

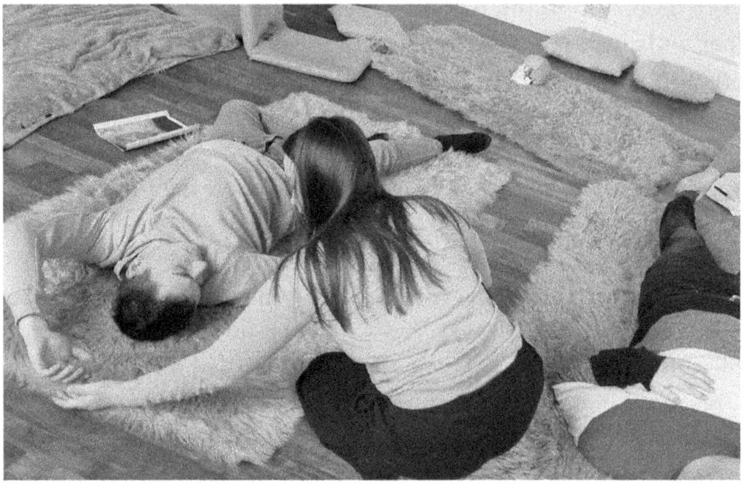

FIGURE 5.2: Natasha Martin: experientially studying touch. Photographer: Amanda Williamson.

of another person is incredibly soothing and releases emotional holding in the fascial matrix, the topic of the last chapter. 'Touch is perhaps the oldest and still most reliable healing modality that we possess' (Smith 2005: xii). It is also the primary sense that underlies our development in the embryo and indeed as we grow and develop into adults. We continuously touch the exterior world in every moment of our lives and the world touches us. There is never a moment when we are not touching or being touched by the world. Often our sense of touch falls beneath conscious awareness and hence somatic movement dance supports participants to connect to their somatosensory system.

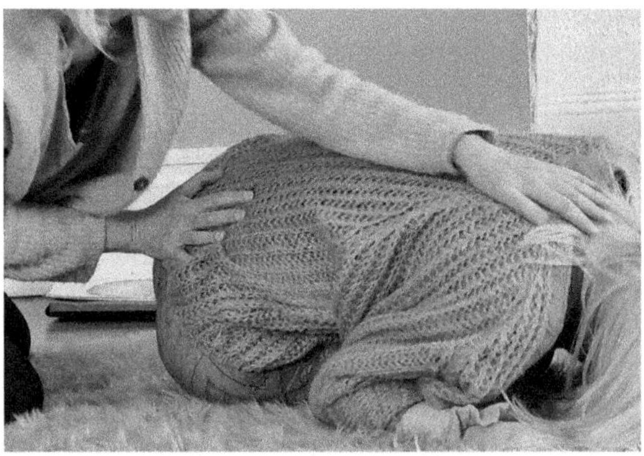

FIGURE 5.3: Movingsoma students training in touch. Photographer: Amanda Williamson.

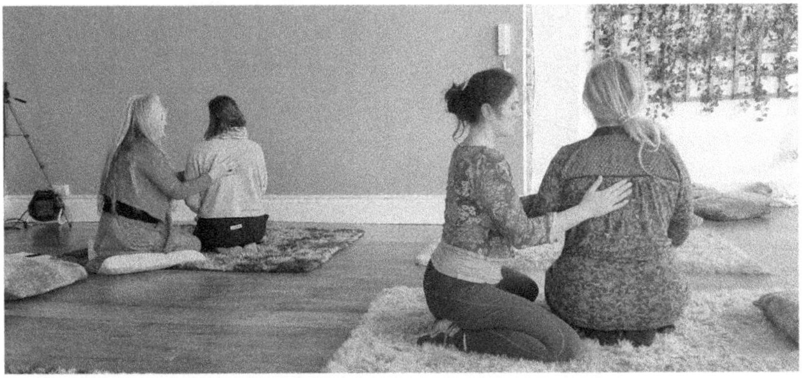

FIGURE 5.4: Movingsoma students training in touch. Photographer: Amanda Williamson.

Touch is deeply transformative when facilitated through presence, heart attunement, non-doing and breath support, rather than imposition and manipulation. In essence, we invite participants back to their first language of growth, development, enfoldment and emergence. 'The power of touch is etched into our brain and every cell in our body seeks relationship. In a healthy environment, touch means safety, assurance, nutrition and familiarity' (Sumner and Haines 2010: 19).

> The human subcutaneous connective tissue has a special sensory system for affective touch, which are responsive to gentle skin contact, stroking, and social touch. This system is also connected to the brain, again to the insula, the centre of consciousness, self-awareness, empathy, emotions, and social skill.
>
> (Schleip 2017: 45)

This very close connection between your skin and brain starts during your embryonic development. In the third week of your embryological development your cells start to reorganize through a process known as gastrulation. Gastrulation starts on day 15. It is the extraordinary process where the cells rearrange themselves from a simple sphere-shaped ball into a multi-layered cellular structure. No one knows how this happens, or why the cells possess such self-regulatory directive intelligence. It is deeply mystical. While our dominant cultural values tend to devalue the mystical and spiritual in favour of science and rationalism, our arrival on this earth is clearly an astonishing mystery that evades even the greatest scientific minds. During the gastrulation process three germ layers are formed; these germ layers are the ancestors of all the developing tissues in the embryo. The three layers are called the 'ectoderm', 'mesoderm' and 'endoderm'. The endoderm is the most internal layer; it forms the lining of the gut and other internal organs. The ectoderm

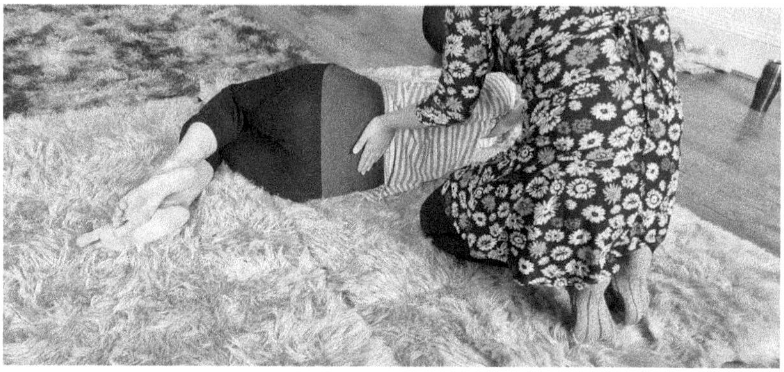

FIGURE 5.5: Movingsoma students. Photographer: Scott Closson.

is an exterior germ layer; it forms the skin, brain, the nervous system and other external tissues. The mesoderm is the middle layer, forming all the muscles, the skeletal system and the circulatory system. Note, the strong connection between the ectoderm, the central nervous and the skin here (note they develop out of the same primitive tissues). In somatic literature, your skin is experienced and explored as the outmost layer of your central nervous system; when you touch skin, you are, in a sense, soothing the central nervous system.

> This close association between the skin and the central nervous system could not have a more concrete anatomical and physiological connection [...] because the skin and brain develop from exactly the same primitive cells. Depending on how you look at it, the skin is the outer surface of the brain, or the brain is the deepest layer of the skin. Surface and innermost core spring from the same mother tissue, and throughout the life of the organism they function as a single unit, divisible only by dissection or analytical abstraction.
>
> (Juhan 2003: 35)

In some sessions a specific method might be offered, such as the process shared in Chapter 2, where the practitioner supported the client to release holding in the sympathetic chain, by attuning to the heart and solar plexus, and particular vertebral levels. In other sessions, touch may be offered in improvisational processes, where the therapist places her hands on the body of other, and invites them to soften and loosen hypertonicity, and disentangle thirsty matted myofascial tissues.

Attuning to other person's body is the most tender skill. It is an embodied skill that can be difficult to learn. Co-regulatory touch and myofascial softening might look easy to the outsider, because it is so soft, fluid and easeful. However, the ability to sense Self in relation to Other, attune to another person's living system, while staying in contact with your body experience and heart requires practice (over a lifetime). The ability to listen, receive, follow, be guided or gently guide, is a serious talent. The skill to move into a transpersonal space (of breath and heart) and offer your living presence to another person is extremely hard. There are many embodied skills and concepts underlying co-regulatory touch and myofascial softening. These are wonderfully sensitive skills, full of care for Self and Other. Some of these are:

- Staying in contact with your own breath and heart as you touch.
- Bringing your presence to another person, while staying in contact with your interoceptive awareness.
- Softening in your synovial, cartilaginous and fibrous joints to enhance your proprioception as you touch.
- Softening in your joints so you can move effortlessly and fluently with Other.
- Attuning to another person's system, listening, receiving, opening and offering.
- Becoming a fulcrum so the client can reorganize their tissues on your tissues.
- Listening to Other, following, supporting and enhancing their movement expression, and sensory–perceptual imaginative trails and pathways.
- Moving as one – attuning your systems, where there is no leader or follower, but an intuitive flow of movement creating a state of non-duality.

Before you touch, it is important to contact your heart and breath, calming your nervous system and creating a coherent heart-field. Previously noted in Chapter 4, touch is electric, and when we touch, an electromagnetic signal is received by the body of other. If our heart-rhythms are coherent, our touch will have a positive effect on Other. If our heart rhythms are incoherent, our touch is likely to deregulate Other. Hence, underlying the therapist's touch is her own heart, breath and easeful parasympathetic state, which enables her to bring a relaxed peaceful presence to her client. As she engages and listens to the participant's living tissues, she maintains her vagal tone moment-by-moment. At the heart of co-regulatory touch and myofascial softening is bringing your calm presence to another person. Notably, bringing heart and presence to Self is a prerequisite to bringing presence and heart to Other (Williamson 2020e). Being present with another person is impossible if you are not present with your breath and heart – bringing compassion to Self throughout your cells via heart-sensing, will deeply affect the process and quality of practice. If you are disengaged from your own body experience and breath, your touch is likely to be detached and insensitive.

In co-regulatory touch and somatic unwinding, we are not diagnosing or correcting, but rather supporting the participant's system to release restrictions through following their own self-regulatory movement, initiated from and supported by touch. As the practitioner touches, they are invited to keep their joints soft, receiving the quality and energy of the participant's psyche (body–mind) through their synovial joint system. The practitioner also keeps soft so they can move effortlessly, following the participant's movement pathways and improvisational trails. Both client and therapist are fine-tuning and receiving the world of their somatosensory system. It is important to approach touch through this lens, rather than imposing concepts of esoteric healing through your hands. Healing is offered through your presence, heart field, attunement, receptivity, calmness, gentleness and openness with another human being. Touch that does not demand anything is very different to touch that is imposing, manipulative, diagnostic and end-gaining.

Co-regulatory touch and myofascial softening further involves:

- two living systems coming together, resting in each other's living tissues with breath awareness
- receiving the living presence of each other's being and energy
- sensing the energy, vibration and quality of each other's living system
- sensing tissue motility, pulses and fluid flows (the aliveness of living tissue).

When working in a therapeutic context, co-regulatory touch often involves the therapist following the participant's movement. The participant leads and the therapist follows. At other times, the therapist gently guides or leads, offering movement pathways that invite the fascial tissues to loosen, release, extend or reach, for example. Often the therapist and participant merge together and move as one. No one is following and no one is leading. In this case, two living systems have become one, and often this creates an experience of non-duality. Underlying touch and myofascial

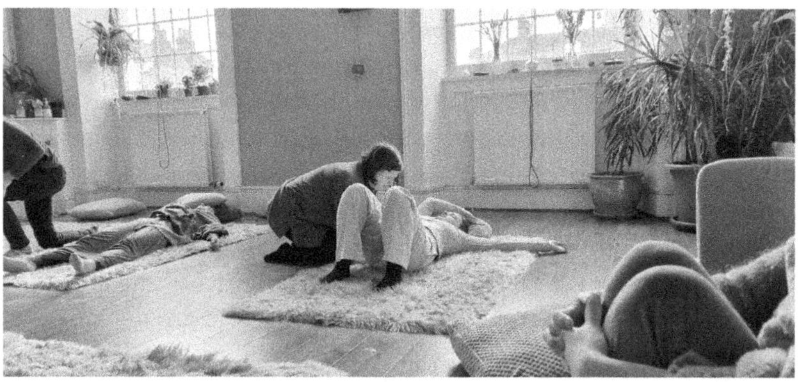

FIGURE 5.6: Movingsoma students training in touch. Photographer: Amanda Williamson.

unwinding is the concept of unravelling matted places of restriction, inviting fluency and ease.

It is important to share with students the difference between objective and subjective touch. There are two main sensory pathways that receive touch. These are called *The spinothalamic tract* and *The dorsal column-lemniscal pathway*. Both receive touch and carry this information to the central nervous system. They are however different. *The spinothalamic tract* is an ascending sensory pathway through the spinal cord. It is responsible for the transmission of pain, temperature and crude touch to the somatosensory region of the thalamus (Bengochea 2021). As Upledger further explains, 'The spinothalamic tract transmits exteroceptive sensations which arise from stimuli outside the self' (2008: 84). This pathway 'transmits pain, temperature, and objective touch' (Upledger 2008: 84). In contrast, the dorsal column-lemniscal 'carries conscious proprioception sensations which arise within the body, including the position of the musculoskeletal components at rest, kinaesthetic sense of the body in motion, and the vibratory sensation' (Upledger 2008: 84). 'It also has tactile discrimination fibres which define the subjective tactical self, including that of texture and pressure' (2008: 84). In short, *The spinothalamic tract* carries sensory information received from outside of your body, and transmits crude touch, and thus is considered objective touch. In contrast, the dorsal column-lemniscal pathway is a refined inner part of the somatosensory system, which receives a wealth of information internally and thus is considered subjective touch. Both systems are of course important when touching, but it is the latter sensory pathway that I really focus on when I train somatic movement dance therapists. As the therapist touches, she

> attunes to her dorsal column-lemniscal pathway (the sensory information arising within her own body). She sense-perceives information through her proprioception and the position of her body (her joints), her own movement (her kinaesthetic sense) and the vibrations and energies within her.
>
> does not focus solely on her hands when touching another person as if they are an object, but rather focuses on receiving the other person's presence through her internal somatosensory system and her hands.
>
> is not actively touching and manipulating, but rather receptively receiving the presence of another person's being and movement through her dorsal column-lemniscal sensory pathway.

When the practitioner offers touch, she is not feeling the other person's body through her hands and fingers only, or feeling them like they are an object, separate from herself. Rather she is sensing another person through her own internal somatosensory system. As she touches, she receives sensory information from within, and through receptive hands. She stays in contact with her own proprioception (keeping her joints soft). She stays in contact with her own interoception (breath and the organ body). When she touches, she listens to her own system, as well as Other. Thus, co-regulatory touch requires a dual listening. Co-regulatory touch could be defined as the ability to sense the living-breathing energy and presence of another person's tissues through your own living system. As she comes into contact with the participant's body she can feel the shape, tonus, texture, vibration, energy and the quality of their tissues, plus small vibrations and micro movements and adjustments.

Co-regulatory touch and myofascial unwinding is about awareness, consciousness and wholeness – bringing to consciousness parts of our being that have dropped below the threshold of awareness or have become tangled and matted with stress. As we collect and integrate parts of our ourselves back into our sensory–motor cortex, we are likely to feel more whole. Many people suffer from sensory amnesia in our fast socio-economic world and become dissociated from the exquisite intelligence of their somatosensory system. Sensory amnesia can be defined as the loss of feeling in the body, or the inability to feel the body, or parts of the body. While hidden, and often in the shadows of the unconscious, our tissues are alive with vibration, energy, proprioceptive and interoceptive intelligence – our fascial tissues are full of fluid that need to circulate and replenish. When practitioners touch, they may also direct their awareness to replenishing dry and stagnant fascial fluids. Through touch, they can sense the tiniest of vibrations, energies, and the tonus and hyptonicity of tissues, and encourage fascial release.

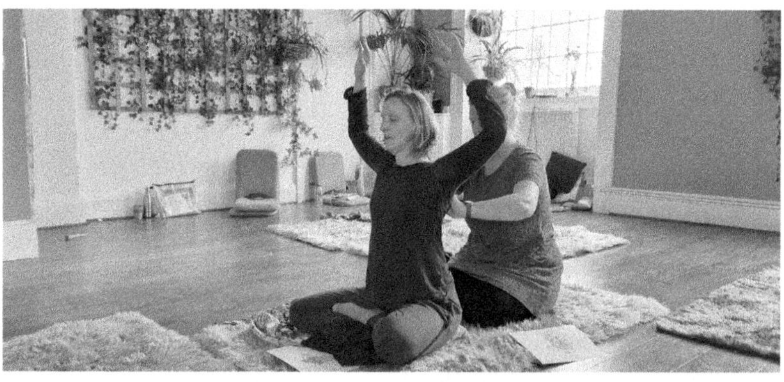

FIGURE 5.7: Movingsoma students training in touch. Photographer: Natasha Martin.

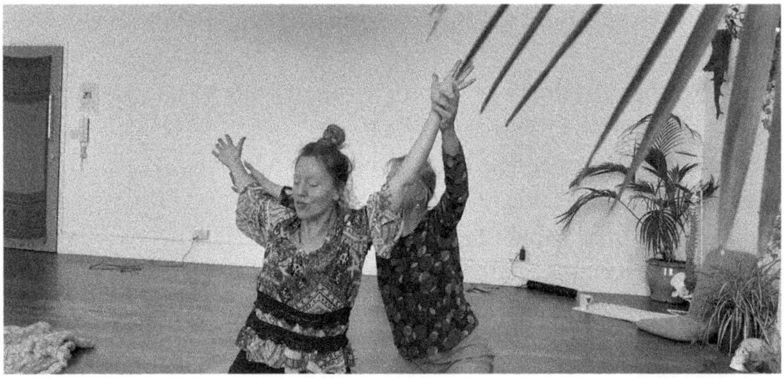

FIGURE 5.8: Karin Rugman and Amanda Williamson. Photographer: Scott Closson.

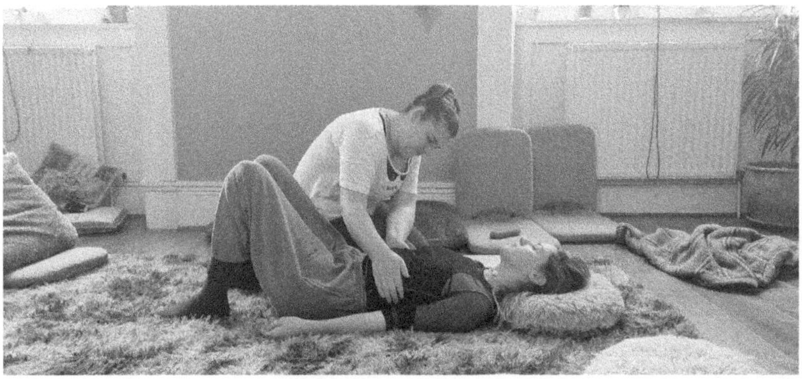

FIGURE 5.9: Celine Parsons and Sylvia Gregory: exploring touch. Photographer: Amanda Williamson.

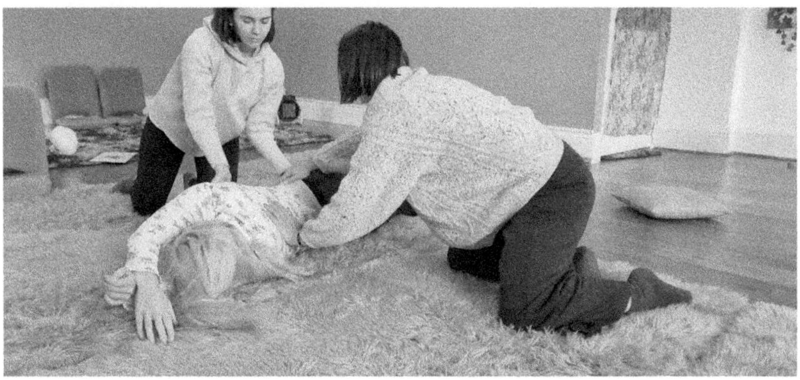

FIGURE 5.10: Movingsoma students exploring touch. Photographer: Amanda Williamson.

Co-regulatory touch and myofascial softening may further involve:

Attuning to the movement of breath through your tissues and the movement of breath through the tissues of Other.
Attuning to the heart of Self and the heart of Other: moving with awareness of each other's heart-field.
Attuning to the fluid being of Self and Other (arterial and venous blood, synovial fluid in the joints, cerebrospinal fluid and lymph).
Sensing the fluidity and viscosity of subcutaneous, deep fascia and visceral fascia under the skin and surrounding the bones and organs.

6

Sense–perceiving the Craniosacral System

> *I attend a somatic movement dance therapy session every Saturday. Over the weeks we have tried all different forms of movement, therapy and meditation together, all of which are proving invaluable to my recovery/rehabilitation. Last weekend we tried a process rooted in cranialsacral movement therapy – I have been blown away by the results as not only have I been pain free in my back – which is unheard of! I set about a project to replace my turf in my garden which involved a lot of strenuous activity and I have suffered no aches or pains whatsoever in my back as a result. I am absolutely amazed by how I have felt this week thanks to this treatment. Would highly recommend going if you struggle with pain or are recovering.*
>
> (Paula Anderson)

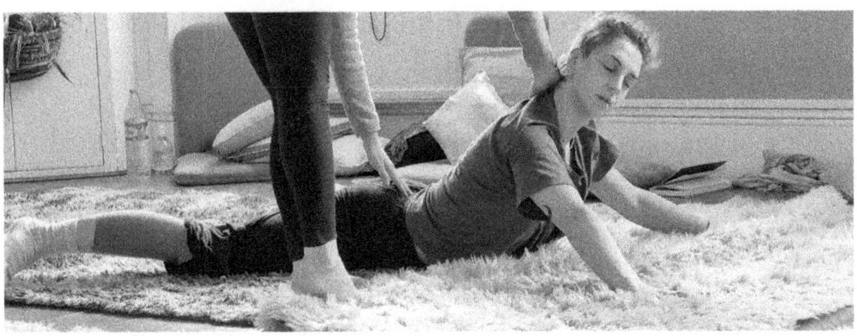

FIGURE 6.1: Jessica Cotton: sense–perceiving her spinal dura. Photographer: Amanda Williamson.

> *You may not know it, but your head is expanding right now. In another few seconds it will start shrinking. If it's already shrinking, then it will start expanding again in just a moment. You won't see such a change in the mirror, and chances are good you could go the rest of your life without noticing it and never lose a good night's sleep. But if you've ever suffered from such things as migraine headaches, temporomandibular joint (TMJ) dysfunction, ringing in the ears, dyslexia, depression, or any number of chronic aches and pains through-out your body, then the fact that your head expands and contracts at a rate of 8 to 12 times a minute could become quite important to you.*
> (Upledger et al. 2008: 65)

In the beginning of Chapter 3, we explored the occiput as a primary fulcrum of support and soft tissue reorganization, with brief reference to the other cranial bones. In this chapter, we will take an in-depth look at the cranial bones and sutures in relation to the craniosacral system. The craniosacral system is a subtle and rather beautiful circulatory system flowing along the midline within the human body. It is often confused with the *craniosacral division* of the parasympathetic nervous system. In Chapters 2 and 3, I shared how the craniosacral division refers to the parasympathetic nerves emanating from the cranium and sacrum. In contrast, the craniosacral system refers to the production, circulation and reabsorption of cerebrospinal fluid within the dural tube that surrounds your brain and spinal cord. While the craniosacral division and craniosacral system are different, they do however share a similar geography. Both involve sense–perception of the caudal–cranial axis. Thus, it is very likely, that when we explore the craniosacral system in the studio, we also invite the parasympathetic division of the autonomic nervous system into expression.

The craniosacral system comprises the bones of the midline (the cranial bones, vertebral column, sacrum and tail-bone), the soft tissues of the meningeal layers (the cranial and spinal dura) and the cerebrospinal fluid (the fluid that is produced in the ventricles of the brain created from arterial blood). In this chapter, I will attend to all these areas discretely and offer some practice-based processes that support participants to attune to this system.

In traditional anatomy, the cranial bones are considered fused, hard and solid. This mechanistic perception of the cranium has haunted western medical descriptions until the ground-breaking fathers of osteopathy, such as Andrew Taylor Still (2017) and Dr William Sutherland (1990) proposed otherwise. Dr Sutherland advanced A.T. Still's ideas of *living anatomy* and suggested that the cranium is not solid, but rather moves slightly to accommodate the production, circulation and reabsorption of cranial fluids (in the order of one- or two-sixteenths of an inch). Sutherland researched how the cranial bones often become compressed leading to dysfunction in many other areas of the body. He published extensively on the following ideas.

> The cranial bones are not solid and fixed. There is motion (however micro) in the bones because the sutures are full of blood, nerves, and fascia
> There is expansion and contraction in the hemispheres of the brain
> There is motion in the membranes covering the brain and spinal cord
> There is a fluid wave within the cerebrospinal fluid that bathes the brain and spinal cord
> There is a subtle motion in the tailbone (sacrum) that is related to the movements within the cranium.
>
> (Adapted from Sutherland 1990)

Somatic movement dance therapy, along with other bodywork modalities, such as cranio-osteopathy, is not invested in the idea of a rock-solid cranium. Rather, in alignment with cranio-osteopathy, the cranium is considered and sense–perceived as bio-tensile. Bio-tensility means there is a degree of motility (however micro) between the cranial bones. Thus, the sutures (fibrous joints) between the cranial bones are not fixed and fused. These movements are not large, but rather in the range of micro-millimetres. All the bones in the cranium (*the occiput*, *the temporal bones*, *the parietal bones*, *the frontal bone and the sphenoid*) are connected by fibrous joints called sutures. Fibrous joints have far less mobility than *cartilaginous* or *synovial* joints, but within this progressive anatomical and physiological framework, fibrous joints are sense–perceived to move slightly (Upledger 1997, 2001, 2008). Upledger shares, 'the misfortune about bones fusing together had its basis in the study of anatomy laboratory cadavers that were old and embalmed' (Upledger 2001: 12). After Sutherland's observations, other osteopaths, such as John E. Upledger continued to explore how the skull bones move 'rhythmically' in 'response to the rise and fall of cerebrospinal-fluid pressure' (Upledger 2001: 8). 'The skull-bone motion is a response to the rise and fall of cerebrospinal-fluid pressure and volume within its semi-closed hydraulic compartment [...] formed by the watertight outer layer of the meningeal membranes, the dura mater' (Upledger 2001: 8).

Upledger shares that in Gray's anatomy (the bible of anatomical reference books), the 'bones of the skull are [viewed as] immobile'. He additionally writes, 'Many doctors agree, implying that any therapy based on movable skull bones must clearly be a nonsense' (Upledger 2008: 67). He further notes, that 'osteopathic physicians, and physicians who do practice craniosacral therapy disagree with this accepted view of cranial immobility' (Upledger 2008: 67). Dr Sutherland put forward the idea that if the cranial bones become stuck, wedged and immobile, this in turn affects the diaphragmatic respiratory mechanism. To paraphrase Upledger, Sutherland noticed a very sudden change in breathing patterns when the cranial bones were prevented from moving (2008: 67–68). As such, Sutherland believed that 'cranial respiration was the primary respiration mechanism of the body, and that breathing was secondary' (2008: 67–68). Advocating that the movement of the cranial bones is a primary respiration raises the importance of coming into conscious relationship with the restorative motion and the motility of the cranial bones in the somatic studio.

Disassociated from the body in the West, it is common for participants to be unaware of the micro-movements taking place between their cranial bones. It takes a great deal of practice and curiosity to feel this motion. One is invited to shift one's perception of the human body from solid, armoured and hard into a fluidic bio-tensile frame of reference. Progressive anatomists thus 'share the opinion with craniosacral practitioners and osteopaths that the cranial sutures do not touch and necessarily solidly adhere with age, but allow subtle movement like, for example, the craniosacral rhythm' (Agustoni 2003: 62).

Much of my research is fully immersed in the idea that the cranial bones and their motion are a key to health. This chapter is dedicated to building a sensory–perceptual relationship with the cranial bones and the craniosacral system, which takes a great deal of sensitivity, attunement and slow-time empirical investigation to sense. The movement of the cranial bones is one of the most delicate and sensitive areas to study. This chapter introduces how the cranial bones move, and the relationship between this movement and the production, circulation and reabsorption of cerebrospinal fluid. Before we move into practice, I will begin with an overview of the craniosacral system. Because I share the craniosacral system in a rather objectified manner, let us take a pause before we begin, and remember, this delicate system is a living part of us. It is a very deep primal part of our being, flowing along our midline.

Different layers and densities of the craniosacral system

The craniosacral system is composed of different layers and densities of tissues, specifically bone, soft tissue and fluid. In health, all these elements move and work together to protect the brain and spinal cord. Learning about this system through experiential anatomy and physiology requires bringing awareness to the following:

- All the cranial bones and the sutures.
- The entire vertebral column, from C0 all the way to the sacrum and the coccyx.
- The meningeal tissues (the dura mater) that surround the brain and spinal cord, commonly referred to as *the cranial dura* and *spinal dura*, or *meningeal system*. These soft tissues protect the brain and spinal cord, and cerebrospinal

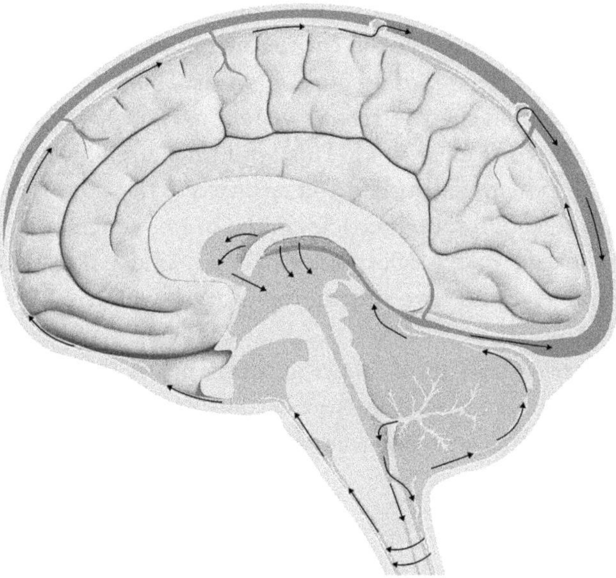

FIGURE 6.2: The ventricles.

fluid flows within this dura mater in a space called *the subarachnoid space*. These tissues protect the entire CNS.

- The ventricular system within the brain (four rather beautiful fluid cavities that produce cerebrospinal fluid). Cerebrospinal fluid is the white fluid that circulates around the brain and spinal cord. The ventricular system transforms arterial blood into CSF.

In the studio, all these elements can be contacted and sense-perceived, but I note early, the best way to introduce the craniosacral system to participants is through sense-perception of their cranial bones, sutures, vertebral column and sacrum (tailbone). Cerebrospinal fluid is rather elusive and hard to sense-perceive at first, whereas our bones are, of course, easier to contact.

What is cerebrospinal fluid?

> Cerebrospinal fluid provides the medium within which the central nervous system exists. It also provides nutrients and drains away unwanted waste products from the brain and spinal cord. The free unrestricted flow of cerebrospinal fluid is therefore essential to proper healthy function of the central nervous system and consequently to integrated healthy function generally.
>
> (Attlee 2012: 49)

Cerebrospinal fluid is a vitally important fluid, moving like a wave, along your midline. It bathes and nourishes the entire central nervous system and removes waste and toxins. It is the guardian angel of your CNS. Note, it is a circulatory system. It is produced in the ventricular system in brain where arterial blood is transformed into a white clear fluid. This fluid then circulates around the brain and spinal cord. It is then reabsorbed and returned to the venous blood. Cerebrospinal fluid is produced in four ventricles in the brain, which you can view in the image above. These four ventricles look extremely unusual in shape. They look rather like an underground cave system, full of fresh water.

> The ventricle system is a system of cavities and canals deep within the central nervous system. These cavities and canals are spaces within the nerve tissue of the brain and spinal cord. The ventricular system consists of four ventricles connected by various communicating channels.
>
> (Attlee 2012: 45)

Rest your awareness on the image of the ventricular system in Figure 6.2. Approximately 600 millilitres of cerebrospinal is produced a day in these ventricles. Note, you have two lateral ventricles located in both sides of your cerebral hemisphere, and a third ventricle situated in between your right and the left thalami. The third ventricle is connected to the lateral ventricles above via *the foramen of Monro*. The fourth ventricle receives the flow of CSF from the third ventricle via *the cerebral aqueduct*. The fourth and last ventricle lies within the brainstem, between *the pons* and *medulla oblongata* (this is another key reason why sensing the occiput and brainstem is important in the studio). CSF moves out of the fourth ventricle into the brain and down and around the spinal cord. This remarkable fluid seeps into the brain tissues. Noted in Chapter 3, it moves down through the foramen magnum and around the spinal cord. As it moves it purifies the brain and spinal cord, 'carrying out its nutritive and cleansing functions' (Attlee 2012: 49). CSF provides protection for the brain and spinal cord, but also nourishment because it has a 'rich composition – including glucose and various proteins and substances dissolved in salts like sodium, calcium, magnesium and potassium' (Agustoni 2003: 10). We produce a fair amount of cerebrospinal fluid a day, as Attlee shares below.

> The total volume of cerebrospinal fluid contained within the ventricles and subarachnoid space is approximately 150 millilitres (a quarter of a pint). The choroid plexi produce around 600 millilitres of cerebrospinal fluid each day, enabling the body to replace and replenish its cerebrospinal fluid four times every day.
>
> (Attlee 2012: 49)

How do the cranial bones move in response to the production, circulation and reabsorption of cerebrospinal fluid?

The cranial bones flex and extend to accommodate the production, circulation and reabsorption of cerebrospinal fluid. In order to explore how the cranial bones flex (expand) and extend (contract), we need to attend to the connection

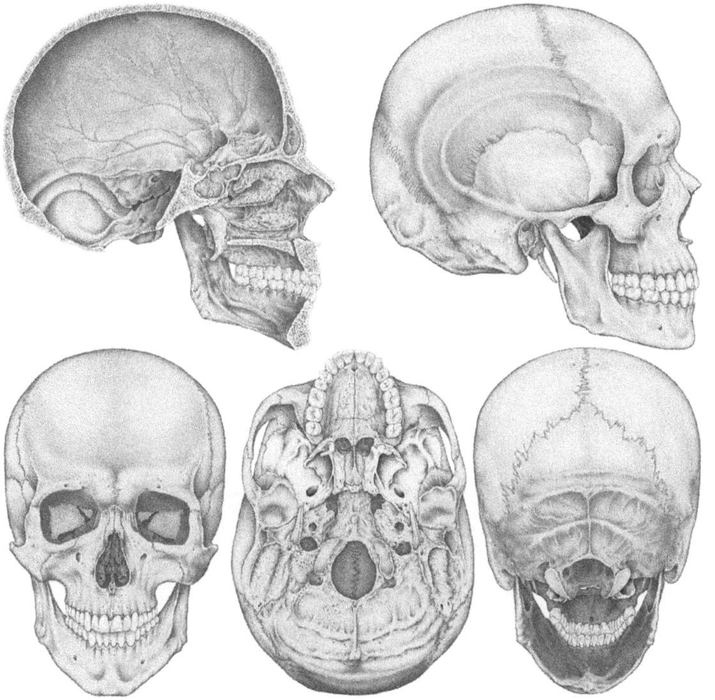

FIGURE 6.3: The cranial bone.

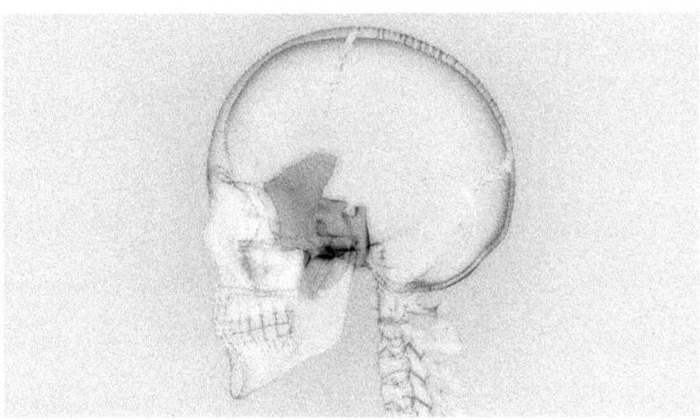

FIGURE 6.4: The sphenoid bone and sphenoid-basilar synchondrosis.

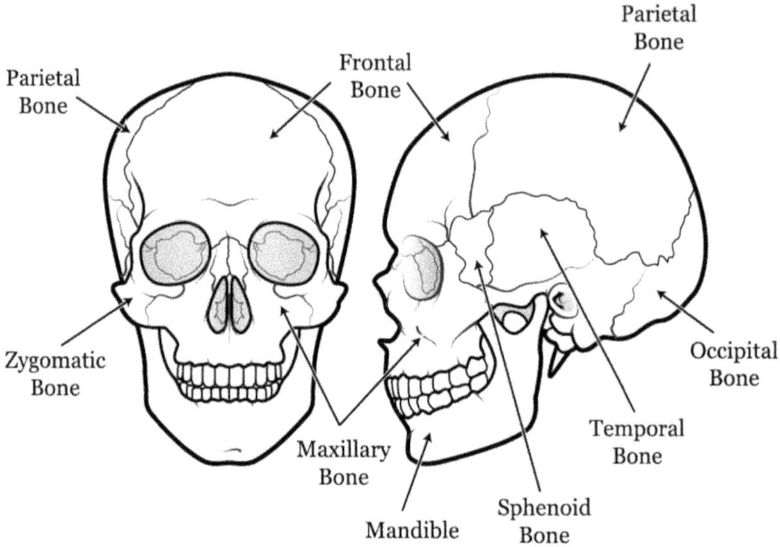

FIGURE 6.5: The cranial bones.

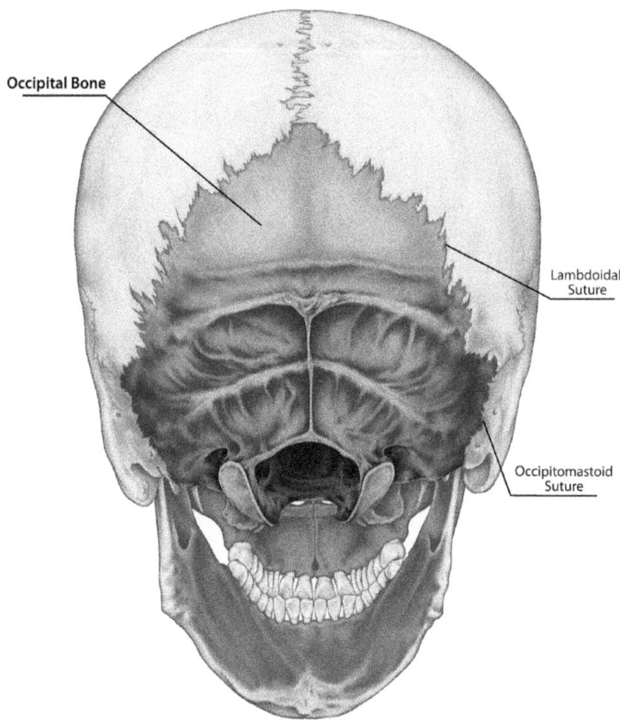

FIGURE 6.6: The occipital bone.

between the sphenoid bone and occipital bone first. Noted briefly in Chapter 3, these bones are joined together by the *sphenoid-basilar synchondrosis*. This joint is considered the 'the pivotal fulcrum around which the whole bony craniosacral system revolves' (Attlee 2012: 180). Noted also in Chapter 3, the atlantooccipital joints provide a key landmark that we can sense–perceive to balance and float the occiput on C1. The sphenoid–basilar joint provides another key landmark, balancing and moving in response to the flow of cerebrospinal fluid. The occiput and sphenoid (joined by the sphenoid–basilar joint) flex and expand in response to the filling and emptying of cerebrospinal fluid. The sphenoid–basilar joint is a cartilaginous joint. All the other joints (sutures) in the skull are fibrous joints. Note, a cartilaginous joint has more mobility than a fibrous joint. As the cerebrospinal fluid fills the cranium, 'the sphenoid moves with the front part of the cranium, arching forward and down (together with the frontal bone)' (Attlee 2012: 184). This is called flexion and expansion. At the same time, 'the occiput moves back, mediating this movement' (Attlee 2012: 184). As the cerebrospinal fluid empties, 'the sphenoid bone and occiput move back into place. This is called extension and contraction' (Attlee 2012: 184). All the other cranial bones move in response – isn't this wonderful to know? At the same, and in synchronicity, the sacrum also flexes and extends. The sacrum rocks forward in the flexion phase (the expansion/filling), and back in the extension phase (the contraction/emptying) phase (Attlee 2012: 171–72). The occiput, sphenoid and sacrum, plus the entire vertebral column flex (expand) and extend (contract) together in response to the production, circulation and reabsorption of cerebrospinal fluid. Note that, 'flexion indicates that the apex of the sacrum is moving anteriorly' and 'extension indicates that apex is moving posteriorly' (Attlee 2012: 172). For clarity, below I offer Attlee's full description of how all the cranial bones move in relation to cerebrospinal fluid. The most important thing to note is the cranial bones are mobile and fluid, rather than fixed and solid.

Sphenoid bone

During rhythmic motion, the sphenoid bone moves with the front part of the cranium, arching forward and down (together with the frontal bone) during the expansion phase, coming back up again during the contraction phrase, hinging around the sphenoid-basilar synchondrosis.

(Attlee 2019: 184)

The occipital bone

This forward and down movement is the opposite of the movement of the occiput and back of the head, thereby creating the flexion/extension movement at the inferior surface of the sphenoid-basilar synchondrosis.

(Attlee 2019: 184)

The frontal bone

During the expansion phase of motion, the frontal areas arcs forward and down towards the face (following the movement of the sphenoid into flexion). During the contraction phase, the frontal area comes back and up.

(Attlee 2019: 210)

The temporal bones

The temporal bones open out into external rotation during the expansion phase. They come back into internal rotation during the contraction phase.

(Attlee 2019: 196)

The parietal bones

The two parietals flare (during the expansion phase of motion) and narrow (during the contraction phase of motion) hinging around the sagittal suture.

(Attlee 2019: 217)

The sacrum

The sacrum, being a single midline structure, responds to the expansion and contraction of rhythmic motion by rocking forward and back into flexion (during the expansion phase) and extension (during the contraction phase).

(Attlee 2012: 171)

The dural tube and how it connects to your cranial bones and vertebral column

Along your midline, the cranial bones, plus the entire vertebral column flex (expand) and extend (contract) together. This is because the membranous tube that contains the flow of CSF is attached internally (within) the cranial bones, and to C2 and C3 in the cervical spine, and at S2 at the sacrum. As the fluid fills and empties within the membranous tube, the bones also move and respond. Let us take a deeper look at the membranous tube that contains the flow of CSF and attaches internally to the bones along your midline.

The membrane system is a continuous tissue sheath or tube that surrounds the entire brain and spinal cord. While it is a continuous tissue sheath running from the cranium to the sacrum, the tissue membrane within the cranium is often referred to as *cranial dura*, and the tissue membrane within the vertebral column is often referred to as *spinal dura*. Sometimes it is useful to differentiate the cranial and spinal dura to sense–perceive the attachment points of the membrane within the vertebral column (C2, C3 and S2), or the attachments within the cranium (at the frontal bone, the two parietal bones, the two temporal bones, the occipital bone, the sphenoid bone and the ethmoid bone). However, the cranial and spinal dura are one continuous sheath or fluent tube. Together the cranial and spinal dura are often referred to as the dura mater or dural tube. As Sumner and Haines share:

> The dura mater of the cranial and spinal cavities is a continuous structure made from one sheet of collagen fibre. This offers an intelligent system creating postural balance for the axis of the body and beyond. Any reorganisation in the dura as a result of a state of balance will affect the whole unit of function of the cranial and spinal dural enfoldment. Its holistic nature means that any trauma to part of the system will inevitably have an effect on the whole.
>
> (Sumner and Haines 2010: 128)

'The meningeal system or dura mater envelops the whole brain and spinal cord in each of us' (Upledger 2001: 2). It is composed of three layers of membrane. The three layers are called: *the dura mater* (this is the outer most layer, meaning tough mother); *the pia mater* (this is the inner most layer, meaning soft mother); and *the arachnoid layer* that lies between the dura and pia mater. However, between the pia mater and the arachnoid layer is *a subarachnoid space* – this is the space where cerebrospinal fluid flows and circulates around the brain and spinal cord (Upledger 2001; Attlee 2012).

> If these layers stick together in an area, the result is pain. Where the pain locates depends upon where the membranes are stuck together and whether or not nerves are involved or 'pinched' in the stuck areas. Pain can be local or referred to a distance.
>
> (Upledger 2001: 2)

The above quote is highly significant in this chapter and influences my practice in the studio. For example, later in this chapter, I will share a process of sense–perceiving the internal attachment points of the dural tube and moving these areas into fluency to release pain and restriction. Noted in nearly all books on craniosacral therapy, the word mater is from the Latin mother, and its etymological root reflects the protective and nurturing nature of the dura mater. The dura mater, the most outer layer, is tougher and stronger; it attaches to the bones from within the cranium, and to some of the bones within the vertebral column (outlined above). As Sumner and Haines shared above, the intercranial membranes are often restricted. 'Tensions within the membranes can have widespread effects, both locally and distantly, both within the cranium and down the spine, impinging on nerves and nerve roots, constricting blood vessels' and 'restricting the movement of bones' (Attlee 2012: 34).

Note that, within the cranium the dural membrane is attached internally to the: frontal bone, the parietal bones, the temporal bones, the occipital bone, the sphenoid bone and the ethmoid bone. By softening and easing the cranial bones, we can start to release tensions beneath the cranial bones in the dura mater. More specifically, the cranial dura has a number of enfoldments that attach within the cranium to specific cranial bones. These are:

> *Falx cerebri*: to the ethmoid bone (at the crista galli), frontal, parietals and occipital
> *Falx cerebelli*: to the occiput
> *Tentorium cerebelli*: to the occiput, parietals, temporals, sphenoid
> *Diaphragma sellae*: to the sphenoid
>
> (Attlee 2012: 32)

As Attlee notes, 'the influence of these membranous attachments plays an integral part in the rhythmic motion of the cranium, establishing fulcrums around which the individual bones express their expansive and contractive movements' (Attlee 2012: 32–33). By softening and easing the cranial bones, with a focus on the occipital bone, temporal bones, parietal bones, ethmoid bone and sphenoid bone we can start to unwind tensions and imbalances within the intracranial membranes. When we sense–perceive the cranial bones floating on the dura below and augment the motility of the cranial bones through soothing, tender, delicate and highly attuned self-regulatory movement in gravity, we can make contact with all these internal fulcrums.

To support practice, note again, the spinal dura is attached from within the vertebral column to the following:

> The foreman magnum: the dural tube is attached firmly around the circumference of the foreman magnum
> The cervical vertebra: The dural tube attaches to the cervical spine internally to C2 and C3
> The sacrum: at S2
> The coccyx: 'via the filum terminale – a thin filament of membrane (comprising all three layers of membrane) which passes down from the lower end of the spinal cord to attach to the posterior surface of the first coccygeal segment'.
>
> (Attlee 2012: 33)

By softening and easing the vertebral column, with a focus on C2, C3 and S2, we can start to unwind tensions and imbalances in the spinal dura. All the attachment points noted above can be attuned to, offering places of loosening, easing and softening through self-regulatory movement. As Agustoni shares 'by relaxing the cranial bones and sutures, the internal meningeal tissues surrounding the brain and spinal cord start to relax' (2003: 42). Thus, 'the external bones and the internal soft tissues are in a reciprocal relationship' (2003: 42).

Cerebrospinal fluid has a rhythm that can be sense–perceived in the motion of the cranial bones, the vertebral column, the sacrum and tailbone. Shared in Chapter 3, the foramen magnum notably provides the attachment for the dural tube. The membranous dura is firmly attached around the entire circumference of the foramen magnum. The dura around the foramen magnum marks the beginning of the spinal membranes, or spinal dura that runs all the way to the sacrum and the coccyx. If you glance at Figure 6.7, you can observe the dural tube dropping all the way from the foramen magnum to the sacrum – and in fact – the coccyx (the filum terminale). Sensing into the foramen magnum and initiating movement from the attachment points of the cranial and spinal dura is a wonderful way of bringing balance to the craniosacral system. Agustoni further reflects on the importance of the connection between the dural tube and the attachment points below,

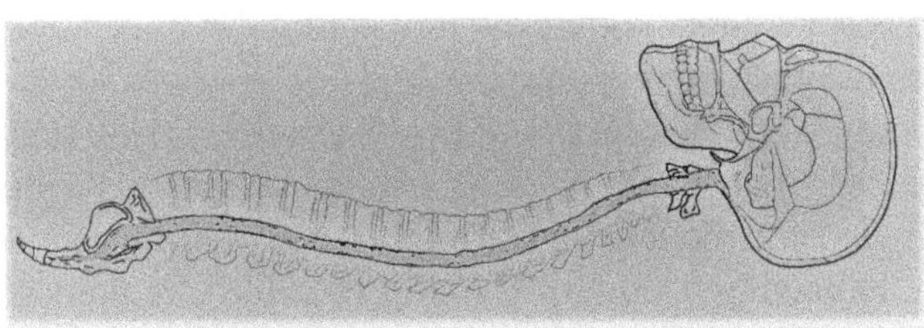

FIGURE 6.7: The dural tube. Image and art by Tony Preston.

> The connection between sacrum, spine, and occipital bone is of central importance for the cranio-sacral system. The spinal dura mater (dura mater spinalis), which covers and protects the medulla, is fastened at the great foraman magnum, in the area of the second (C2) and third (C3) cervical vertebra and at the sacrum. The craniosacral rhythm is transmitted via the occipital bone, the connective tissue, and the spinal dura mater downward to the sacrum and the pelvis.
>
> (Agustoni 2003: 42–43)

The slow rhythm of cerebrospinal fluid

> Everyone has several kinds of rhythms in their body. There is the cardiac rhythm, in which the heart beats 60–80 times per minute. Then there is the respiratory rhythm of your breathing, in which you inhale and exhale 15–20 times per minute. Underneath those rhythms is another one called the CranioSacral Rhythm (CSR). In this rhythm your head gently expands and narrows, and your spine gently lengthens and shortens in an effort to exchange and circulate cerebrospinal fluid. It does this 6–12 cycles per minute. The membranes that surround your head and spine act as a little hydraulic pump that draws this clear fluid out of your blood, bathes the brain and spinal cord with it, and then returns it to the blood supply. In this way the cerebral-spinal fluid is filtered and renewed.
>
> (Upledger 2008: 29)

Explored further in Chapter 7, sense–perceiving the free flow of fluids within the body is a defining educational and therapeutic principle inherent in the somatic movement paradigm. It is one of the most significant differences between the bodywork we offer, compared to other restorative health modalities that use a bio-mechanical model, such as those found in sports science. In bio-mechanical models, the focus is on muscles, bones and nerves, and an overly external mechanical perception of the human body. In somatic movement practices, much focus is on internal fluid, fluctuating within the human organism (Conrad 2007; Cohen 1993). The health of our body relies on different, but interrelated fluid systems that exchange and support each other in constant circulatory motion.

Note in Upledger's quote above, the flow and pulse of cerebrospinal fluid is much slower than other rhythms in your body. CSF cycles six to twelve cycles per minute, compared to the beat of our hearts which is 60–80 times per minute. Sensing the craniosacral rhythm involves attuned sensory-perceptual awareness that develops over time. Following the importance of autogenic self-regulatory improvisation, defined in Chapters 1 and 2, this tide-like fluid and energy are sensed with more ease when you have shifted into parasympathetic ease-and-release. You might feel this rhythm when you least expect it, but especially when you have dropped into a relaxed state of being, a physiological state where you can receive subtle movements within you. Developing a sensitive relationship with the craniosacral rhythm takes practice. This rhythm is usually far beneath conscious awareness. It is a gentle delicate rhythm that can be augmented through somatically attuned movement all along your midline.

A short detour into embryology: The primal midline

We need to take a slight detour into embryology in order to share how important and foundational the craniosacral system is – and thus our midline is. When we bring awareness to the craniosacral rhythm, we are attuning to a fluid midline and an energy of pre-birth, commonly referred to as 'the fluid midline' or 'the primal midline' in many vitalistic therapies. Our sacred midline starts to develop in the third week of our embryonic development. How lovely this is to share with students! This is a period of development and emergence when we are essentially water beings. Thus, when we contact this rhythm, we use images of tides, waves, the ocean and still water to guide somatic touch and movement in the studio. 'The embryo is a water being that congeals over time' (Shea 2010: 5). As the embryo develops 'it becomes denser' in the 'ebb and flow' of embryonic fluids (Shea 2010: 5). Sense–perceiving the craniosacral rhythm is sometimes a watery embryonic experience. We are contacting a fluid line, prior to our experience of gravity; thus, the midline is a very ancient water source of our emergence and becoming. Sumner and Haines beautifully introduce the complexity of the primal and fluid midline below.

> The primal midline starts life as a surge of cell reorganisation in the ectodermal layer of the embryonic disk at the start of the third week after conception. A primitive streak appears from the caudal end of the disc, rising up over a day to produce a pit half way up the length of the disk. This uprising movement is a movement that typifies the expression of the primal midline throughout life [...] By day 17 after conception there is a hollow tube formed in the mesoderm that will become solid and be the reference for the neural tube and the gut tube. Therefore, the notochord is the first midline tube to be formed and the primitive streak is the first expression of midline motion. Over the next few days the action of differential growth means the primitive streak diminishes as the notochord becomes more prominent. It's as if the primitive streak represents an energetic surge or directional intention that creates a chain reaction of midline formations. The primitive streak is there for a day and gone the next, while the notochord becomes the first axis of the developing body.
>
> (Sumner and Haines 2010: 49–50)

To further elucidate Sumner's writing above, the primitive streak and the developing notochord can be viewed as a foundational life-force and emerging midline that we can return to in the studio when we feel stressed, disorganized and muddled. Of profound significance, with the arrival of the primitive streak the rostro-caudal (head to tail) axis of the embryo develops (Webster and Wreede 2016: 14). It is a faint beautiful line, and it is a mystery why this line appears and where it comes from. It first appears at the caudal end (the tail) of the embryo and grows up cranially. The primitive streak, noted by the writers above, is an energetic surge that lays the foundation for other midline formations. The primitive streak is transient, appearing only for a day, and therefore the notochord is considered the first substantial axis of the developing embryo. Sumner and Haines further share:

> It's understandable that this process could be viewed as a mystical expression which reveals the fundamental movement of life often referred to by the yogis as kundalini, the kabbalists as shekinah, the Taoists as thrusting chi. The notochord is the central energetic channel of the body system that underpins all other channels and body physiology. The notochord, like the primitive streak, dissolves and becomes the energetic phenomenon at the core of the system. The vertebral bodies form around the notochord as do the body of the sphenoid and the ethmoid [...] This is taken therefore as the line of the primal midline. The midline is a fulcrum for all development and healing.
>
> (Sumner and Haines 2010: 60)

Sumner and Haines differentiate between two aspects of the primal midline, one located in your bony craniosacral system and the other located in your fluid sacral cannel. Below is a description of both midlines, which we will return to at the end of this chapter.

> The fluid posterior midline: it starts as a neural grove; it is located within the spinal cord through the lamina terminalis at the front of the third ventricle.
>
> The primal anterior midline: it passes through the coccyx, sacrum, vertebral bodies and cranial base ending at the sphenoid body/ethmoid. A continual (therefore non-tidal) uprising surge, it follows the path of the notochord.
>
> (Sumner and Haines 2010: 50–51)

Of super heightened note, the flow and motility of the craniosacral system is considered primary – i.e., if the cranial bones and sacrum are not moving in rhythmic response with the internal flow of cerebrospinal fluid, then the pulmonary respiratory system is hindered (Sutherland 1990). Thus, the craniosacral system, and its fluid rhythm, is considered more formative than pulmonary respiration; this is why the craniosacral system is often referred to as 'primary respiration' (Upledger 2010: 5). Sumner and Haines write, 'our ability to be in relationship to primary respiration can be seen as our ultimate resource' (Sumner 2010: 60).

Cerebrospinal fluid circulates along your midline – from your cranium all the way to your tail (your sacrum/coccyx). The importance of this system can be seen in many ancient traditions – kundalini energy rising is the most obvious. Essentially it is a surge of life-force moving from sacrum to the cranial bones – a surge that appears in the third week of our embryonic development, noted above. This rhythm often evades sensory-perceptual awareness in the early stages of studio practice. Frustration can cause this rhythm to drop further out of sensory-perceptual reach – approaching this fluid requires slow-time being, love, patience and a non-judgemental approach towards Self and other – and the lightest of touch and reverence. I use the word reverence because the cranial bones and their motion are usually beneath our collective and personal consciousness. These amazing bones, and their gentle motion, feel so relieved and soothed when they are acknowledged, named, touched or held. The cranial bones call for touch and appreciation – just as people need to be witnessed, acknowledged, touched, appreciated and nurtured by others.

Many practices in the field of somatic movement contact the craniosacral system indirectly. For example, releasing, tipping and pouring the weight of the cranium (shared throughout this book) is likely to support the flow of cerebrospinal fluid. Gravitational movement explorations that contact the intelligence of spinal mobility, integrating the fluency of the cervical, thoracic, lumbar and sacral spine, are likely to assist the flow of craniosacral fluid. When participants augment the fluidity of their vertebral column, it is likely to change the fascial viscosity of the dural tube and its attachments. As participants curl and uncurl, the spinal nerves that exist on each side of vertebrae (that are covered in fascia) are likely to find ease. Freeing restricted nerves also contributes the free flow of CSF.

'The craniosacral system supports many other body systems' such as 'circulation (arterial and venous blood), the nervous system, endocrine system (hormonal system), lymphatic, respiratory system, and musculoskeletal system' (muscles, connective tissue, fascia, ligaments, tendons and joints) (Agustoni 2003: 10). Of note, any relaxation activity offered in the studio that supports the regulation of the autonomic nervous system is likely to support the craniosacral system. 'Relaxing strengthens our autonomic nervous system through its parasympathetic elements and thus supports our self-regulation and regeneration from inside our bodies' (Agustoni 2011: 10). Upledger shares that craniosacral work

> improves fluid movement in all systems throughout the body. By doing this it enhances the supply of nutrients to cells; the removal of toxins and waste products

from the tissues; the circulation of immune cells, thus enhancing the body's natural defences against disease producing bacteria and viruses; the delivery of fresh blood to organs and tissues; and the movement of cerebrospinal fluid.

(Upledger 2001: 65)

Sensing the cranial bones

Settling into awareness I map the contours of my skull.
Occiput releasing, surrounding tissues easing,
melting into gravity.
Parietal bones soften and breathe gently into my hands.
Frontal bone lets go of thoughts and unnecessary clutter.
Temporal bones pulse with rivers of vitality and lifeforce.
I offer myself comfort and ease through a deep listening.
Sensing into the hidden caverns within, a bright light shines at the centre
like a jewel in the mountain.
It glistens and glows, Illuminating the beautiful sphenoid bone.
I am in the presence of the pituitary and hypothalamus.
Gentle waves of light and life vibrate into the vast landscape of body.

(Karin Rugman, poetic embodied reflections after sense–perceiving and moving with awareness of her cranial bones)

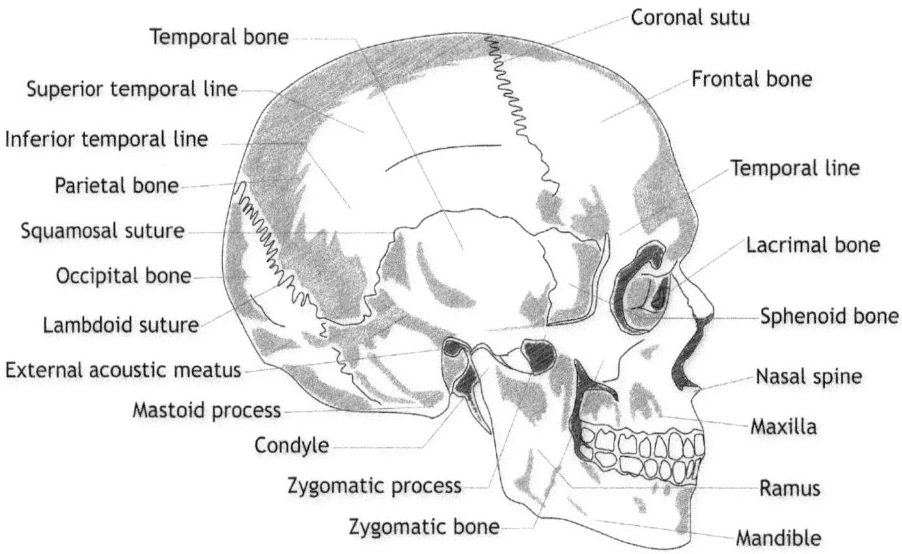

FIGURE 6.8: The cranial sutures.

The easiest way to introduce participants to the craniosacral system is through the bones first; specifically, the cranial bones, vertebral column, sacrum and tail bone. Bone is a denser tissue, and we can feel our structure readily, in contrast to the allusiveness, lightness and spatiality of the CSF. Through the bones, we are inviting participants to make sensory contact with their 'primal anterior midline' that 'passes through the coccyx, sacrum, vertebral bodies and cranial base ending at the sphenoid body/ethmoid' (Sumner and Haines 2010: 50). Below I offer a pathway into the craniosacral system through gravity, soft-tissue-rolling and touch. How we touch the cranial bones will affect our experience and consciousness of these bones. Our intention is to bring awareness to their living presence – their aliveness, floating motility, beingness, sensitivity and intelligence. These bones are a living part of our being. They love care, attention, communication and relationship. The more you sense–perceive your cranial bones through your hands, lightly, listening to their quality and living beingness, the more motility you will feel.

I invite participants to build an intimate relationship with their cranial bones, know where they are, name them, and sense–perceive their self-regulatory intelligence through touch and movement. Each bone has a different quality and even a different emotionality. I use the word emotionality because each bone feels vastly different, and often participants feel very emotional when they start to build a relationship with the living tissues of each bone. Usually perceived as hard and solid, in practice they become living beings, motile and alive. Below I share brief examples of participants contacting their cranial bones.

Each bone can be sense–perceived by releasing the weight of the occiput into the hands of the therapist, into one's own hands, or into the floor. Naming the bones, albeit through a male-centric western anatomical language, as well as sense–perceiving their aliveness, acknowledges their living presence in a mechanistic world that devalues the intelligence of our living tissues and separates us from our living source.

Rather than perceiving the cranium as a solid object that encloses your brain tightly, it is useful to re-perceive each cranial bone as floating lightly on the dura that surrounds your brain. Sumner and Haines write extensively on how the bones of the cranium float because they are in a fluid relationship with the membranes, and cerebral spinal fluid below them. As Sumner and Haines exquisitely express, the 'cranial bones are islands in a sea of membrane and fluid' (Sumner and Haines 2010: 130). They further write

> bones are never alone. In fact nothing in the body is ever alone because there is always connective tissue close by. In the case of the neurocranium and the spinal column it's the dura mater membrane. The vault bones have a particularly strong relationship to it as they grown out of a layer of membranes themselves. These bones are literally part of the dura mater and move in a strong synchrony with it.

The bones are also in a strong relationship to fluids. The meninges contain cerebrospinal fluid and the bones can often feel like they floating on water, and being pushed around like flotsam and jetsam. A true experience of the bones of the neurocranium would be to acknowledge the relationships to membranes, fluids and nervous tissue. In addition the bones themselves are highly fluid and have an internal space. There is a constant flow of blood. The movements are fluid-like even though they are discrete structures.

(Sumner and Haines 2010: 130)

Cupping the occiput
I notice the heaviness and weight of my burdens.
They slowly melt and release into my hands.
I feel the embrace of my ancestors behind me
supporting me and
guiding me forward.
There to catch me when I falter.
Drawing from my roots,
a strong impulse of life force.
I am here.

As I greet my parietal bones
and breathe into my hands,
I feel the comfort of the womb.
A warm, safe space of deep listening.
I expand into its edges
and feel reassured and calm.
Encased in love.

Sensing my temporal bones,
my head floats.
A lightness of being,
widening and expanding.
Breathing into growth and certainty.

Vision of forest in frontal lobe.
Dark greens and blues cascade
and swirl in my sight.
Long dark tunnel,
like a cavernous trail
in the heart of a mountain.

Leading me somewhere?
My hands become eyes
that look out toward the future.
Light and space,
I become an eagle
soaring high in the luminous sky.
Catching the breeze and
drifting on its edges,
I feel freedom
and peace.

(Karin Rugman, reflective writing after sense–perceiving her cranial bones)

Example of practice: Soft-tissue-rolling around the cranium: Sensing the sutures and bones

When we rest the occiput in gravity, and start to tip and pour the cranium, we roll onto the other cranial bones, such as *the temporal bones*, *the parietal bones*, *the sphenoid bone* and the *frontal bone*. Each of these bones are connected by fibrous sutures. 'The places where the edges of these skull bones come together are actually very specialized joints' (Upledger 1997: 146). We have been taught that the cranial bones are fused together. This idea is deeply embedded in our socio-historical collective consciousness. However, noted earlier, there is slight movement in the sutures, and these tiny movements are essential to health. As Upledger notes, 'the sutures are full of elastic fibres, and collagen tissue, nerve and blood vessels – they are very much alive' (Upledger 1997: 149). They are not white, dried up and solid as seen in the craniums of skeletons. Further, 'the motions are very small, on the order of one – or two-sixteenths of an inch' and 'very difficult to see with the human eye' (Upledger 1997: 148). And further, the dura mater (below the bones) weaves up into the living sutures, and thus, the dura mater tissue is connected to the sutures. There are four primary sutures, full of nerves and blood vessels, that are useful to sense–perceive when you soft-tissue-roll your cranium in gravity. When participants are invited to tip, pour and roll their cranium in gravity (always with breath awareness and with the body fluidly following), they are transmitting a gentle pressure across the following main sutures:

The lambdoid suture is the joint between the parietal bones and the occipital bone.
The squamous suture is the joint between the parietal bones and the temporal bones.
The coronal suture is the joint between the frontal bone and the parietal bones.

The sagittal suture is the joint between the two parietal bones.
The occipitomastoid suture separates the occipital bone and mastoid portion of temporal bone.

Participants are also transmitting a gentle pressure across the many sutures surrounding the sphenoid bone. For example:

- *The sphenofrontal suture* is the cranial suture between the sphenoid bone and the frontal bone.
- *The sphenoparietal suture* (this is the suture between the sphenoid bone and the parietal bones).
- *The sphenosquamosal suture* (this is the suture between the sphenoid bone and the squama of the temporal bones).
- *The pterion* (this is where the frontal, parietal, temporal and sphenoid bones join together. You can locate this place on the side of the skull, just behind the temples).

All the joints in the body are vital to integrated health, and the sutures in the skull are no exception to this rule. It is the space between the bones and their fluid articulations, whether fibrous, cartilaginous or synovial that supports softening, ease, release. The cranial sutures feel complicated to learn at first, but participants soon become familiar with them through self-touch and self-regulatory movement.

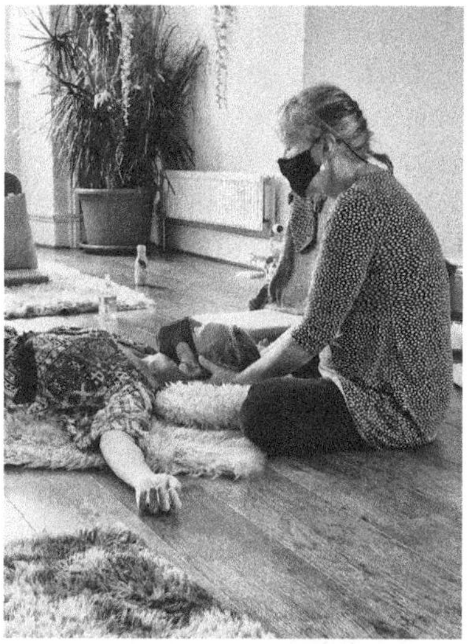

FIGURE 6.9: Amanda Williamson and Karin Rugman: sensing cranial bones and sutures. Photographer: Natasha Martin.

The occipitomastoid suture and the squamous suture

Invite participants to roll onto and release the weight of their cranium into your hands (palms). Encourage them to slowly tip, pour, yield and soften (rest) their cranium in your hands. Allow the participant to use your hands as a fulcrum. Share with them that they can drop the weight of their cranium into your hands, tip, glide and slide, roll and rest – respond in relation to your touch. Invite them to sense their occipital bone and then tip slowly onto their temporal bones and parietal bones. Here they are crossing the occipitomastoid suture and the squamous suture. Invite them to notice when they are transmitting pressure across the occipitomastoid suture

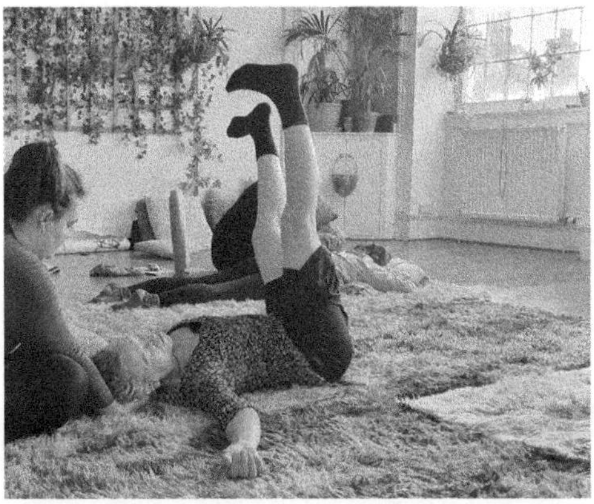

FIGURE 6.10: Celine Parsons and Amanda Williamson: soft-tissue rolling the cranial bones. Photographer: Sylvia Gregory.

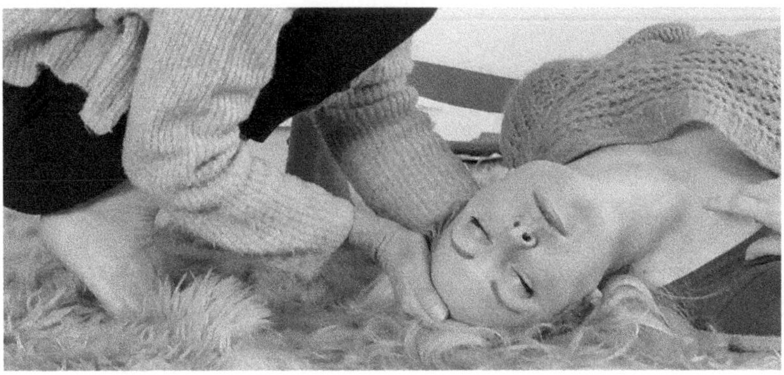

FIGURE 6.11: Sarah Pinch and Hazel Rose. Photographer: Amanda Williamson. You can invite clients to soft-tissue roll their cranium in your hands. Invite them to use your hands as a fulcrum, self-regulating how they want and need to move.

and the squamous suture. As participants tip and pour, invite them to rest in their temporal and parietal bones, noticing if there is a difference in the sense–feeling between these bones. Invite them to sense–perceive when they are crossing sutures. Never force, but rather invite them to listen to the intelligence of these bones, and if they want to rest, soften or still. Sometimes the cranial bones call for rest, sometimes for a little pressure – sometimes they enjoy a continuous soft-tissue-rolling on the floor or in hands. If you work gently and attentively and only invite movement that feels delicious you can gently decompress the bones.

The lambdoid suture

When participants gently tip their head backwards, they are moving from their occipital bone onto their parietal bones, and in doing so, are transmitting a gentle

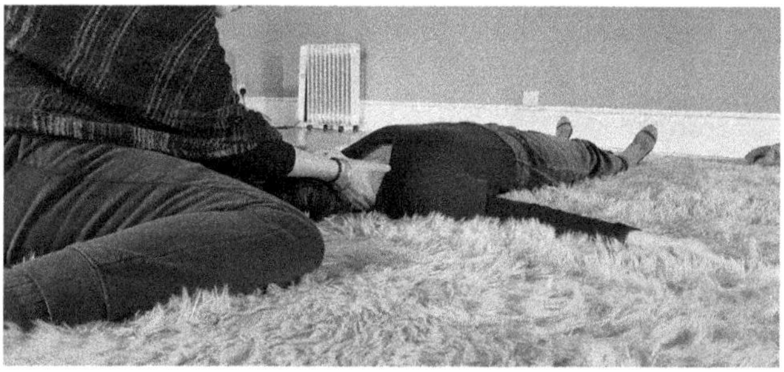

FIGURE 6.12: Movingsoma students: sensing the Lambdoid suture. Invite a softeness tenderly contacting these bones. Photographer: Amanda Williamson.

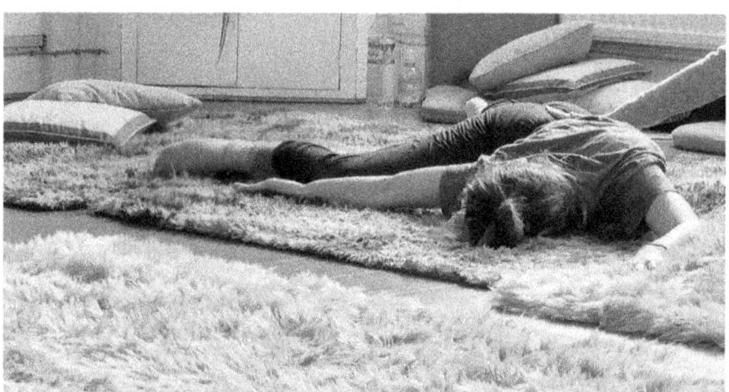

FIGURE 6.13: Jessica Cotton. Photographer: Amanda Williamson. Your client may roll away from you in order to self-regulate, especially when sensing the frontal bone, and the sagittal and coronal sutures.

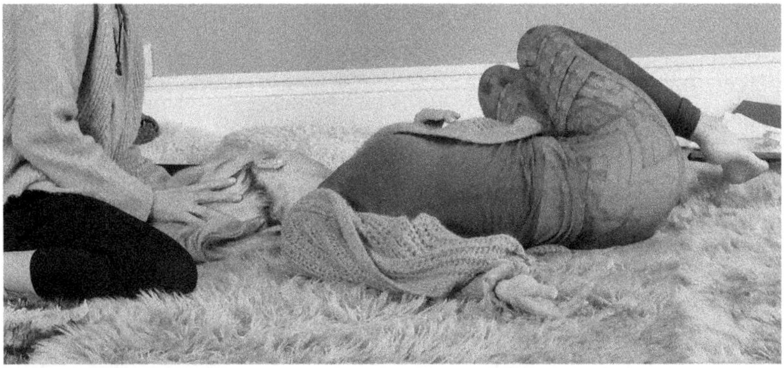

FIGURE 6.14: Movingsoma students: sensing their cranial bones and sutures: Photographer: Amanda Williamson.

pressure across the lambdoid suture. Invite participants to enjoy gently tipping back onto their parietal bones, crossing the lambdoid suture. Invite them to sense–perceive the occipital bone and the parietal bones in your hands, noticing a difference in sense–feeling between these bones. Encourage them to see if they can sense the transitional tissues of the lambdoid suture. Keeping the cervical spine soft and responsive and the rest of the body tenderly following.

The coronal suture

Invite participants to tip, pour and roll around onto their frontal bone. This journey will take time. Invite the rest of the body to follow, softly spiralling, curving and unwinding. Invite participants to sense–perceive their frontal bones in gravity, and the transitional tissues of the coronal suture between the frontal bone and parietal bones.

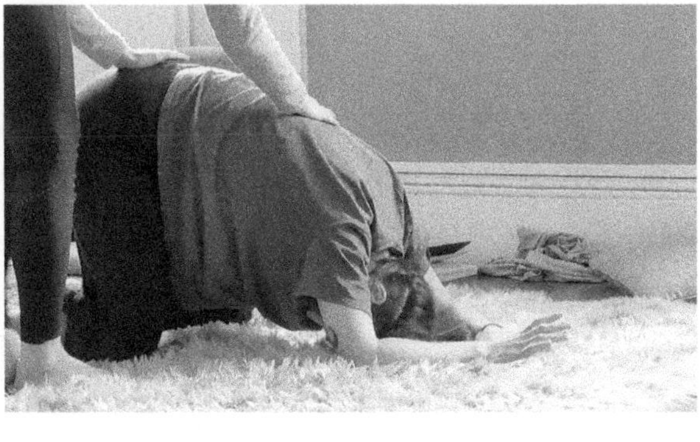

FIGURE 6.15: Your client may roll away from you in order to self-regulate, especially when sensing the sagittal suture. Photographer: Amanda Williamson.

The sagittal suture

Sense–perceiving the coronal suture necessitates gently rolling the cranium in gravity, with the body following, often taking participants into usual positions. The sagittal suture is harder to sense if you are new to movement. Invite participants to roll lightly from their frontal bone onto their parietal bones and sense–perceive the long sagittal suture. Invite the mover to explore all their cranial bones, with the body following.

> I found it interesting that when I attend a somatic movement session, I love my head being touched the most. My head feels heavy with repetitive thoughts, looping worries (self-castigation is my main thinking), making me anxious. When my head is held, oh my goodness, wow, what a relief. It's a process where I feel renewed and so light, that I feel fun again and connection with others. I feel trust, when you hold my head. Trust in humans, not fear of them. This work has helped my depression, which is on-going and I need to find ways to live again, in pain. Hold my head please! Let's do this process again. It's magical. I know it's science too, but I expand, release, and just feel such care during cranial bone work. I know you care for me, because you are attending so gently to me.
>
> (Clare Wiley)

Example of practice: Releasing the intercranial membranes and loosening the dural membranes

Invite participants into soft-tissue-rolling around all their bones and the major sutures. Invite participants to follow easeful pathways that feel comfortable and delicious, never forcing too much pressure on the bones. By softening and easing the cranial bones, we can start to release tensions beneath the cranial bones in the dura mater. The cranial dura has a number of enfoldments that attach from within the cranium

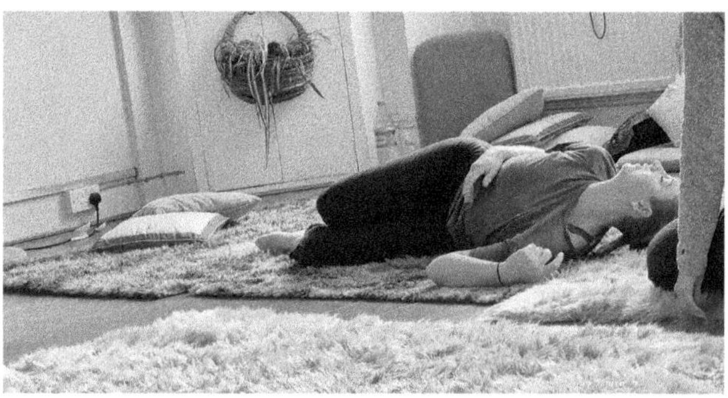

FIGURE 6.16: Soft-tissue rolling around the cranium with co-regulatory support.

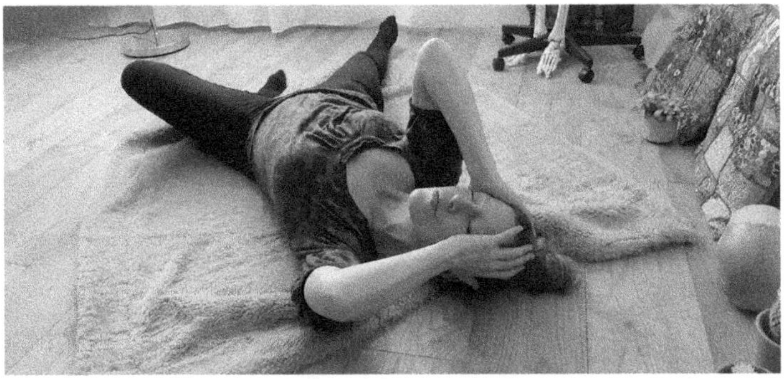

FIGURE 6.17: Amanda Williamson: self-touch, tender, kind and gentle. Sensing bones calling for touch. Photographer: Scott Closson.

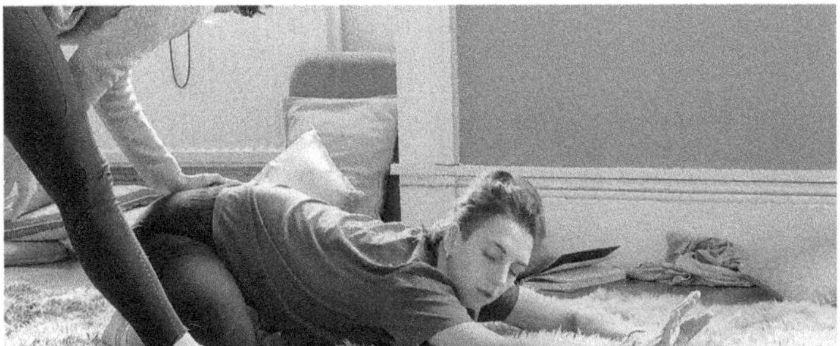

FIGURE 6.18: Jessica Cotton: sense–perceiving the dural tube in the sacrum and tail bone. Photographer: Amanda Williamson.

to specific cranial bones. As you soften, breathe, and roll, you can release restrictions in the Falx cerebri, Falx cerebelli, Tentorium cerebelli, and the Diaphragma sellae.

Notice which bones are calling for self-touch, connection, love, care, breath, sound, toning and humming.

Sometimes the bones like to follow your hands, or someone else's hands, surging and pouring their weight and fluid content into hands. At other times they like to rest and soften into your hands. Listen to their self-regulatory intelligence.

Example of practice: Loosening the dural membranes

We noted earlier that the fascial membrane, commonly called the dural tube is a continuous sheath that surrounds the brain and spinal cord, and the brain and spinal

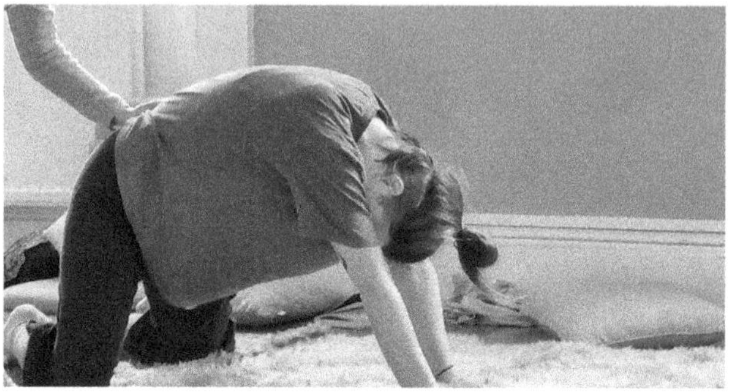

FIGURE 6.19: Jessica Cotton, sense–tracking her dura. Photographer: Scott Closson.

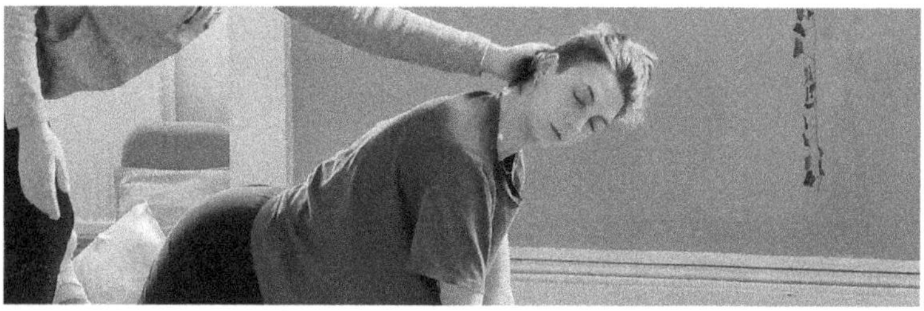

FIGURE 6.20: Jessica Cotton: sense–perceiving the dural attachments at C2 & C3. Photographer: Amanda Williamson.

cord floats in cerebrospinal fluid. We also noted that this continuous membrane is attached to the cranium (within), attached to the vertebral column (within) at C2 and C3 (in the cervical spine) and attached within at S2 (in the sacral region). Additionally, we noted that this fascial sheath is made of collagen and can get restricted, just like any other soft tissue in the body. Therefore, I often invite participants into self-regulatory movement that loosens the spinal dura mater, via head-to-tail play, and with a particular focus on the internal attachment points. The practice I share in the figures 6.18, 6.19 and 6.20, invites participants to drop their awareness into the following areas, sense–perceiving how these areas need to move and loosen:

- the foramen magnum
- C2 and C3
- the sacrum at S2
- the Coccyx (the filum terminale).

> This way of working is a safe space, full of light and nature where I can unfurl and begin settle into a slower more natural rhythm, drop to gravity and come home to

my body. As someone without a dance background I've found this process very liberating. Both the space and my experiences during our sessions have been profoundly nurturing and healing. The work is inspiring, helping me to develop a deeper awareness of my joints, tissues and nervous system and gain new perspectives. When we work on the cranial bones, a lightness and playfulness of spirit arrives, as well as a soothing feeling through all of me.

(Ellen Wright)

Example of practice: Sensing–perceiving the posterior midline

Earlier I shared Sumner and Haines's description of the anterior and posterior midline. I will refer to it again below for clarity.

> The fluid posterior midline: it starts as a neural grove; it is located within the spinal cord through the lamina terminalis at the front of the third ventricle.
>
> The primal anterior midline: it passes through the coccyx, sacrum, vertebral bodies and cranial base ending at the sphenoid body/ethmoid.
>
> (Sumner and Haines 2010: 50)

We remember that both these midlines developed from the primitive streak and later the notochord in our early embryonic development. One is bony and the other is fluid. So far in this chapter, in terms of practice, we have focused on the anterior midline, and the cranial bones and sutures, which is the bony aspect of the craniosacral system. We have also focused on releasing restrictions in the cranial and spinal dura. In the last part of this chapter, I share coming into sensory relationship with the posterior midline, which can be felt through a slightly different orientation to the spinal cord, CSF fluid and the soft membranes surrounding it. In this process, you are sensing your spinal cord, floating in the dural tube. The spinal canal passes down within your vertebral column, and thus you are moving your sense–perception from bones into fluid. It is a qualitatively different experience to sensing the bones along the midline, although a sense of fluency should define both experiences. Softening in mouth, releasing in the jaw, sensing an opening in the neural cavity, and moving your awareness to the front of your spine, surrounded by soft tissues helps to contact the posterior midline.

> I was taught spirituality was without me, above in the sky, and therefore praying always reached, looked beyond the body. The monotheistic religion I grew up in badly damaged me - it split me in two. The cranial processes invite me to pray through

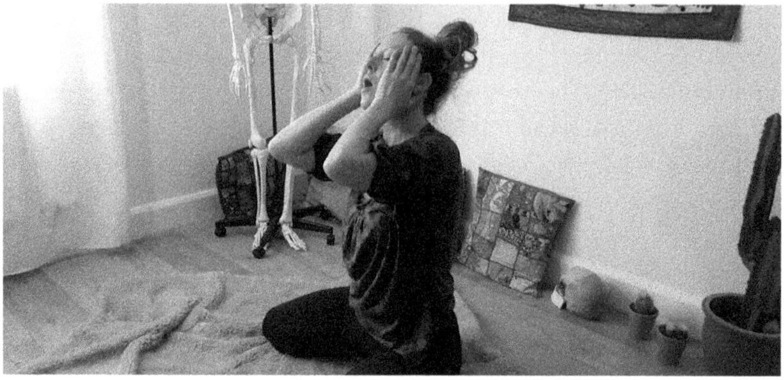

FIGURE 6.21: Amanda Williamson: sense–perceiving her neural cavity and posterior midline. Photographer: Scott Closson.

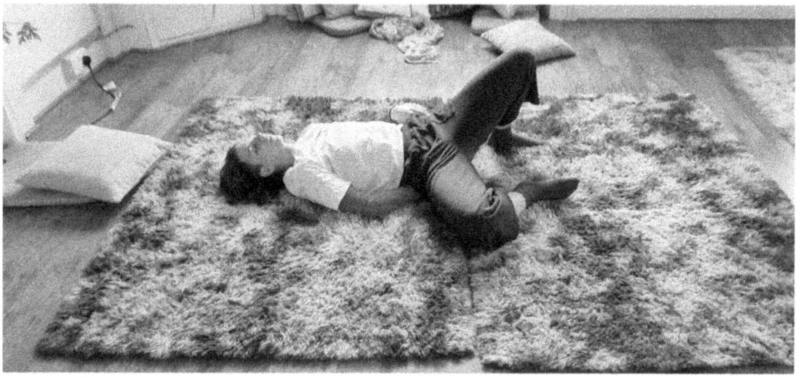

FIGURE 6.22: Jessica Cotton: sense–perceiving her fluid posterior midline. Photographer: Amanda Williamson.

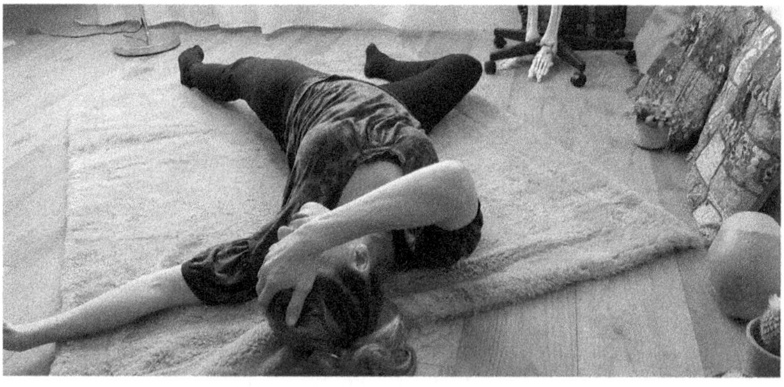

FIGURE 6.23: Amanda Williamson: sensing her fluid midline. Photographer: Scott Closson.

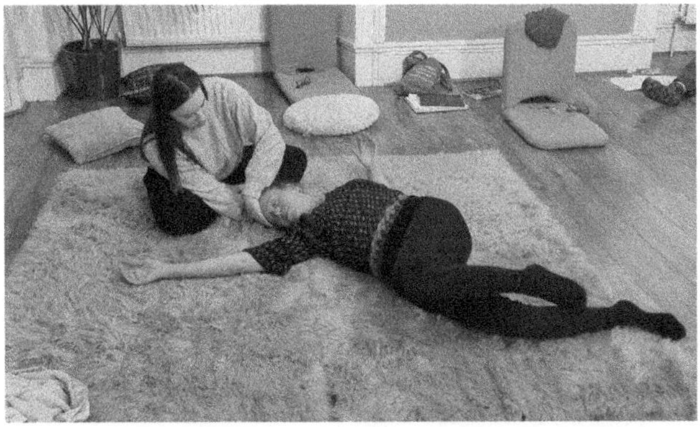

FIGURE 6.24: Natasha Martin and Amanda Williamson: sensing her cranial bones. Photographer: Sylvia Gregory.

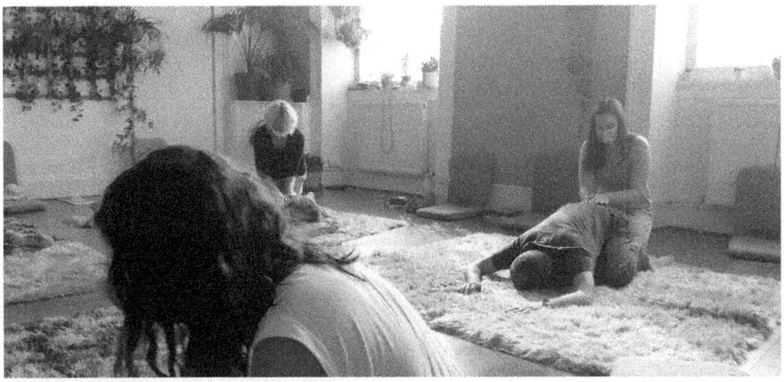

FIGURE 6.25: Movingsoma students: sense–perceiving the sacrum. Photographer: Scott Closson.

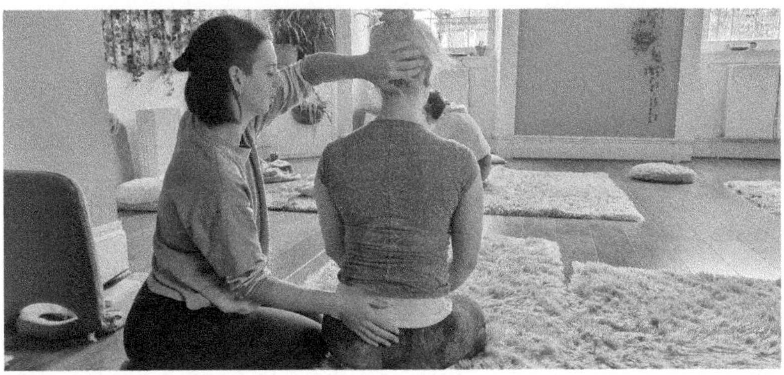

FIGURE 6.26: Sarah Pinch and Jessica Cotton: sense–perceiving the occipital bone and sacrum. Photographer: Amanda Williamson.

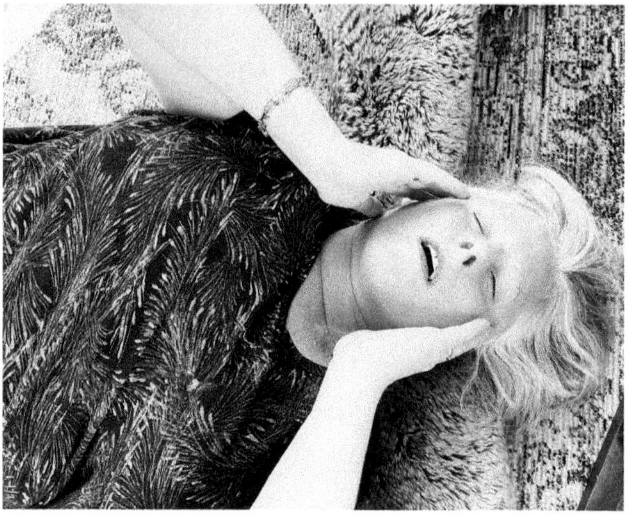

FIGURE 6.27: Vanessa Tucker: sensing her fluid posterior midline. Photographer: Amanda Williamson.

> my body, not with words, but nonverbally with sensation, image and movement. In order to sense the divine, I understand now, that going within is paramount to my health and spirituality. When I settle along my midline, I feel safer and balanced and it helps me stay balanced on a rough day. Instead of ascending, I descend. What deep peace I felt as you held my cranial bones. Knowing you were there for me and you didn't rush was so healing. Time became sacred as I dropped into sensation with you witnessing me. Oh and when I say divine, I mean that life-force breathing within me that I can sense and feel - therefore now I communicate with the divine through sensing, not words.
>
> (Sally Augate)

Key offerings and learnings

Before we move onto Chapter 7, exploring fascial fluidity, I offer some key learnings from this chapter.

- The cranial bones are presented as solid and hard in western anatomy.
- In progressive anatomy and in many vitalistic health modalities they are perceived as floating on the dura and there is a small degree of motility between the bones; thus, the sutures as not fused, but rather alive and living.

- There is often restriction in the cranial and spinal dura: attuned movement can ease and release constrictions in the dura.
- Soft-tissue-rolling *around* the cranium with the body tenderly following and responding is an efficaious self-regulatory and co-regulatory practice.
- Soft-tissue-rolling around the cranium transmits gentle pressure across living sutures, decompressing and reorganizing the cranial bones.
- Movement attuned to the sacrum and cranial bones can assist the flow of CSF and loosen restrictions in the dura.
- Sensing the cranial bones floating on the dura below is vital to decompressing and releasing the bones.

7

Soft-tissue-rolling and Fascial Health

I was amazed that the pain went in my lower back and upper back after class. I had no idea that my fascial tissues might be struck and dehydrated. When I learned about about my trapezius (where it is and which tissues are underneath it) it changed my relationship to my back pain. I learned to soften all my tissues and glide and slide the layers but with such attention. I rubbed my tissue layers into ground and created gentle compressions all around my trapezius and thoracic–lumbar fascia. Gosh what a difference. As I roll my tissues actually tell me where to go. I notice areas of pain, I dwell in these areas and listen to how my fascial tissues need to express out to shift the pain. It looks so simple, but as roll my tissues, especially my trapezius, rhomboids, latismisum dosi, and those long muscle tissues running up my spine, I release. I bring myself blood flow and I replenish my own body. Much more happens, I have dreams too, as I release. When I leave, I have very little pain. I really had no idea every muscle was covered in fascia and the tissues get struck and stressed. I had no idea, before I came here, that fluids constantly move in my tissues. I had no idea that movement can move this fluid. I only ever thought of blood, not lymph, or fascia. Eye-opening education.

(Tom Whisker)

In 2007, Bonnie Gintis published her exceptionally beautiful book *Engaging the Movement of Life: Exploring Health and Embodiment through Osteopathy and Continuum*. The book linked Emilie Conrad's modality 'Continuum Movement' (2007) with approaches used in Osteopathy, particularly motility (the free flow of fluids within the human body). She noted how Continuum and Osteopathy share the principle of supporting the free movement of fluid through the body (Gintis 2007). Sense–perceiving internal bio-flows and augmenting their biological reality is observantly a defining practice-based element of many somatic movement modalities internationally, and indeed found widely in the application of somatics into dance techniques and performance contexts. Emilie Conrad's modality 'Continuum' advanced the importance of the fluid body within the wider paradigm of somatic movement (Conrad 2007), but she was alone. One only has to witness, for example, Contact Improvisation (Pallant 2006), or Bonnie Bainbridge Cohen's work (1993), as well as the many different but interrelated approaches to release-based dance techniques taught in universities, to discern how fluency and motility is an international embodied concern (Brodie and Lobel 2012). Cohen's and Conrad's work on phylogenetic movement and our watery ancestry from the single cell to a multi-cellular organism has had a particularity profound influence on the somatics milieu. However, preceding Conrad and Cohen, earlier pioneers, such as Ida Rolf (1977) and Don Hanlon Johnson (1977) had already made profound connections among cranio-osteopathy, internal motility and the somatics movement in the 1970s. Spirals, circles, non-directional and free-flowing movement underpinned by sensing internal bio-flows inspires many practitioner's work across Europe, the United States, New Zealand and Australia. In fact, I note, it is extremely hard to facilitate somatic movement dance without sharing the healing power of sense–perceiving and augmenting motility in the studio. The body is reperceived and experienced as a watery bio-tensile organism (a fluid fascial matrix), rather than an armoured hard solid angular structure. This re-focusing and reframing is emblematic of the somatic movement dance field at large, and witnessed in cognate bodywork practices, such as craniosacral therapy and cranio-osteopathy.

My own work is underpinned by attuning to bio-flows. When you invite participants into interoceptive awareness, for example, they are connecting with breath, heart and the organ system (the fluid body) which is suspended in the visceral fascia. Thus, a key aspect of interoceptive awareness is in fact attuning to the fluid body. But more than this, improvisation underpinned by somatic awareness (a key characteristic of the field), naturally arguments the fluid systems, particularly the fluency of fascia, the focus of this chapter, which is approximately 70% water.

The somatic movement field has been highly influenced by Ida Rolf (1977) and her classic 'gel-to-sol' model. Emile Conrad was a key somatic movement practitioner who further pioneered the gel-to sol-model. The gel-to-sol model refers to changing the viscosity of fascia through movement and energy (Conrad 2007). It is further important to note, the somatic movement field dance did not grow in isolation but developed alongside other modalities that pioneered fluency and motility, such as craniosacral therapy and cranio-osteopathy (Shea 2010, 2016; Upledger 1997, 2008, 2001). In progressive anatomy and bodywork (which includes somatic movement dance education and therapy), there has been profound shift in consciousness, from perceiving the body as a solid hard angular structure (essentially a pully and lever system), to reperceiving the body as soft, fluidic and bio-tensile.

We are essentially water-based beings, and this realization supported the development of many unique approaches to somatic movement and dance. Gintis shares our water-based reality below:

> Within the human body, the brain is 85% water. Blood is 93% water. Muscle is 75% water. Even bone, which seems so hard, is about 22% water. Muscle bone, and other connective tissues have a unique capacity to bind and release water, shifting from a state of relative gel to sol, changing density and resilience. The lowest content in the body is found in tooth enamel, which is only about 2% water.
>
> (2007: 93)

The shift in my own life from being a hard, armoured, bound and restricted person, to becoming softer, fluid and receptive (and heart-centred) certainly occurred during my own training in somatic movement education and therapy, in Massachusetts. Fluidity and attuning to internal fluid systems was an incredibly special and highly significant aspect my training. As Gintis shares, 'Bio-logical systems are primarily fluid-based, so that most nutrients, waste products, and other things that need to be transmitted are exchanged most freely through fluid' (2007: 91–92). Our fluid systems move, circulate and transform below the threshold of our awareness, but can be enhanced through slow-time sensory-perceptual movement awareness. For example, and explored in Chapter 6, the flow of cerebrospinal fluid, which is approximately 99% water, can be enhanced by moving with awareness of the caudal–cranial axis (the head–tail connection) and decompressing the cranial bones. We noted in Chapter 6, this is because the circulation of cerebrospinal fluid retains its rhythm and flow in relation to the movement of the cranial bones, the vertebral column and the sacrum. Another example of augmenting fluid flow through sensory-perceptual movement awareness is supporting the lymph, which is approximately 95% water, to return to the heart. This can be supported by attuning to breathing and sensing the movement of the thorax and diaphragm in particular, or enhanced through gentle light self-touch, guiding this centripetal fluid from the nodes back towards the heart. Another wonderful example of enhancing bodily fluids through movement is supporting crystallized, stiff and dried out fascia, which is approximately 70% water, to soften into fluency via soft-tissue-rolling in gravity, breaking up adhesions and resolving trigger points. This is the gel-to-sol model in action. Acknowledging, experiencing and empirically investigating our fluid nature – our water-based reality – is key to releasing tensions, restrictions, torsions and pain. Where tissues are restricted, there is pain, such as adhesions in the fascia, which block circulation.

Fascia started to interest me when I became crystallized and absolutely stuck. After working at the computer for decades involved in lecturing, heading up degree programmes, editing and publishing, I suddenly lost the ability to move my arms. I had noticed a range of strange pains across my scapulae and throughout my arms for a number of years, but one day, unexpectedly, I couldn't lift my arms at all – and the pain was unbearable. This experience, while frightening, became my greatest teacher about the living reality, fluency and viscosity of fascia. I was not alone in my experience. Several of my clients who work in education, or who have computer-based jobs were also experiencing pain in their back, arms and neck. Increased mobility and release from trigger point pain was very notable after class, especially after working in gravity for long periods of time, sense–perceiving the fascia and inviting the viscosity of the fascial matrix to change. I was elated when I healed my arms through an empirical investigation into fascia, touch, pressure, energy and somatic movement. After this experience, fascia became central to my work. Below I share some efficacious and gentle ways of working with fascia in the studio, which I note are very different from fascial training programmes that take a more masculinist functional approach (Myers 2014, 2017). But first, let us read some theory about the intelligence of our all-encompassing fascial matrix. I have divided this chapter into the following parts, offering an extensive overview of fascia, as well as practice-based enactments in the studio.

What is fascia?
Mechanoreceptors in fascia
Trigger points and adhesions
Soft-tissue-rolling in gravity: releasing trigger points and easing pain
Sense–perceiving different layers of fascia
Different pressures
Relational touch and fascial unwinding
Tender and receptive fascial unwinding and relational touch

What is fascia?

> Most thinking in the West for at least half a millennium, has been based on a microscopic lens. We keep examining things by breaking them down into smaller and smaller parts, to examine each part's role. Introduced by Aristotle, but epitomised by Isaac Newton and René Descartes, this mechanical type of approach has led, in the physical medicine field, to books filled with geometric angles, levers, and force vectors based on drawing each individual muscle's insertion closer to the origin.
>
> (Myers 2014: 2–3)

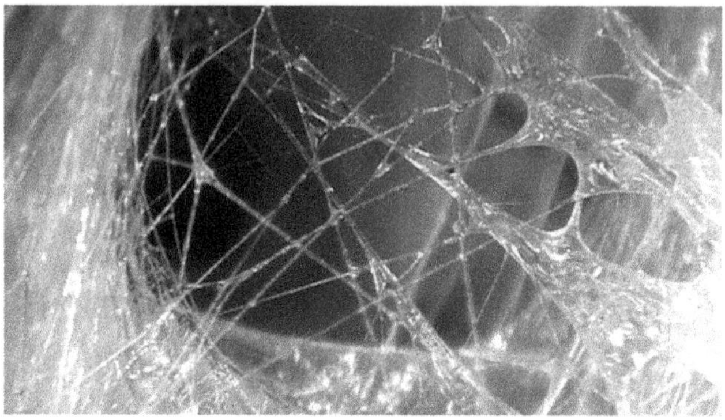

FIGURE 7.1: Fascia.

Western anatomy and physiology are a taken-for-granted truth (a naturalized and normalized perception of the human body). Historically, the naming and classification of the human body were developed through the dissection of corpses in the West (Johnson 1995, 1993), and I add, primarily by men. The great anatomists we read about in history are all men, such as *Andreas Vesalius*, *Charles Estienne*, *Jacopo Berengario*, *Bartolommeo Eustachi* and *Leonardo Da Vinci*, for example (Rifkin et al. 2006). The human body has been drawn, dissected and named largely through an androcentric lens and worldview. This way of perceiving the human body is so deeply enculturated into our intellect and living tissues it is hard to imagine, or indeed experience, the body in a new way. As Myers notes, in classical anatomy, the 'naming of parts of the body imposes an artificial, human-perceived distinction on an event that is unitary' (Myers 2014: 15). He further reflects:

> [A]natomy is, after all, separating the parts with a blade. From Galen through Vesalius and beyond, it was tools of hunting and butchery which were applied to the body, and presented to us as fundamental distinctions we now take for granted. These knives (later scalpels, and then lasers) quite naturally cut along the often bilaminar connective tissue barriers between different tissues, emphasising logical distinctions within the extracellular matrix, but obscuring the role of the connective tissue syncytium considered as a whole.
>
> (Myers 2014: 15)

In contrast, the discovery of fascia supported progressive anatomists and therapists to approach and experience the body in a radically new way, inviting traditional classifications to melt, soften and dis-armour. When we develop sensory awareness of the transanatomical, subanatomical and omnidirectional fascial matrix, we enter a world of de-differentiation, connectivity, volume, radiality, spirality, viscosity, fluency and water. The discovery of fascia and its incredible properties marks a tectonic shift in how we can approach the living and moving body.

> Every bone, every muscle, every blood vessel, every nerve, every organ is enveloped in fascia – and yet the fascia is not separate pieces of membrane – it is one continuous unbroken sheet of fascia, extending throughout the body, forming interconnected pockets of fascia enveloping every structure.
>
> (Attlee 2012: 262)

Fascia envelops and weaves throughout every part of our being, as Attlee further explains below.

> Not only is fascia enveloping every structure in the body, but also it penetrates deeply into the tissues. Every muscle is enveloped in fascia, and each bundle of muscle fibres within the muscle is wrapped in fascia. And more than this, each individual muscle cell has its own fascial sheath – every miniscule fascial sheath being connected into the surrounding fascia and thus to the whole body. In the same way every nerve is enveloped in a fascial sheath (epineurium); every bundle of nerve fibres is enveloped in fascia (perineurium); and every individual nerve cell, microscopically thin, has its own individual fascial sheath (endoneurium).
>
> (Attlee 2012: 263)

The experiential study of fascia is 'transanatomical' and 'subanatomical' (Avison 2015). It is transanatomical because it is the largest organ in the body, enveloping all the discreet parts and systems that traditional anatomy dissected and classified. It is subanatomical because fascia 'penetrates deep into the internal structure of cells, right into the nucleus of the cell, via receptor molecules known as integrins' (Attlee 2012: 263). When we contact fascia in the studio we are coming into relationship with the largest organ in the human body 'running from the top of your head to the soles of your feet. It weaves through every structure in your body' (Fenster 2020: 3). However, it is not just longitudinal, as Fenster's quote above implies, it is an omnidirectional radial organ, with volume and bio-tensility (Avison 2015). Fascia is best perceived and experienced as a *continuum* that enfolds and nurtures every part of you.

> Historically, doctors thought of fascia largely as inert packing material – a biological version of Styrofoam peanuts. Surgeons, for their part, simply cut the fascia out and tossed it away, viewing it as 'the stuff that gets in the way of the good stuff'.

> Even anatomists missed the big picture because they generally work on cadavers that are preserved, a process that turns the soft, delicate, water-permeated web-work of fascia into dry, brittle sticks. In recent years, we've discovered that the fascia isn't just inert 'filler'. Instead, it's a single, interconnected web of tissue that surrounds and penetrates every organ, every muscle, every bone [and every nerve and cell]. We now know that fascia runs throughout the entire body and that it's incredibly biologically active.
>
> (Fenster 2020: 3–5)

Very notably, 'fascia contains 10 times more sensory nerve endings than your muscles, making it one of the body's most powerful sensory organs' – 'this explains why problems in the fascia are often the real cause of pain, blamed solely on your muscles' (Fenster 2020: 12). Because of the large number of sensory nerve endings in fascia, more recently anatomists have realized 'pain primarily arises in the fascia and not in the muscle fibers' (Schleip 2017: 33). Given this important discovery, one can begin to sense how crucial sense–perceiving your fascia is in the studio and how learning to regulate pain through augmenting the fluency of fascia is vitally important.

Fascia is a deeply intelligent integrative part of your being. 'It allows the parts of your body [organs, bones, nerves, muscles, blood vessels] to glide under, and around each other' (Fenster 2020: 12). As you dance, 'the layers of your fascia glide when you move' – 'in fact, when your fascia is healthy, it can glide up to 75 percent of its length' (Fenster 2020: 12). Further, fascia 'holds everything in place' and without it 'your skeleton would just be a pile of bones, and your organs would pool together indiscriminately' (Fenster 2020: 12). Fascia is thus a biotensegrity structure that holds you together. Notice when you are upside down soft-tissue-rolling in the gravity, you do not fall apart. 'Tensegrity creates internal forces that suspend everything in place' (Fenster 2020: 13). As Fenster (2020) and Myers (2014) reflect, your bones and organs are suspended and float in your fascia. This is a radically different way of perceiving the skeletal-muscular and organ system.

Fascia is primarily made of collagen and elastin, which bind together to form various tissues (Schleip 2017: 21–22). The fascia in the body exists in different densities, such as wet fluid collagen, to large fibrous sheets of myofascial tissues that you can feel (Myers 2014; Fenster 2020). Fascia is the most curious and paradoxical organ. As Avison notes, fascia is a 'matrix that surrounds everything, connects everything, yet paradoxically disconnects everything' (Avison 2015: 6). On the one hand, it enfolds us from outer to inner, 'from the finest level of detail within us, between the cells, to the outer most layer of skin in which we are wrapped' (Avison 2015: 5). On the other hand, it differentiates us, because fascia manifests through different densities and tissues, such as muscles, ligaments and tendons. Notably, in some places, fascia 'is so fine it cannot be seen by the naked eye, while in other places it forms thick, layered sheets making up a named entity such as the thoraco-lumbar fascia, which supports the lower and mid back' (Avison 2015: 5). Fascia 'occupies the incredibly complex world of the "in-between" and forms a single, body-wide, tensional network in all dimensions' (Avison 2015: 7). Avison further notes the entire body could also be perceived as totally and completely 'made up of variations of fascia', for example,

> bone is a calcified form of fascia at its thickest, hardest and most compressed, while cartilage comes next, with high hyaline content, then ligament, then tendon, then myofascia containing numerous muscle fibres. It is the main building material in our bodies, varying in thickness and density, extending even to the softest and most delicate of membranes.
>
> (Avison 2015: 5)

Fascia offers us an antithesis to western anatomical differentiation. *Differentiation* is the naming and classification of discreet body parts and systems, which is certainly important in the studio. *De-differentiation* is an approach where the moving body is reperceived as one continual fluid fascial matrix. Somatic movement dance educators and therapists can offer processes underpinned by de-differentiation in the studio, viewing all the tissues in the body as interconnected and in conscious communication.

Often you will read about three layers of fascia. In reality, these layers are artificial distinctions because the fascia that lies beneath your skin is connected to the fascia that enfolds your muscles, organs, nerves and blood vessels. It is a global organ, and therefore, experiencing fascia as an omnidirectional radial web is rather more accurate. Keeping this in mind, it is however useful to explore classified layers of fascia and apply them to practice.

Below your skin, for example, you have a layer of fascia called the *superficial fascia*. It is a subcutaneous layer composed of loose connective tissue. Notably, it is connected to the skin, and equally weaves into the muscles below. Hence, it is not really a separate layer, but rather the outermost landscape of your fascial matrix. It is rich in vascular supply, nerves and receptors. It is made of loosely packed interwoven collagen and elastic fibres. *The deep fascia* below envelops all the bones, muscles, nerves and blood vessels. It is a tougher layer of connective tissue. Below the deep fascia, we meet *the visceral fascia*, sometimes called *parietal fascia*, which nurtures, enfolds and suspends all the organs. At the supermolecular level, we also find a layer termed *the extracellular matrix* (ECM). This is a rather magical level that creates the connective tissue in the first place (it is a generative source). 'The term extracellular matrix [...] is applied to the sum total of extracellular substance within the connective tissue' itself (Myers 2014: 2–3). The extracellular matrix is a,

> dynamic supermolecular webwork extending into every nook and cranny of the body: a nuclear matrix within a cellular matrix within a connective tissue matrix. In essence, when you touch a human body, you are touching an intimately connected system composed of virtually all the molecules within the body linked together.
>
> (Myers 2014: 15)

Further, the extracellular matrix

> binds every cell in the body to its neighbours and even connects [...] the inner network of each cell to the mechanical state of the entire body [...] Part of its connecting nature may lie in its ability to store and communicate information across the entire body.
>
> (Myers 2014: 16–17)

When we approach fascia in the studio, we invite participants to let go of western anatomical classifications of the human body. The somatic movement field grew in antithesis to mechanistic models; thus, reperceiving the body through a spirilloid voluminous non-linear lens is certainly not new to the field. Entering the world of fascia is best achieved by initially letting go of your longitudinal axis. We are not merely anterior/posterior, inferior/superior, up/down, back/front or medial/lateral – we are omnidirectional, radial, spirilloid, curvaceous, round and full of volume. Gravitational self-regulatory improvisation supports people to let go of their verticality and decades of emotion held in the fascia. Gravity, noted throughout this book, is a deep healer; it offers us manifold opportunities to change the viscosity of our fascia, as we tip, pour, roll, melt, yield, press, stretch, reach, and glide and slide across the floor. In such a process, we are also exploring our biotensegrity, noticing how our organs, bones and joints adjust and reorganize themselves rather magically within our fluid matrix.

If you are inactive, your fascial tissues stick together. This often causes a thickening in the collagen fibres. Thick and stuck fascia, in turn shapes your posture, and no less, your sensory experience. Healthy alignment is as much to do with loose gliding slippery fascia, as it is the alignment of bones and muscles (Fenster 2020). Dehydration, chronic stress and/or a sedentary lifestyle all affect posture and alignment (Fenster 2020). Of note, the hydration of the fascia has a significant influence on all the tissues it wraps and envelopes. Therefore, if your fascia is tight, dehydrated and full of adhesions, you are likely to feel pain and tightness, and this will affect the health of all your internal structures and tissues – and of course how you are feeling. Chronic sympathetic holding, muscular contraction, tight tonus and pain in fascia are common in clients. Constricted fascia decreases the blood supply, causes pain, limits neural flow, and restricts mobility and range of motion. When we are stressed and sympathetically charged, our muscles and fascia contract. If a lion is chasing us, we need muscle contraction to run fast. However, in our globalized westernized technocratic culture, we are not running from lions, but rather fleeing from multiple stressors that edge us towards fight-and-flight. While we are not terrified of predators, we are still trying to survive the world, and emotion and stress are held in the fascial matrix as Fenster shares: 'Fascia is physically affected by emotional stress, which helps to explain the tightness you feel when you are tense. This is a two-way street because fascial structures and tightness, in turn, can cause stress and anxiety' (2020: 15).

Mechanoreceptors in fascia

> Our richest and largest sensory system is not the eyes, ears, skin, or vestibular system but in fact our muscles with their related fascia. Our nervous system receives its greatest amount of sensory input from our myofascial tissues. Yet the majority of these sensory organs are so small that until recently little has been known about them.
>
> (Schleip 2003a: 15)

The fact that 'the central nervous system receives its greatest amount of sensory nerves from our myofascial tissue, providing more sensory input than our eyes, ears or skin' (Attlee 2012: 260), alerts us to just how important fascia is in terms of afferent sensing in the studio. Fascia sends an incredible amount of information back to the central nervous system through its sensors and nerve endings. The fascial system has primarily developed to convey 'mechanical information fast – through the interplay of tension and compression, along the fibrous net, the gluey proteoglycans, and even through the cells themselves' (Myer 2014: 32). It

> provides an essential communication system throughout the body. It acts as a liquid crystalline matrix carrying highspeed messages via electrical charges. These communications travel much faster than the nervous system, transmitting information regarding tension and injury to all parts of the body.
>
> (Attlee 2012: 260)

Fascia is a fast communicator, but slow to change and remodel, as Myers notes:

> The timing of the fascial system is interesting in that it has two rhythms; at least, two that are of interest to us. On the one hand, the play of tension and compression communicates around the body as a mechanical vibration. This is roughly equivalent of 720 mph (1100 kph), which is more than three times faster than the nervous system. So contrary to conventional wisdom, the fibrous net communicates more quickly than the nervous system.
>
> (Myers 2014: 33)

Earls and Myers further note that compared to other body systems, such as the nervous and circulatory system,

> the fascial network is at once faster to communicate (720 mph for mechanical information verses 150 mph for the nervous system transmission) but slower to respond than either the neural or vascular. The fascia's remodelling response is measured in days and weeks, rather than seconds or minutes. It is slow to accept changes initiated from the outside [...] This makes the fascial system a repository of much of the patterning for chronic issues.
>
> (Earls and Myers 2017: 20)

Fascia is a sensory organ feeding a wealth of information back to the central nervous system about 'motion, changes in position, pressure, shear motion or stretching' (Schleip 2017: 32). Thus, the sensory receptors in fascia play a large role in our proprioceptive abilities. The fascia of the 'musculoskeletal system is now considered in its own right a sensory organ and a body-wide information system' (Schleip 2017: 33). Notably, sensory receptors 'are far more numerous than the nerve fibres that cause muscle movement, namely motor neurons' (2017: 33). Further, 'the number of different sensors and nerve endings in the fascial components of a muscle exceeds by far the number of sensory neurons of the muscle itself' (2017: 33).

Collectively these sensory receptors are known as *mechanoreceptors*. We can observe in the list of sensory receptors below just how connected the fascia is to our proprioception, and additionally, to our autonomic nervous system (Schleip 2003: 32). When we melt, release, stretch and soft-tissue-roll in gravity (applying different degrees of pressure, force and energy), and explore relational touch (applying different pressures and energies to the fascia), or shake, jiggle, bounce and swing (following our improvisational paths in the studio), we are stimulating the *mechanoreceptors* below.

> *Pacinian corpuscles* are programmed to react to rapid changes, to vibration, or to sudden impulses. These particles need dynamic alterations in motion or force.
>
> *Ruffi corpuscles* specialise in long alternating, and sustained, and in rather quieter, steady stimuli, such as massage or slow stretch.
>
> *Golgi receptors* are unresponsive to passive movement stimulation; they only react when the stretched muscle fibres are active at the same time. They are situated in or near the tendons and are able to reduce muscle tension when the tendons are under high strain. In this way they protect the tendons and the joint from being over loaded.
>
> *Interstitial receptors* are connected to the autonomic nervous system, which controls unconscious processes and movements, such as digestion. In addition to pressure and shear motion, they can signal pain and temperature: they are also the most common type of receptor.
>
> (Schleip 2017: 32, original emphasis)

Fascial unwinding through consciously aware movement undoubtedly plays an important role in releasing sympathetic holding, and gently supports clients to shift into a parasympathetic state. This is because particular sensory receptors such as Ruffini receptors 'tend to induce a lowering of sympathetic nervous activity' (Schleip 2003a: 144). Additionally, as Schleip notes, clinical findings generally evidence that 'slow deep tissue techniques tend to have a relaxing effect on local tissues, and, indeed, on the whole organism' (Schleip 2003a: 144). Further, this 'makes substantial and profound two-way connections with the autonomic nervous system' (Attlee 2012: 260). The fascia is densely innervated by mechanoreceptors, which are responsive to different types of movement, vibration, energy and pressure. Stimulation of Ruffini and interstitial mechanoreceptors 'induces profound changes in the autonomic nervous system, with an increase in vagal activity, which results not only in changes in local fluid dynamics and tissue metabolism, but also global neuromuscular, emotional, cortical and endocranial changes, leading to muscle relaxation' (Attlee 2012: 260). There are many ways to bring conscious awareness to fascia in the studio. When you invite participants to settle, soften, yield, compress, decompress, pressure and unwind their tissues in gravity, the viscosity, elasticity and plasticity of the fascial tissue starts to change, in turn supporting deep relaxation.

> Research has shown that stimulation of fascial mechanoreceptors triggers changes in the autonomic nervous system, as well as global muscle relaxation. In other words, deep mechanical pressure to these areas causes a person to be more relaxed. Therefore, it appears that deep manual pressure– specifically if it is slow or steady – stimulates particular fascial mechanoreceptors, which results in an increase of vagal activity.
>
> (Schleip 2003a: 141)

Hence, applying different degrees of pressure within the fascial matrix can potentially reduce hyperarousal in the sympathetics. Research has shown that the receptors in the fascia have an 'autonomic function', meaning 'stimulation of their sensory endings leads to change in heart rate, blood pressure' and 'respiration' (Sumner and Haines 2010: 142). There is thus a sensitive feedback mechanism between the myofascial tissues and the autonomic nervous system. As Schleip's research has shown, 'any intervention on the fascia is an intervention on the autonomic nervous system' (2003a: 108). Practices of softening, loosening, yielding and melting into gravity – and tipping, rolling, sliding, gliding, pressuring, lengthening, stretching, compressing, decompressing and releasing the fascia are extremely effective in not only changing the density of fascia, but also in reducing sympathetic arousal. *Thixotropy* is a term you hear when studying fascia, and it refers to changing the state, density and viscosity of your fascia. Movement explorations such as those I share below could be called practices of thixotropy. Another term you hear when studying fascia is *piezoelectricity*, which refers to how pressure produces an electrical charge in the fascia.

Trigger points and adhesions

Your fascial net will have undergone immense stress throughout your life, often holding tension, stress, postural torsions and asymmetries. Fascia creates our shape and posture. Our posture is negatively affected if our fascia is dry, our fibres are torn, matted-up, and full of torsions, asymmetries and painful adhesions. Noted earlier, research has shown that when we feel stressed our fascia tightens, and of course when we feel bound, tight, compressed and constricted it heightens our anxiety (Fenster 2020). As Fenster shares, 'stress causes your fascia to contract, leading to tightness, knots, and poor hydration – so one of the best things you can do for your fascia is to dial down your stress' (Fenster 2020: 146). I would add here, one of best things we can do in the studio for our 'mental health' is to loosen, refresh, enliven, liquify and melt the tension in our fascial matrix.

The relationship between stress and our facial matrix is often in a negative cycle, but one we can break and re-pattern slowly in the somatic studio.

We must note, fascia is filled with water, that often gets toxic over time. Movement and touch has the potential to drive water through the fascial tissues, increasing circulation and removing toxins (Fenster 2020). When we sense into the fascial web we are coming into relationship with a liquid organ that can change in viscosity through different types of movement, energies, forces and pressures (Fenster 2020; Schielp 2003a, 2003b). This is especially exciting for somatic movement dance therapists who are trained to lead sessions that invite participants to explore a wide range of movement qualities, with attuned attention to different rhythms, dynamics, forces, speeds, qualities, pressures and energies. Therapists are also trained in specialized touch, and again, it is very exciting to work with the knowledge that different qualities of touch and degrees of pressure can influence the viscosity and liquidity of fascia.

In the world of fascial therapies, foam rolling is used as a technique to 'ease chronic or exercise-related pain' – commonly referred to as 'self-myofascial release (SMR)' (Fenster 2020:105). Fenster shares that the benefits of rolling are: 'less chronic pain; less pain after exercise; more energy; better flexibility; greater range of motion; reduced stress and improved circulation' (Fenster 2020: 107). Foam rolling enlivens and rejuvenates fascial tissues, 'driving water into the fascia and increasing circulation' (Fenster 2020: 108). Different degrees of pressure are applied in order to resolve trigger points, push toxins out and support adhesions to heal by increasing circulatory flow through damaged tissues (Fenster 2020: 105–28). Fascial knots, restrictions, trigger points, areas of pain and tightness are resolved through using foam rollers, applying variant pressures and durations of pressures to the fascial tissue. In somatic movement dance practices, we do not use objects to support fascial release, although some practitioners use rollers if they are integrating myofascial rolling techniques into their somatic movement practice. However, we do offer soft-tissue-rolling in gravity for long periods of time. Soft-tissue-rolling in gravity is emblematic of my practice.

When participants are invited to soften into gravity, they often feel pain. The pain receptors in the fascial tissues are calling for ease, release, unwinding, dissolving, compressing, decompressing, squeezing, stretching, lengthening, expanding or loosening. Through slow-time self-regulatory movement in gravity, we can listen to these sensory receptors and follow how our living tissues need to express and find a resolution. When we drop into gravity with breath awareness, we may notice we feel bounded, restricted and stiff. Sometimes participants will experience points of pain called trigger points. Trigger points are often caused by toxins.

> Like every other organ in your body, your fascia suffers when you're exposed to toxins in food, air and water. Toxins inflame your body, damage your cells, dehydrate you, and deplete your nutrients, and all of this impacts the fascia.
>
> (Fenster 2020: 39)

As Fenster shares, 'over time, the fascia accumulates toxins such as lactic acid and pyruvic acid' (Fenster 2020: 28). Often trigger points and pain are caused by not drinking enough water. Therefore, it is important to share the water-based nature of fascia with participants.

Trigger points love to be gently rolled-out, softened, pressured a little, squeezed and decompressed. Squeezing literally 'allows the fascia to replace old water with new' (Fenster 2020: 28). Toxic points need to be released and fresh water invited to flow back into the tissues. Fenster notes, squeezing the tissues is particularly effective in replenishing the fascial tissues and releasing trigger points. He also shares that pumping movement will replenish places of restriction and toxicity.

> When you move, the resulting pressure on your fascia pumps water out of it, sweeping out toxins along with it. Then when you rest your fascia, fresh water gets pumped back into it, cleansing and hydrating it and feeding it the nutrients its needs.
>
> (Fenster 2020: 28)

However, it is not just squeezing and pumping that is effective in supporting healthy fascia, but rather following self-regulatory movement arising from the first-person sensory perception of your fascial matrix. Your fascial net is unique to your life journey, story and lived experience. Working with a one-size all fits mentality is not something I do, but rather, I invite participants to attune to the proprioceptive and interoceptive intelligence within their own fascial matrix.

Another reason for pain is adhesions. Adhesions are collagen fibres that have become injured and these areas

> begin to grow in a tangled, crisscrossing pattern as they attempt to patch the damaged spot [...] as a result, knots and adhesions can form, trapping toxins, restricting your movement, and leading to loss of function and even extreme pain.
>
> (Fenster 2020: 30)

Tigger points and adhesions can be attended to through somatic sensing and following pathways of ease. Equally, attending to movement globally can help to resolve trigger points in a localized area. My point is being, we don't need to approach fascial pain in a mechanical way, with a one size fits all mentality – with only a few types of movements, working-out the body at a distance from our sensory-perception. Rather, we invite the mind to rest and focus in the intelligence of fascial tissues, listen deeply and follow easeful pathways, resolving pain sense–perceived from the first-person perception of our living tissues. From this deep listening, many types of movement qualities, dynamics, speeds, forces, spatiality, rhythms and planes of action will emerge. Each person is uniquely resolving their own stiffness and easing out how their body has been impacted by the exterior world.

Because somatic movement dance is rooted in sensing, feeling, perceiving and improvisational action, participants involved in this modality are at a huge advantage in terms of resolving their own pain, relieving trigger points and supporting the healing of adhesions through increasing circulatory flow in their fascial net. When we don't move, our fascia literally 'dries out, stiffens, gets sticky, and even becomes toxic' (Fenster 2020: 28). Overuse of fascia through repetitive patterns causes adhesions or *microtraumas,* where the fascia becomes 'tangled, matted, and thickened, with excess of collagen threads going in every direction' (Fenster 2020: 29). As Fenster shares, 'motion is lotion, and the fascia needs to move in many different directions everyday' (Fenster 2020: 29). Many people who attend sessions, and who are new to somatic movement therapy have congested, constricted and stagnant fascia. I have also had terrible problems with my fascia, crystallizing and dying out through grief and depression, pulling down and twisting through existential depression caused by menopause, tightening through high levels of socio-economic stress, holding in childhood trauma, and institutional pressures enslaving my soul (losing contact with my inner Self).

> Fascia essentially consists of the primary substances of life: protein and water. The most common extracellular substance in the body is collagen [....] Water is crucial as a medium for cellular metabolism. As a consequence, various techniques used to treat fascia focus on the water content and on exchange of fluid.
>
> (Schleip 2020: 18, 21)

When we explore fascia, we are primarily coming into a relationship with water and collagen. The qualities of collagen are 'strong, but bendy' and 'the fibres are long, spiral-shaped and hollow' (Sumner and Haines 2010: 143). 'The fibre mimics a copper coil and perhaps the fluid charges up with potency because of the fibres electrical nature. In healthy fascia there is a quality of shimmering electric-fluid potency that is unique' (Sumner and Haines 2010:143). Healthy fascia is smooth, slippery and flexible. When fascia is hydrated and healthy, it provides a smooth slippery surface for muscles and organs to slide over. Wet collagen is responsible for this fluid gliding. I would posit that one of the reasons why somatic movement dance is so transformational is because gravitational improvisational processes change the viscosity of fascia, even when the facilitator is not focusing consciously on fascia as an explicit sensory inroad. Soft-tissue-rolling and decompressive practices break up adhesions, release trigger points and support the healthy gilding and sliding of internal structures. Thus, practice can support solid fibres that have become knitted together to become fluid i.e., the sol-to-gel continuum is augmented. Emilie Conrad's work, along with the earlier pioneer, Ida Rolf, both attended to the sol–gel continuum. Moving from a dense gel to a fluid sol state underpins much of their work. Balancing the sol-to-gel continuum refers to how different fibres that make up the fascial network can change state, from solid fibres to a gel-like fluid – this is when pain is eased and released.

Fascia becomes healthier when you are conscious of breath during movement. Underling all somatic movement dance work is breath awareness, enhancing the flow of oxygen through the tissues as participants move (Eddy 2016). Additionally, the move-and-rest cycle is something researchers endorse for fascial health (Fenster 2020). Scientific research has evidenced that fascia needs both activity and rest (Fenster 2020). The balance between rest and activity lies at the heart of somatic movement; thus, somatic movement pedagogies are already enacting the importance of the move-and-rest cycle in extremely detailed and creative ways (Eddy and Williamson 2014b).

Soft-tissue-rolling in gravity: Releasing trigger points and easing pain

Movement processes that support organismic ease, relieve stress and soothe pain lie at the heart of somatic movement dance practices. Somatic practitioners are trained to support people to move with different qualities, rhythms, forces, energies, tempos and through different planes of action. All movement is of course good for the fascia, but deep-body listening, sensing into the proprioceptive and interoceptive intelligence of your own fascia is highly effective in self-regulating pain and discomfort. Noted earlier, but worth remembering, fascia is the largest sensory organ in the human body, with ten times more nerve endings than found in muscles. Thus, attuning afferently to the fascia and efferently following pathways that feel delicious, nutritious and life-giving supports participants to resolve trigger points, thus self-regulating pain.

When I work with fascia, I always start in gravity and with autogenic self-regulatory movement first, as described in Chapters 1 and 2. Inviting participants into parasympathetic ease will soften and release holding in fascia and lay the receptive ground for other types of energetic movement enactments on the fascia. Parasympathetic awareness, especially bringing the vagus nerve into a state of health, also reduces inflammation, which is a key to pain relief (Henton 2020). Parasympathetic release prepares a receptive calm nervous system that enables participants to attune to their fascia with enhanced sensory-perceptual movement awareness, in a tranquil state. Sensing pain, while feeling anxious will only serve to create more pain and holding. Thus, I note, once more, parasympathetic release is absolutely essential in restoring health and helping participants manage pain. Soft-tissue-rolling in gravity helps to resolve knots, trigger points, adhesions, and eases tightness, stiffness and restriction. Below, I offer a short practice-based example. For readers new to this field, the process shared below would take an hour and 30 minutes with reflective drawing and writing post moving. These are not quick-fix exercises, but rather slow-time sensuous processes, that invite participants to linger, play and care for their fascia over time, a life-long practice of self-regulating impacts, hurts and assaults, and thus experiencing more agency. Below is a list of ways you can start to invite participants to attend to their myofascial tissues, which you will notice, formed the bedrock and seabed of this book.

Surrendering the weight and mass of body tissues into gravity, contacting moment-by-moment breath awareness

Sense–perceiving the bones floating in a sea of connective tissue: resting the bones in the soft fascial tissues that surround and enfold the bones.

Sense–perceiving the organs and inner fluid body floating in a sea of connective tissue: resting the organs in the elastic fluid fascia that suspends and nurtures the organs.

Using the floor as a fulcrum, which you can pivot around, twist, press, pressure, compress, decompress and release the fascia, attending to trigger points and adhesions.

Increasing circulation and fluency through the tissues via undulating, waving and rippling through the fluid body.

Increasing circulation and fluency through the tissues via gliding, sliding, rolling and pouring your weight along the floor.

Using the floor as a fulcrum, where you can push, tip and weight bare, stimulating the strong fascia around the joints, ligaments and muscles.

Using the floor as a fulcrum around which you reach, pull, extend, expand and stretch, inviting stiff fascial tissues into fluency.

Example of practice

Invite participants to settle into gravity, with breath awareness. Bring awareness to the soft tissues surrounding and enveloping the bones. Invite the bones to settle, rest and soften into the fascia enfolding the bones. Rest in the afferent sensation of soft fluid tissues surrounding and enveloping bones. This is a qualitatively different experience to sensing hard bones lying on the floor. Invite the image of the bones floating in a sea of connective tissue into your awareness.

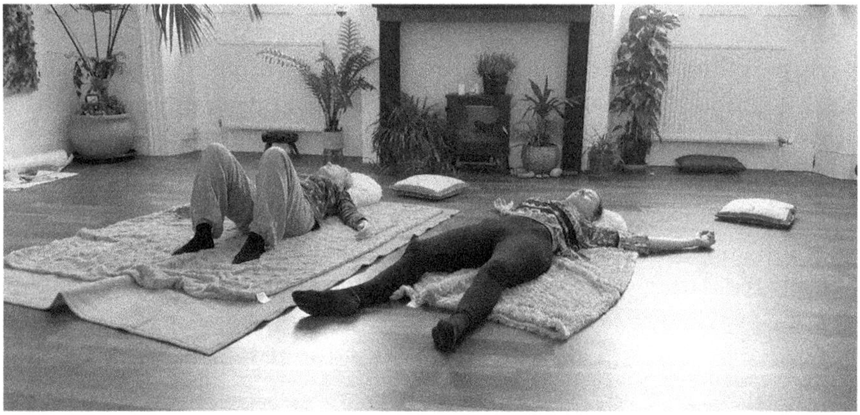

FIGURE 7.2: Karin Rugman and Amanda Williamson: sensing their bones floating in a sea of connective tissue. Photographer: Scott Closson.

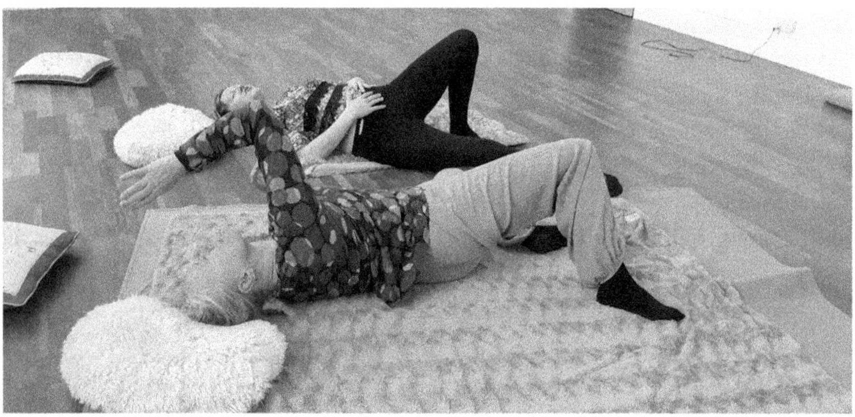

FIGURE 7.3: Karin Rugman and Amanda Williamson: sensing bones moving in soft-tissue. Photographer: Scott Closson.

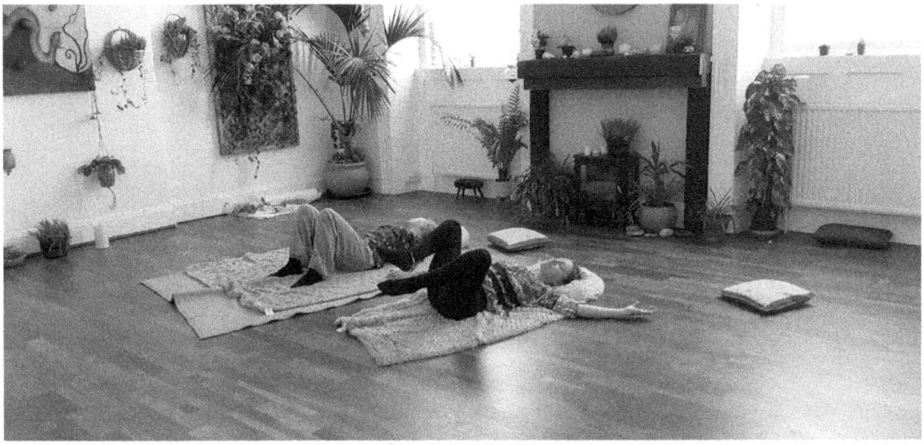

FIGURE 7.4: Amanda Williamson and Karin Rugman: settling their tissues. Photographer: Scott Closson.

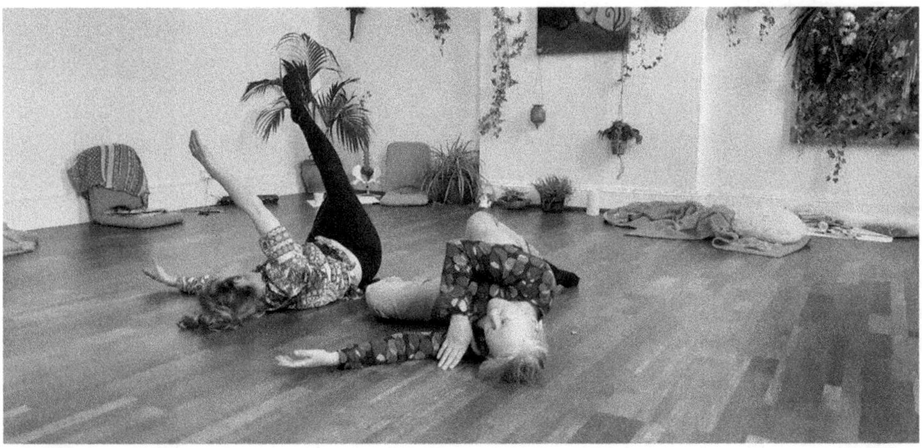

FIGURE 7.5: Karin Rugman and Amanda Williamson: sensing and reaching bones through soft-tissue. Photographer: Scott Closson.

Release the weight of the cranium and play gently with the caudal–cranial axis, innervating the parasympathetic nerves in the cranium and sacrum. Bring awareness to the vagus nerve travelling out of the cranium into the body. Invite breath awareness, noticing the expansion of tissues on the inhalation and the surrendering of tissues on the exhalation. Breathe the vagus nerve into health, attending to the movement of breath in the thorax and diaphragm.

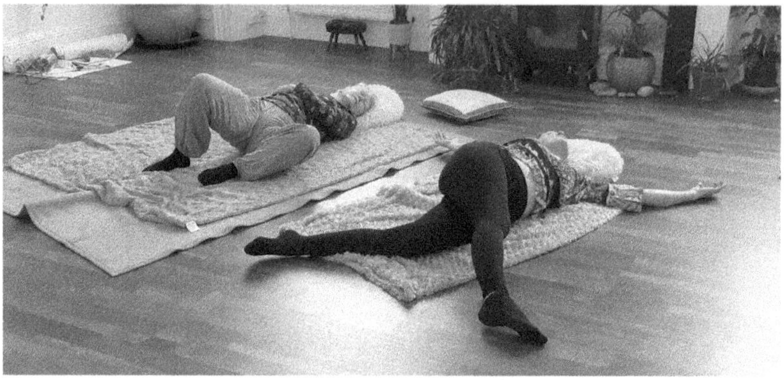

FIGURE 7.6: Amanda Williamson and Karin Rugman: easing fascial restrictions. Photographer: Scott Closson.

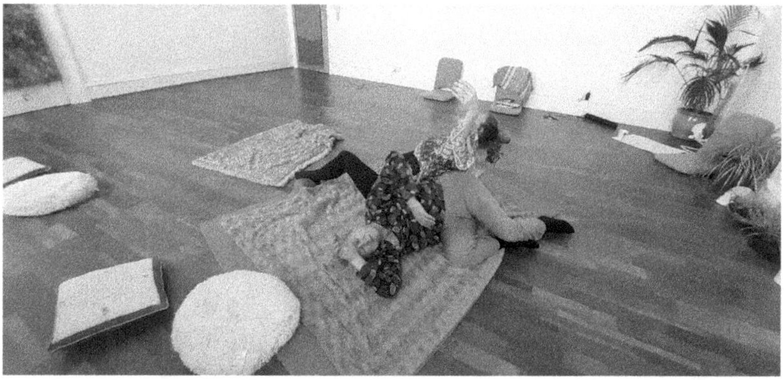

FIGURE 7.7: Amanda Williamson and Karin Rugman: following fascial pathways of ease. Photographer: Scott Closson.

Invite participants to sense how their living tissues need to ease-out, following the living intelligence of their sensory receptors. Invite them to listen to afferent sensation, and follow pathways of easing, softening, melting, releasing, yielding and stilling. Seek pleasurable movement and places to hang-out – to rest, breathe and still in the soft tissues.

Invite participants into soft-tissue-rolling across the floor, gently pushing, tipping, pouring, rolling, softening, melting and yielding the fascial tissues into ground. Invite participants to massage their fascia into the floor as they roll, noticing places of restriction. Sometimes places of restriction call for stilling, shaking, rocking, loosening, pressuring or yielding. Sometimes they call for gentle compression and decompression. Sometimes they call for deep slow stretch, or lengthening and expansion.

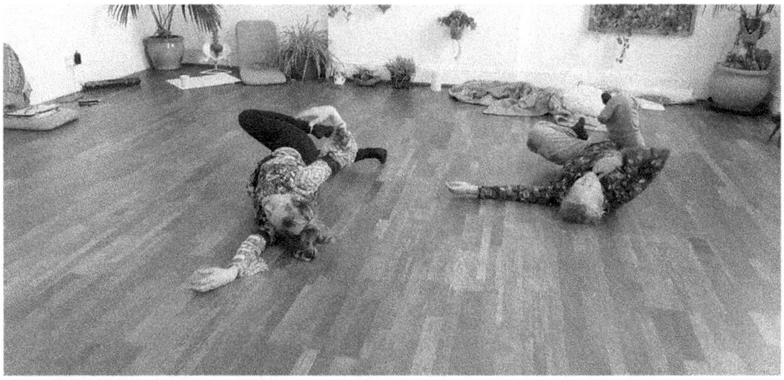

FIGURE 7.8: Karin Rugman and Amanda Williamson: soft-tissue rolling. Photographer: Scott Closson.

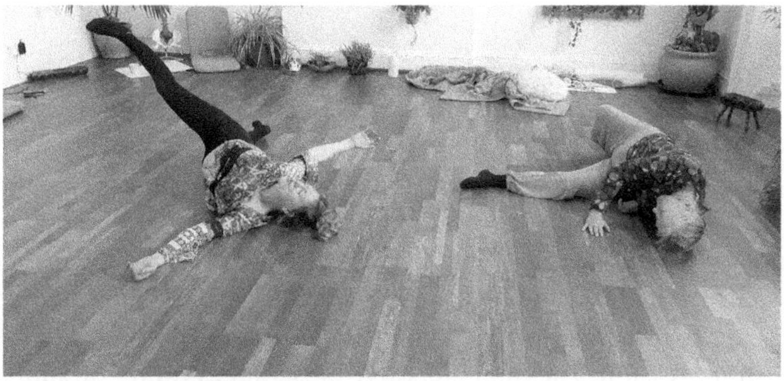

FIGURE 7.9: Amanda Williamson and Karin Rugman: soft-tissue rolling. Photographer: Scott Closson.

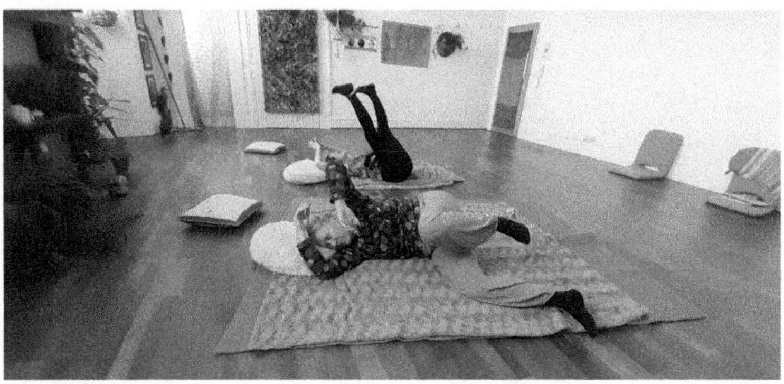

FIGURE 7.10: Karin Rugman and Amanda Williamson: soft-tissue rolling. Photographer: Scott Closson.

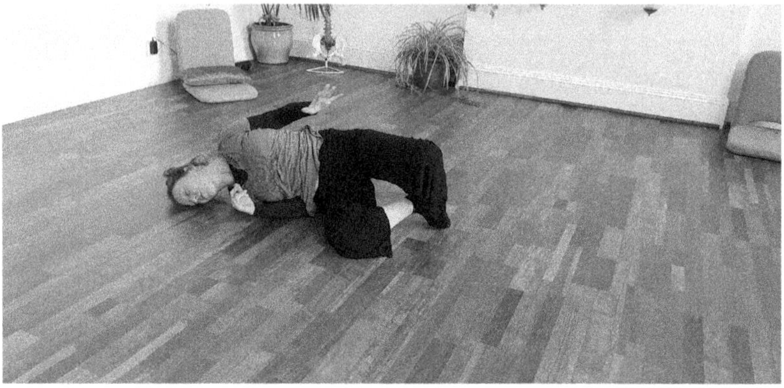

FIGURE 7.11: Amanda Williamson: resolving a trigger point through different degrees of pressure. Photographer: Scott Closson.

Participants might notice trigger points. Each trigger point will call for resolution through a different energy, quality, movement initiation and direction. You might notice participants hang-out in a particular area for a long time, rocking gently, shaking or lingering through a slow sustained stretch. For example, above, I am resolving a trigger point in my scapulae, and the rest of my body is spiralling in response, as I gently compress and decompress the tissues around my shoulders.

Invite participants to hang-out and linger in tissues that are calling for attention and care. Notice what your living tissues desire: do they desire weight, pressure, compression, rocking, shaking, loosening, gliding or sliding. With participants new to practice model the many ways you can soft-tissue-roll in

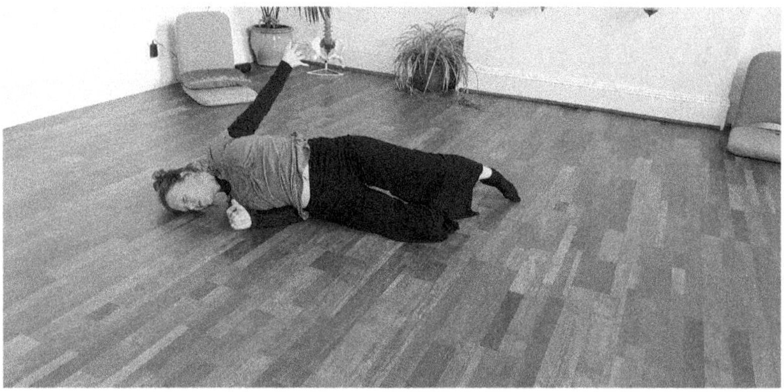

FIGURE 7.12: Amanda Williamson: gently compressing and decompressing. Photographer: Scott Closson.

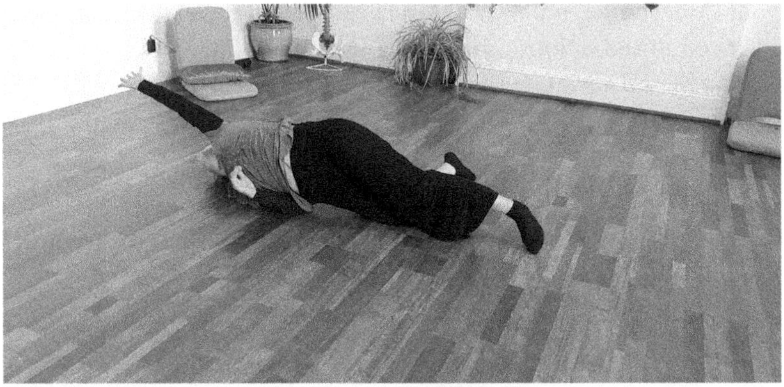

FIGURE 7.13: Amanda Williamson: pushing, reaching and pulling. Photographer: Scott Closson.

response to trigger points, sensing the intelligence of tissues calling for care and attention.

Sense–perceiving different layers of fascia

In practice, it is wonderfully fun, enlivening and indeed freeing to explore different layers of fascia. For example, you can focus on moving with awareness of the loose connective tissue under your skin. You can also attune and move with awareness of the deep fascia that envelops all your bones, muscles, nerves and blood vessels. Additionally, you can move with awareness of your visceral fascia (elastic *parietal fascia*), which nurtures, enfolds and suspends all your organs.

Practice: Sensing the loose connective tissue just under the skin

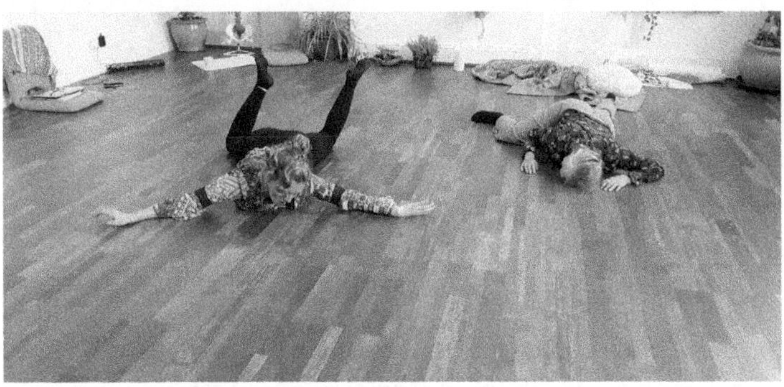

FIGURE 7.14: Amanda Williamson and Karin Rugman: gliding, sliding and resting in soft tissues. Photographer: Scott Closson.

Below your skin, you have a layer of fascia called superficial fascia. It is a subcutaneous layer composed of loose connective tissue. This layer loves to soften, glide, slide, yield, melt and surrender with breath awareness.

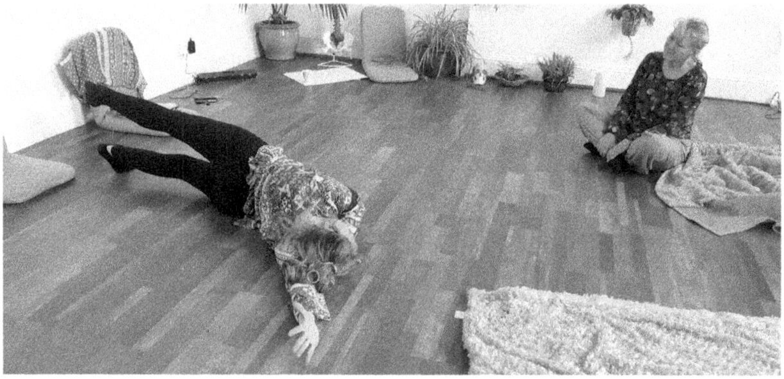

FIGURE 7.15: Karin Rugman and Amanda Williamson: gliding and sliding. Photographer: Scott Closson.

Invite participants to soft-tissue-roll, gliding and sliding, across every surface of their body.

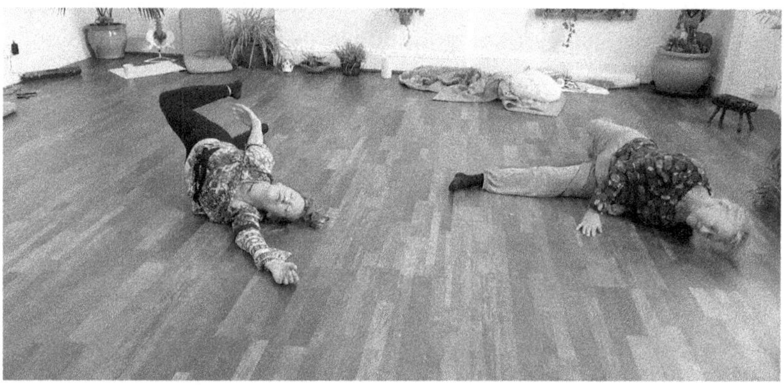

FIGURE 7.16: Karin Rugman and Amanda Williamson: gliding and sliding. Photographer: Scott Closson.

Invite participants to receive afferent sensory information from this subcutaneous layer. Listen to and hang-out in the layer just below the skin. Notice the living presence of the fascia just under the skin. How does this layer want to express?

Practice: The fascia surrounding the muscles, bones, nerves and blood vessels

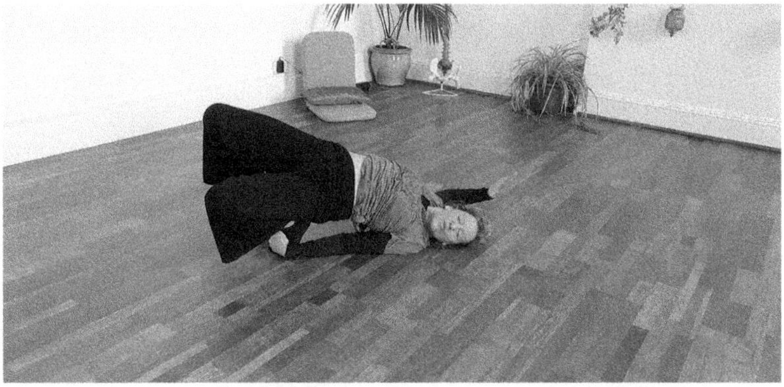

FIGURE 7.17: Amanda Williamson: compressing muscle tissue and sensing bone. Photographer: Scott Closson.

Invite participants to receive afferent information from the fascia surrounding their bones, muscles and tendons. This is a deeper layer of fascia. This layer of fascia has incredible proprioceptive intelligence. Focusing on stretching muscles, stimulating the nerves, or playing with your synovial joints contacts this layer.

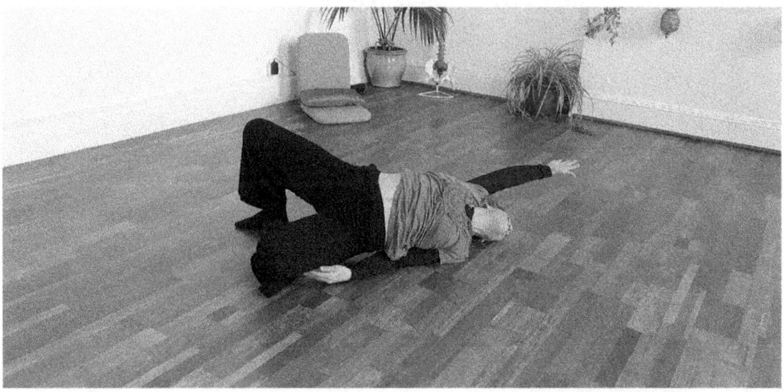

FIGURE 7.18: Amanda Williamson: lengthening and stretching. Photographer: Scott Closson.

Invite participants to sense–perceive the fascia surrounding their muscles, ligaments and tendons: initiate movement from the bones, noticing the soft tissue enveloping every bone in the body. Explore initiating movement through the limbs, inviting the soft tissue surrounding the bones to relax and breathe.

Practice: The visceral fascia surrounding the organs

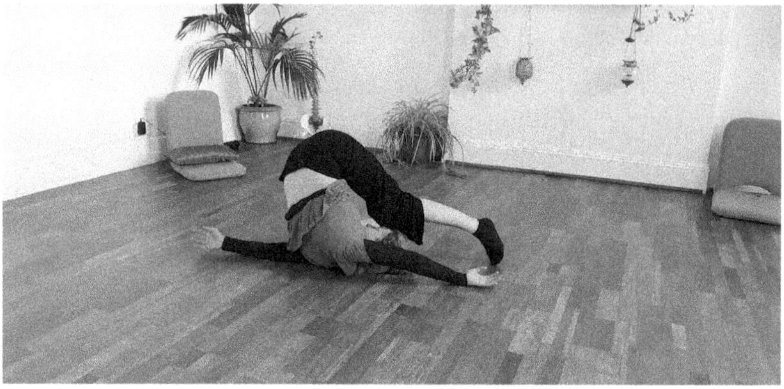

FIGURE 7.19: Amanda Williamson: pouring her organ body. Photographer: Scott Closson.

Invite participants to receive afferent information sense–perceiving their visceral fascia surrounding and suspending all the organs. This is a very fluid layer, where you can sense the organs suspended in fascia. Sensing the heart and releasing in the oral cavity and back of the throat helps to drop awareness into this ocean of fluid and elastic tissue. Opening the airways and softening in the mouth, jaw, throat, thorax and diaphragm helps to sense this layer. Initiating movement from the heart, or any organ helps to sense–perceive this layer.

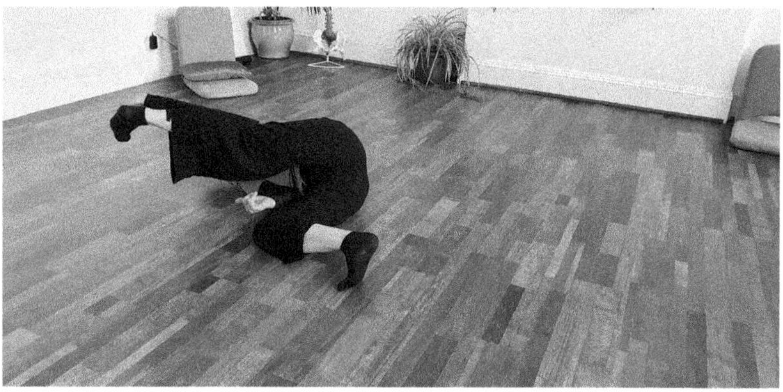

FIGURE 7.20: Amanda Williamson: tipping and pouring the fluid body across the floor. Photographer: Scott Closson.

Tipping, rolling and pouring the weight of the fluid body across the floor also contacts this internal ocean of fascia.

Different pressures

Fascia 'consists of the same components in different proportions – collagen, elastin, and an aqueous or gel-like ground substance' (Schielp 2017: 19). Collagens 'play an important role – they consist of fairly densely packed fibres that literally give the human body and all vertebrates their shape. They are referred to as scaffold proteins or structural proteins' (Schielp 2017: 19). 'Elastin is the second commonest structural protein found in fascial tissue' and as 'its name actually suggests its most important feature [...] is elasticity'. Collagens have 'interesting mechanical characteristics: they are easily extensible, yet very tear resistant – their tensile strength can be greater than that of steel' (Schielp 2017: 20). Most wonderfully, fascia helps to store and release energy because the contraction and stretching of the collagen fibres helps to store and release energy, rather like a spring extending (Fenster 2020). Soft-tissue-rolling in gravity can also argument the strength and elasticity of fascia. We can further support our fascia into health through:

- Contraction, stretching and lengthening: augmenting the release of energy in our collagen fibres.
- Elasticity: augmenting the flexibility and suppleness of fascia: *extending, lengthening, stretching, expanding, enlarging, reaching, opening.*
- Strengthening: augmenting the potency and power of collagen: *pushing, pressing, weight-baring, hanging and pulling.*

Somatic movement dance therapists have an advantage in relation to restoring the health of fascia because they are highly trained in leading somatic movement improvisations. They language, tone and sound participants through a wide range of qualities, temporalities, spatialities, speeds, dynamics, rhythms, forces and planes of action. Fascia does not like repetition – repetitive and habituated movement does not enliven the omnidirectional bio-tensile nature of the fascial net. Therefore, while practices such as yoga are great for fascia, especially because of deep and sustained stretch, improvisational movement augments one of the key scientific findings about fascial research, which evidences that fascia needs to move in new and manifold ways (Fenster 2020: 29). Participants are offered the opportunity to improvise freely attuned to their sensory-perceptual movement awareness. Through attuned fascial improvisations we seek and follow new pathways, augmenting an infinite range of qualities, dynamics, speeds and rhythms. Fascia loves to be enlivened through new pathways and multi-directional sensory-perceptual imaginal landscapes and trails.

When participants have self-regulated their own fascial restrictions, I often invite them to explore a wide range of different movement qualities that stimulate different receptors in the fascia. I usually lead the process through a combination of the following:

slow-sustained stretch, pressuring the tissues, sensitively attuned compressions and decompressions into the floor, shaking, jiggling, loosening, squeezing, releasing, gliding, sliding, contraction, lengthening, weight-bearing, pushing, extension and expansion. Below are some brief examples of what improvisations might look like.

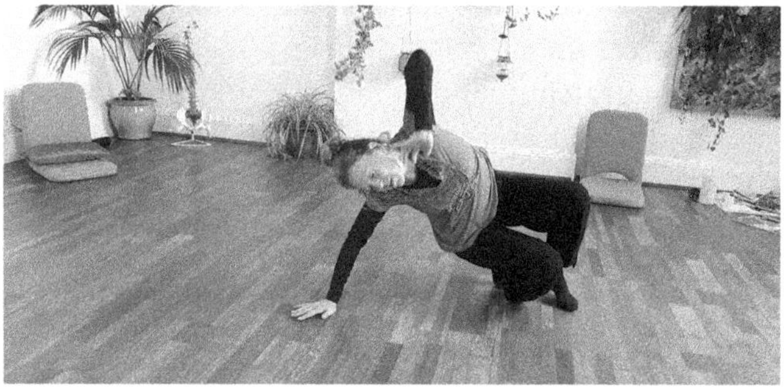

FIGURE 7.21: Amanda Williamson: weight baring. Photographer: Scott Closson.

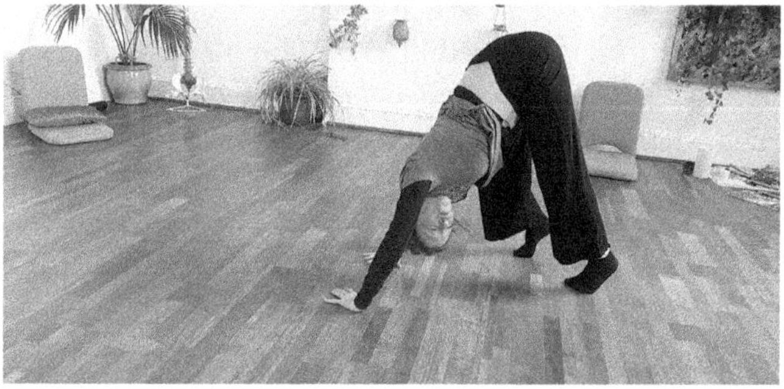

FIGURE 7.22: Amanda Williamson: pushing and pressing. Photographer: Scott Closson.

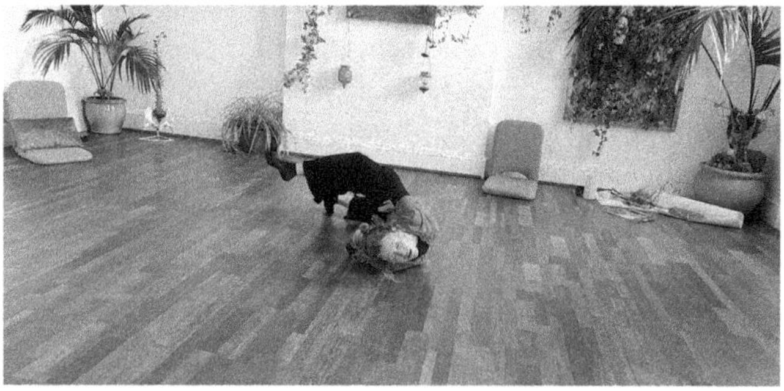

FIGURE 7.23: Amanda Williamson: pushing, surging. Photographer: Scott Closson.

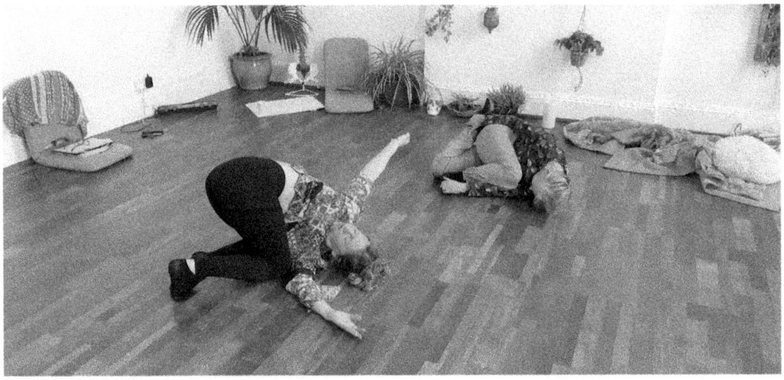

FIGURE 7.24: Amanda Williamson: compressing and decompressing. Photographer: Scott Closson.

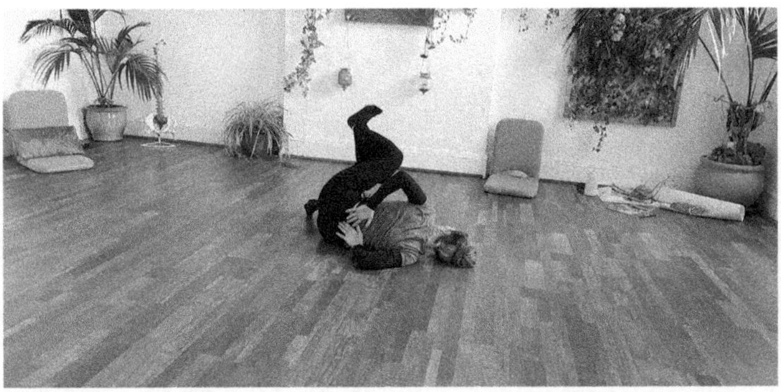

FIGURE 7.25: Amanda Williamson: squeezing and pressing. Photographer: Scott Closson.

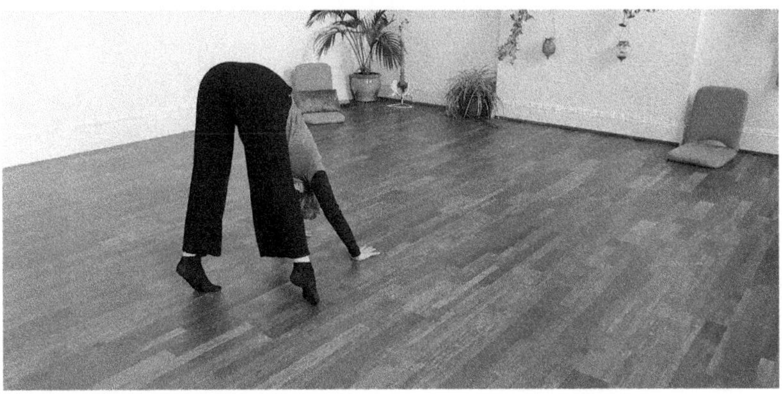

FIGURE 7.26: Amanda Williamson: pushing and strengthening. Photographer: Scott Closson.

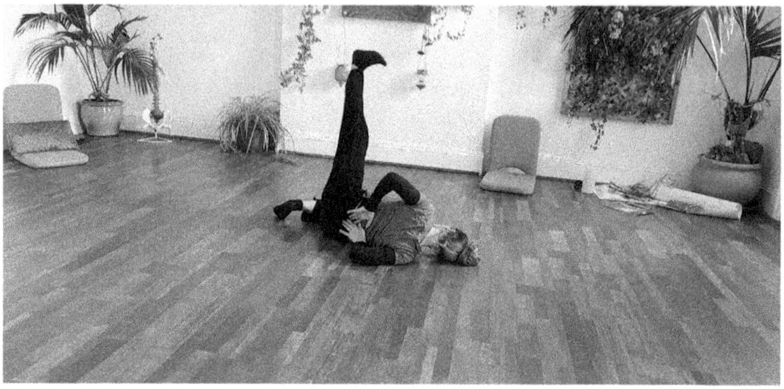

FIGURE 7.27: Amanda Williamson: lengthening and opening and pushing through the heal. Photographer: Scott Closson.

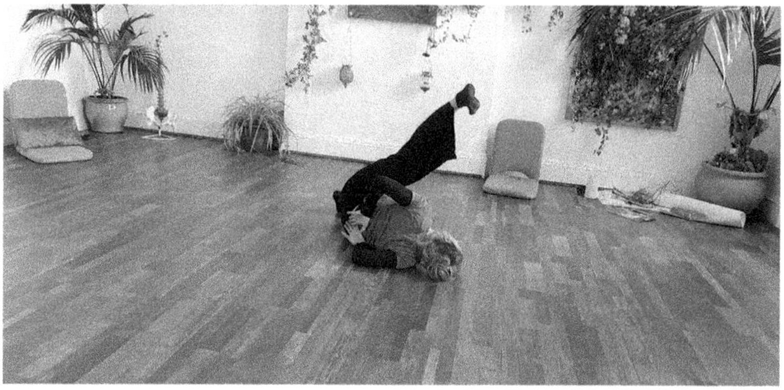

FIGURE 7.28: Amanda Williamson: lengthening and tipping. Photographer: Scott Closson.

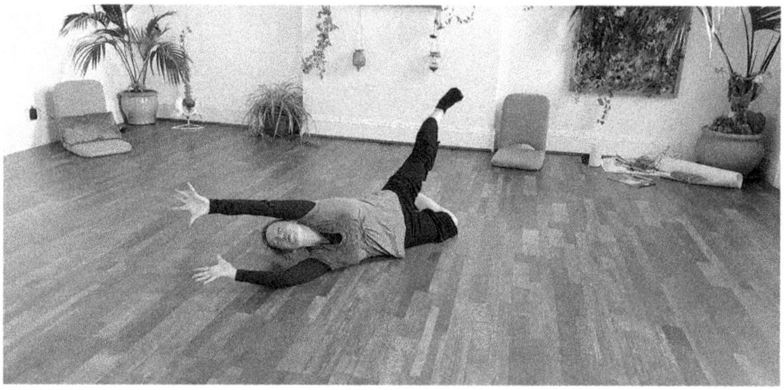

FIGURE 7.29: Amanda Williamson: slow deep sustained stretch. Photographer Scott Closson.

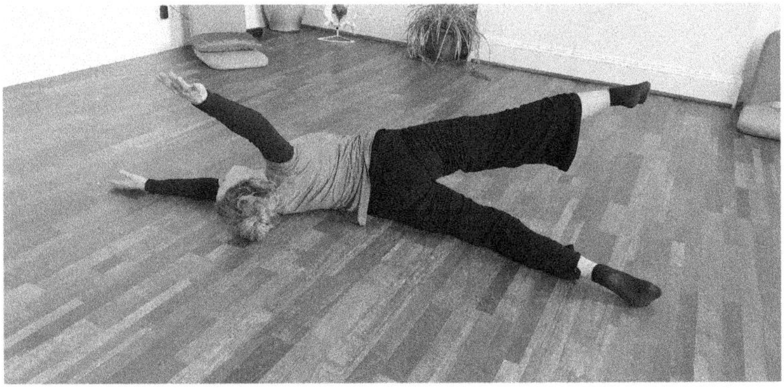

FIGURE 7.30: Amanda Williamson: opening and stretching. Photographer: Scott Closson.

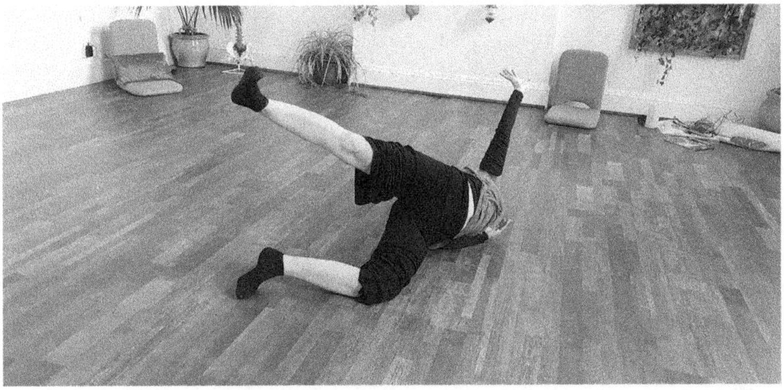

FIGURE 7.31: Amanda Williamson: pressuring, pushing and stretching. Photographer: Scott Closson.

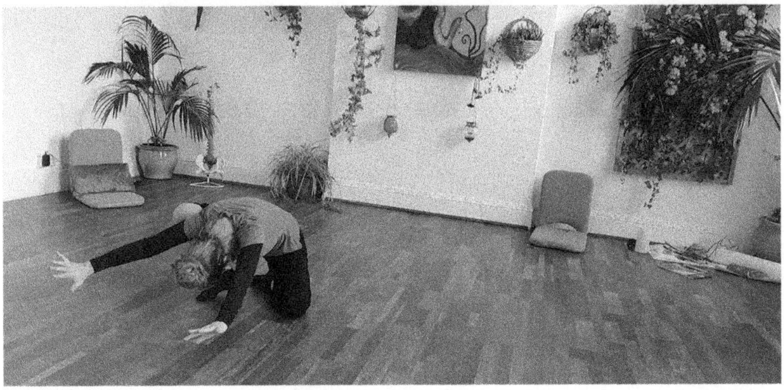

FIGURE 7.32: Amanda Williamson: slow deep strained stretch. Photographer: Scott Closson.

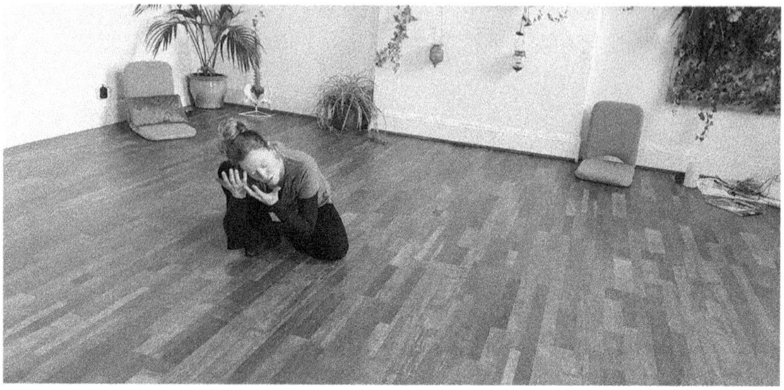

FIGURE 7.33: Amanda Williamson: listening. Photographer: Scott Closson.

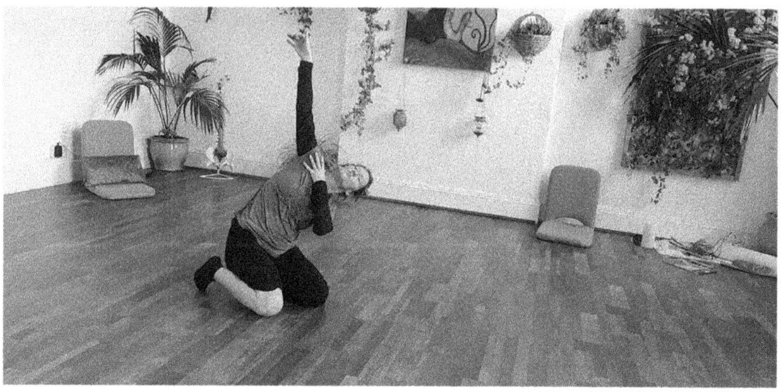

FIGURE 7.34: Amanda Williamson: releasing hyper-tonicity through asymmetric play. Photographer: Scott Closson.

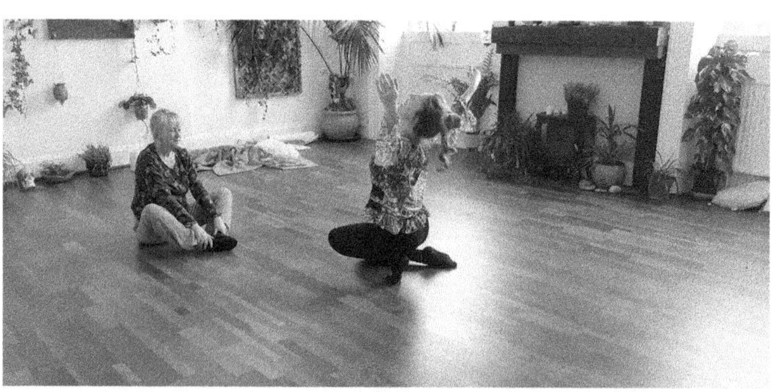

FIGURE 7.35: Karin Rugman and Amanda Williamson: loosening and jiggling. Photographer: Scott Closson.

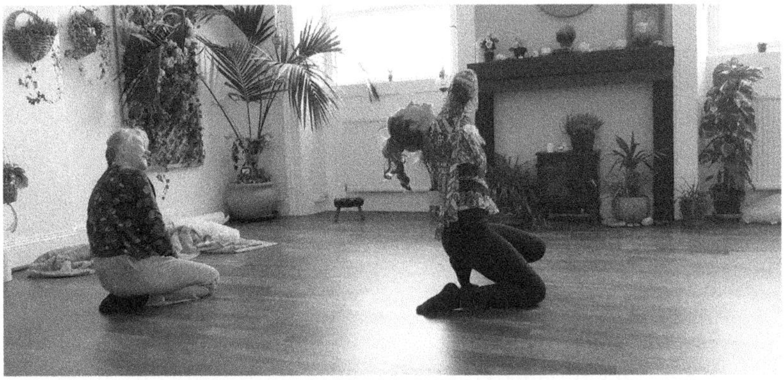

FIGURE 7.36: Karin Rugman and Amanda Williamson: bouncing. Photographer: Scott Closson.

Noted earlier, fascia is subanatomical and transanatomical. Somatic movement dance educators and therapists have an enormous advantage in terms of sensory contact with the fascial web because they invite movement that is omnidirectional and full of volume. We invite the unwinding of fascial restrictions, trigger points or felt tensions from any point of initiation in the body. We do not just focus on the fascia around muscles longitudinally. We initiate and follow the movement from any place within the organism (no matter how unusual). We explore micro-movements, subtle impulses, internal flows and the tiniest tensions felt in the body, undetectable to the outside eye of the therapist, but easily felt by the attuned participant. We invite continuous wave-like rippling movements throughout the organism, which enhances the fluid nature of fascia. Notably, the field is based in movement initiations from very deep fascial systems in the human body. In my case, I spend much time contacting the cranial and spinal dura previously discussed in Chapter 6. Note, this is a hugely different approach from movement systems that simply teach static or sustained stretch. Incredibly effective, is exploring fascial journeys from the surface to the deep internal fascia, and vice versa – moving from the outside in and inside out. In such practices, the subanatomical and transanatomical can be contacted imaginatively and enlivened with omnidirectional awareness.

In the world of fascial therapies, you will come across comments such as this: 'there are two types of stretching which you can use to elongate, hydrate and lubricate your fascia: active stretching (also called dynamic stretching) and static stretching' (Fenster 2020: 62–63). As good as these are, there are in fact many more types of stretching that happen through self-regulatory somatic movement. It is reductive to assume one can only dynamically and statically stretch. Tiny stretches, explored with different energies and qualities are just as important, such as exploring stretching the fingers, or the jaw, the big toes or the eyes, for example. As participants attune to their own tissues, they can sense what needs stretching, and how and where – and with what force, intensity and energy (it is not always the most obvious places that need stretching in the organism).

The soma is thirsty for stretch, but these can be small and gentle, wildly curvaceous, asymmetrical, distorted and spirilloid.

Fascia is a holistic web that connects every part of your body to every other part; thus, 'stretch your leg, and you affect the fascia of your cervical spine' (Fenster 2020: 12–13). Unwind and decompress your feet and you are likely to notice a release right up through the fascial compartments in your legs, the pelvis and back. Somatic movement dance education and therapy is already a post-Cartesian modality that focuses on integration, so exploring the interconnectivity of fascia sits easily with the field's values and pedagogical concepts. Because fascia is one connected organ that is transanatomical, subanatomical and omnidirectional, movement in a localized area can potentially release pain in a distant area of the body. For example, somatic movement work focused on releasing fascial tension in the dural tube, all along the midline from the cranium to the sacrum, might relieve pain in the back and throughout the limbs. Applied pressure and compression in one area, such as the scapular, will create sensations and release in other areas, as the fascial web unwinds, and communicates across its bio-tensile forces. Equally, working globally will affect local areas. It is useful to offer processes that explore how the global influences the local, and how the local affects the global.

Healthy alignment is as much to do with loose gliding slippery fascia, as it is the alignment of bones and muscles. Ida Rolf was well known for describing fascia as an organ of posture (1977). It is not just bones and joints that are involved in posture, but rather the entire fascial net that the bones and organs float in. Your bones would fall into a pile on the floor without the incredible radial and omnidirectional web that gives you volume and tensegrity. Tension in the fascial net caused by dehydration, chronic stress, sympathetic holding and/or a sedentary lifestyle all influence posture and alignment. I offer that spending a great deal of time in gravity helps to remodel the fascia. Not only does this reduce the load placed on the joints (remember the ligaments and tendons are fascia), but the entire skeletal–muscular, nervous and vascular system are enveloped in the fascia (Williamson 2020b). Remodeling the fascial net in gravity is one of the very best ways to undo poor postural habits. People often pull up and stand tall when someone comments on their bad posture as if shoving their head up and shoulders back will resolve bad posture. This is one of the worst responses to the feeling you have bad posture. Pulling yourself up will only add to chronic sympathetic holding, which is likely to be expressed in the fascia through torsions, twists and asymmetries. Fascia needs to be remodelled, released, softened, balanced and the tensional and compressive forces redistributed throughout the fascial net. Working from gravity and then moving through different planes, is one of the best ways to regain good posture. As you soften and release in gravity, sensing your own sensory receptors, slowing-down and inhibiting your motor response, you can choose new fascial pathways of ease and fluency. You can feel where tension is expressed, where trigger points are shouting out (calling for resolution) and where kinks and knots are holding you in a state of pain and discomfort – all affecting your posture.

Spending a great deal of time in gravity, but then inviting participants to move through different planes of action with bio-tensile awareness can relieve strains and knots affecting posture.

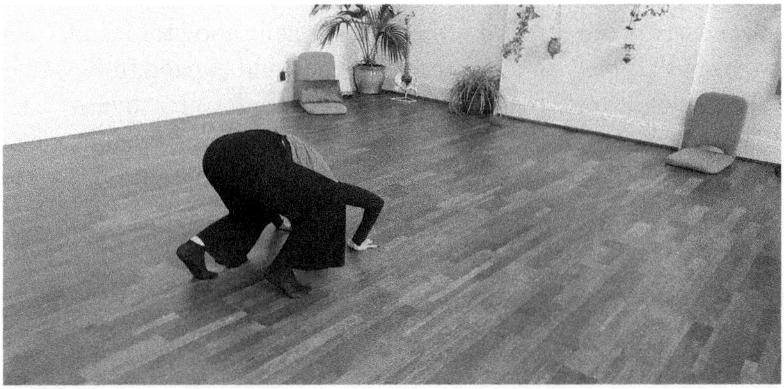

FIGURE 7.37: Amanda Williamson: pushing, pressing, bouncing. Photographer: Scott Closson.

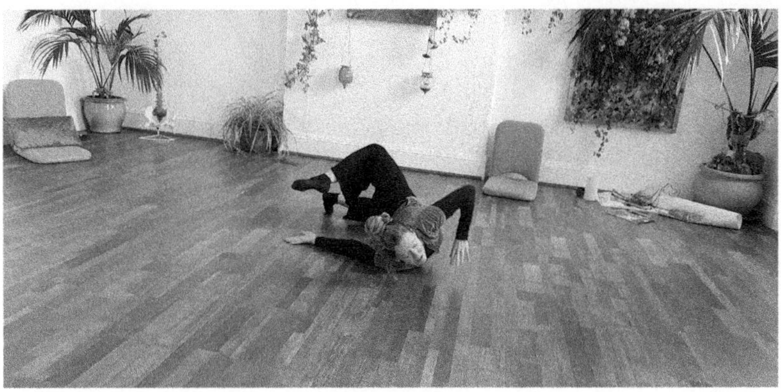

FIGURE 7.38: Amanda Williamson: squeezing and releasing. Photographer: Scott Closson.

Key offerings and learnings

- Rolling in gravity is emblematic of the field: I have come to term this soft-tissue rolling.
- Soft-tissue-rolling and free improvisation underpinned by breath awareness in gravity enhances circulatory flow, releases trigger points and helps adhesions to heal.
- Softening, yielding and melting is good for the fascia. However, it is important to invite participants to explore different pressures, compressions, decompressions, qualities, rhythms, tempos and forces in order to change the viscosity of stuck and tight fascia.
- A combination of shaking, loosening, gliding and sliding, pushing, pressing and pressuring is good for the fascia.
- The balance between rest and activity is especially good for fascia. Craft practices that push, press, pressure, stretch, reach and expand, followed by deep rest. This helps to push toxins out and invites fresh water to move back in.
- The fascial matrix has proprioceptive and interoceptive intelligence: fascial work affects the autonomic nervous system, with different types of pressure inviting the parasympathetic into expression.

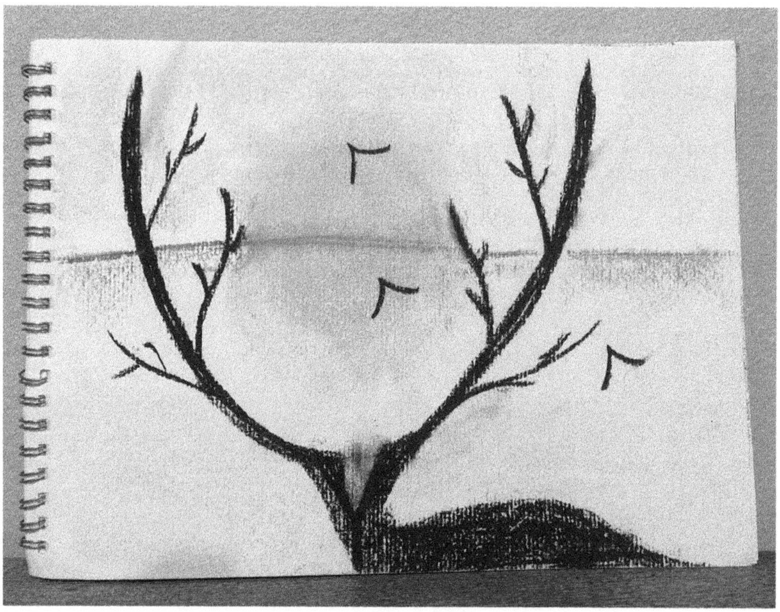

FIGURE 7.39: Mark-making, after moving with awareness of my cranial bones exploration. Photographer, mover, artist: Natasha Martin.

- Fascia holds emotions: thus, working with the fascia, particularly through relational touch and fascial unwinding helps to release emotional holding in the facial matrix.
- Fascia is so deeply interconnected throughout your body that release in one area is likely to support health in other areas.

This way of working has given me a new awareness of my body, the space around me, and a fresh relationship with movement. Being shown how to self-regulate through attuned movement and knowledge of anatomy, has empowered me to take charge of my own well-being. I regularly draw on my experiences from the studio, to find both physical ease and emotional well-being in my day-to-day life. This way of working has transformed my experience of movement into something that is enjoyable, creative, playful and healing. For someone who has a history of chronic illness since childhood, this is a significant shift, and I feel a whole new dimension of physical experience is accessible to me. Had this kind of therapeutic approach been available to me in my youth it would likely have saved me many years of feeling disassociated and avoiding physical activity. I also found being witnessed and held in a safe heart-space incredibly helpful, and the work has given me a tool for expressing and releasing emotion/trauma that needed a non-verbal outlet. I have also learned many things about myself through co-regulation/witnessing others, which was both permissive and humbling. This is not something you have the opportunity to experience very often, and as someone with an over-stimulated awareness of other people's needs, this work has helped me to balance and harness my energy. I feel newly awakened and enlivened. I can draw on this knowledge wherever I am.

(Rebecca Sillence)

Bibliography

Agustoni, D. (2003), *Harmonizing Your Craniosacral System: Self-treatments for Improving Your Health*, Berkeley: North Atlantic Books.

Alberti, F. (2010), *Matters of the Heart: History, Medicine, and Emotion*, Oxford: Oxford University Press.

Alexander, F. Matthias (1932), 'The use of the self', *British Medical Journal*, 1:3728, p. 1149.

Alexander, F. and Coghill, E. (1942), *The Universal Constant in Living*, London: Re-Educational Publications.

Attlee, T. (2012), *Cranio-sacral Integration: Foundation*, London: Singing Dragon.

Avison, J. (2015), *Yoga: Fascia Anatomy and Movement*, East Lothian: Handspring Publishers.

Batson, G. (2014), *Body and Mind in Motion: Dance and Neuroscience in Conversation*, Bristol: Intellect.

Beaulac, A. (2016), *Sitting with Lao-Tzu*, Berekley: Apocryphile Press.

Blum, H. (2015), 'Editorial', *Dance, Movement and Spiritualities*, 2:1, pp. 5–8.

Blum, H. and Williamson, A. (2015), 'Interview with Harrison Blum', *Dance, Movement and Spiritualities*, 2:1, pp. 73–79.

Brodie, J. and Lobel, E. (2012), *Dance and Somatics: Mind-Body Principles of Teaching and Performance*, Jefferson: McFarland & Company.

Cohen, B. (1993), *Sensing, Feeling, and Action: The Experiential Anatomy of Body–Mind Centering*, Northampton: Contact Editions.

Childre, D. and Martin, H. (1999), *The HeartMath Solution*, New York: HarperCollins.

Conrad, E. (2007), *Life on Land: The Story of Continuum*, Berkeley: North Atlantic Books.

Dispenza, J. (2012), *Breaking the Habit of Being Yourself*, London: Hayhouse.

Earls, J. and Myers, T. (2017), *Fascial Release for Structural Balance: Revised Edition*, Berkeley: North Atlantic Books.

Eddy, M. (2009), 'A brief history of somatic practices and dance: Historical development of the field of somatic education and its relationship to dance', *Journal of Dance & Somatic Practices*, 1:1, pp. 13–28.

Eddy, M. (2017), *Mindful Movement: The Evolution of the Somatic Arts and Conscious Action*, Bristol: Intellect.

Feldenkrais, M. (1977), *Awareness through Movement: Easy-to-do Health Exercises to Improve Your Posture, Vision, Imagination, and Personal Awareness*, New York: HarperCollins.

Fortin, F., Gomez, N., Joly, Y., Rabin, L., Rouquet, O. and Smith, L. (2014), 'Conversations about the somatic basis of spiritual experience', in A. Williamson, G. Batson, S. Whatley and R. Weber (eds), *Dance, Somatics and Spiritualities: Contemporary Sacred Narratives*, Bristol: Intellect, pp. 261–82.

Fraleigh, S. (2014), 'Permissions and the making of consciousness', in A. Williamson, G. Batson, S. Whatley and R. Weber (eds), *Dance, Somatics and Spiritualities: Contemporary Sacred Narratives*, Bristol: Intellect, pp. 239–260.

Fraleigh, S. (2015), 'Attunement and evanescence', *Dance, Movement and Spiritualities*, 2:1, pp. 9–25.

Fraleigh, S. (2018), *Back to the Dance Itself: Phenomenologies of the Body in Performance*, Illinois: University of Illinois Press.

Fraleigh, S. (2020), 'Attunement and evanescence', in A. Williamson and B. Sellers-Young (eds), *Spiritual Herstories: Call of the Soul in Dance Research*, Bristol: Intellect, pp. 35–68.

Fraleigh, S. (2025), *Moving Consciously: Somatic Transformations through Dance, Yoga, and Touch*, Illinois: University of Illinois Press.

Francis, R. (2020), *The Un-tapped Vagus Nerve: Self-Healing exercises and Techniques*, Torrazza Piemonte: Amazon Italia Logistic.

Fortin, S. (2014), 'Conversations about the somatic basis of spiritual experiences', in A. Williamson, G. Batson, S. Whatley and R. Weber (eds), *Dance, Somatics and Spiritualities: Contemporary Sacred Narratives*, Bristol: Intellect, pp. 261–82.

Fenster, D. (2020), *Free Your Fascia: Relieve Pain, Boost Your Energy, Ease Anxiety and Depression, Lower Blood Pressure and Melt Years off Your Body with Fascia Therapy*, London: Hay House Publishers.

Frederick, F. (2005), *The Alchemy of Touch: Moving Towards Mastery through the Lens of Zeo Balancing*, n.p.: Complementary Medicine Press.

Fuller, D. (2012), *Osteopathy and Swedenborg: The Influence of Emanuel Swedenborg on the Genesis and Development of Osteopathy, Specifically on Andrew Taylor Still and William Garner Sutherland*, Pennsylvania: Swedenborg Scientific Press.

Gintis, B. (2007), *Engaging the Movement of Life: Exploring Health and Embodiment through Osteopathy and Continuum*, Berkeley: North Atlantic Books.

Goleman, D. and Davidson, R. (2017), *The Science of Meditation: How to Change Your Brain, Mind and Body*, Milton Keynes: Random House.

Hackey, P. (2002), *Making Connections: Total Body Integration through Bartenieff Fundamentals*, New York: Routledge.

Halprin, D. (2002), *The Expressive Body in Life, Art, and Therapy: Working with Movement, Metaphor and Meaning*, London: Jessica Kingsley Publishers.

Halprin, A. and Kaplan, R. (2015), *Moving Toward Life: Five Decades of Transformational Dance*, Middletown: Wesleyan University Press.

Hanna, T. (1980), *Somatic: Reawakening the Mind's Control of Movement, Flexibility, and Health*, Cambridge: Da Capo Press.

Hanna, T. ([1993] 1979), *The Body of Life: Creating New Pathways for Sensory Awareness and Fluid Movement*, New York: Healing Arts Press.

Hannah, B. (2013), *Encounters with the Soul: Active Imagination as Developed by C.G. Jung*, Wilmette: Chiron Publications.

Haplrin, D. (2014), 'Body ensouled, enacted and entranced: Movement/dance as transformative art', in A. Williamson, G. Batson, S. Whatley and R. Weber (eds), *Dance, Somatics and Spiritualities: Contemporary Sacred Narratives*, Bristol: Intellect, pp. 87–114.

Hartley, L. (1995), *Wisdom of the Body Moving: An Introduction to Body–Mind Centering*, Berekley: North Alantic Books.

Hartley, L. (2014), 'Embodiment of spirit: From embryology to authentic movement as embodied relational spiritual practice', in A. Williamson, G. Batson, S. Whatley and R. Weber (eds), *Dance, Somatics and Spiritualities: Contemporary Sacred Narratives*, Bristol: Intellect, pp. 11–33.

Hartley, L. (2020), 'Women, body, earth and spirit: Journeys of descent through myth, embodiment and movement practice', in A. Williamson and B. Sellers-Young (eds), *Spiritual Herstories: Call of the Soul in Dance Research*, Bristol: Intellect, pp. 35–68.

Hayes, J. (2007), *Performing the Dreams of your Body: Plays of Animation and Compassion*, Chichester: Archive Publishing.

Hayes, J. (2013), *Soul and Spirit in Dance Movement Psychotherapy*, London: Jessica Kingsley Publishers.

Hayes, J. (2014), 'Dancing in the spirit of Sophia', in A. Williamson, G. Batson, S. Whatley and R. Weber (eds), *Dance, Somatics and Spiritualities: Contemporary Sacred Narratives*, Bristol: Intellect, pp. 61–86.

Haze, N. and Stomstead, T. (1999), 'An interview with Janet Adler', in P. Pallaro (eds), *Authentic Movement: Essays by Mary Starks Whitehouse, Janet Adler and Joan Chodorow*, London: Jessica Kingsley, pp. 107–120.

Hinton, L. (2020), *The Secrets of the Vagus Nerve Stimulation*, Great Briton: Amazon.

Johnson, D. (1987), 'Body work and being: The deeper significance of somatics', *New Realities*, pp. 20–23.

Johnson, D. (1992), *Body: Recovering Our Sensual Wisdom*, Berkeley: North Atlantic Books.

Johnson, D. (1994), *Body, Spirit, and Democracy*, Berkeley: North Atlantic Books.

Johnson, D. (1995), *Bone, Breath & Gesture: Practices of Embodiment*, Berkeley: North Atlantic Book.

Johnson, D. (1997), *Groundworks: Narratives of Embodiment*, Berkeley: North Atlantic Books.

Johnson, D. (1998), *The Body in Psychotherapy: Inquiries in Somatic Psychology*, Berkeley: North Atlantic Books.

Johnson, D. (2006), *Everyday Hopes, Utopian Dreams: Reflections on American Culture*, Berkeley: North Atlantic Books.

Johnson, D. (2008), *The Meaning of Life in the 21st Century: Tensions Among Science, Religion, and Experience*, Berkeley: North Atlantic Books.

Johnson, D. (2014), 'Preface', in A. Williamson, G. Batson, S. Whatley and R. Weber (eds), *Dance, Somatics and Spiritualities: Contemporary Sacred Narratives*, Bristol: Intellect, pp. x–xxi.

Johnson, D. (2018), *Diverse Bodies, Diverse Practices: Toward an Inclusive Somatics*, Berkeley: North Atlantic Books.

Johnson, H. (1977), *The Protean Body*, New York: Harper and Row.

Juhan, D. (2002), *The Physical and Psychological, and Spiritual Powers of Bodywork: Touched by the Goddess*, New York: Station Hill Press.

Juhan, D. (2003), *A Handbook for BodyWork: Job's Body*, New York: Stanton Hill Press.

Jung, C. ([1933] 2002), *Modern Man and His Symbols*, London: Routledge.

Jung, C. ([1969] 2003), *On the Nature of the Psyche*, London: Routledge.

Jung, C. ([1972] 2003), *Four Archetypes*, London: Routledge.

Kittikong, T. (2015), 'Choreographing the site of impermanence: Performing body with Buddhist philosophy and meditation in movement based performance', *Dance, Movement and Spiritualities*, 2:1, pp. 52–72.

Kieft, E. (2020), 'Soul loss and retrieval: Restoring wholeness through dance', in A. Williamson and B. Sellers-Young (eds), *Spiritual Herstories: Call of the Soul in Dance Research*, Bristol: Intellect, pp. 180–206.

Leaf, C. (2021), *Cleaning up Your Mental Mess: 5 Scientifically Proved Steps to Reduce Anxiety, Stress and Toxic Thinking*, Grand Rapids: Backers Publishing.

Levine, P. (2008), *Healing Trauma: A Pioneering Program for Restoring the Wisdom of Your Body*, Canada: SoundsTrue.

Lipton, B. (2015), *The Biology of Belief, Unleashing the Power of Consciousness, Matter & Miracles*, London: HayHouse.

McHose, C. and Frank, K. (2006), *How Life Moves: Explorations in Meaning and Body Awareness*, California: North Atlantic Books.

McNiff, S. (1998), *Trust the Process*, Boston: Shambhala Publications.

McNiff, S. (2000), *Art-based Research*, London: Jessica Kingsley.

McNiff, S. (2015), *Imagination in Action: Secrets for Unleashing Creative Expression*, Boston: Shambhala Publications.

Myers, T. (2014), *Anatomy Trains: Myofascial Meridians for Manual & Movement Therapists*, n.p.: Churchill & Livingstone Elsevier.

Nagy, M. (1991), *Philosophical Issues in the Psychology of C. G. Jung*, Albany: University of New York Press.

Olsen, A. (2002), *Body and Earth: An Experiential Guide*, Middlebury: Middlebury College Press.

Olsen, A. and McHose, C. (1998), *Bodystories: A Guide to Experiential Anatomy*, Lebanon: University Press of New England.

Pallant, C. (2006), *Contact Improvisation: An Introduction to a Vitalizing Dance Form*, Jefferson: McFarland & Company.

Papadopoulos, R. (ed.) (1992), *Carl Gustav Jung: Critical Assessments*, London: Routledge.

Pert, C. (1997), *Molecules of Emotion*, London: Simon & Schuster.

Porges, S. (2017), *The Pocket Guide to PolyVagal Theory: The Transformative Power of Feeling Safe*, New York: W.W.Norton & Company.

Power, K. (2020), *How to Hack Your Vagus Nerve*, UK: Amazon.

Reed, S. (2020), 'Awakening the spirit through dance, somatics and Scaravelli Yoga', in A. Williamson and B. Sellers-Young (eds), *Spiritual Herstories: Call of the Soul in Dance Research*, Bristol: Intellect, pp. 478–503.

Richard, F. (2020), *The Un-tapped Vagus Nerve: Self-healing Techniques*, Torrazza: Amazon.

Rifkin, B., Ackerman, M. and Folkenberg, J. (2006), *Human Anatomy: The Visual History from the Renaissance to the Digital Age*, New York: Abrams.

Rivers, J. (2020), *Taoism for Beginners: Understand and Apply the Principles and Practices*, UK: Amazon.

Rolf, I. (1977), *Rolfing: The Integration of Human Structures*, Santa Monica: Dennis Landman.

Rosenburg, S. (2017), *Accessing the Healing Power of The Vagus Nerve: Self-help Exercises for Anxiety, Depression, Trauma, and Autism*, Berkeley: North Atlantic Books.

Schleip, R. (2003a), 'Fascial plasticity: A new neurobiological explanation. Part 1', *Journal of Movement & Bodywork Therapies*, 7:1, pp. 11–19.

Schleip, R. (2003b), 'Fascial plasticity: A new neurobiological explanation. Part 2', *Journal of Movement & Bodywork Therapies*, 7:2, pp. 104–16.

Schleip, R. (2017), *Fascial Fitness: How to Be Resilient, Elegant and Dynamic in Everyday Life and Sport*, Chichester: Riva Verlag.

Shea, M. (2010), *Biodynamic Craniosacral Therapy: Volume Three*, Berkeley: North Atlantic Books.

Shea, M. (2016), *Biodynamic Craniosacral Therapy: The Heart of Practice*, Torrazza Piemonte: Amazon Italia.

Smith, F. (2005), *The Alchemy of Touch: Moving Towards Mastery through the Lens of Zero Balancing*, Taos: Complementary Medicine Books.

Snowden, R. (2006), *Jung: Key Ideas: From Analytic Psychology and Dreams to the Collective Unconscious and More*, London: Hodder and Stoughton.

Stevens, A. (1994), *Jung a Very Short Introduction*, New York: Oxford University Press.

Still, A. (2013), *The Philosophy and Mechanical Principles of Osteopathy*, London: Pantianos Classics.

Still, A. (2017), *Osteopathy, Research and Practice*, London: Pantianos Classics.

Stromsted, T. (2014), 'The alchemy of authentic movement: Awakening spirit in body', in A. Williamson, G. Batson, S. Whatley and R. Weber (eds), *Dance, Somatics and Spiritualities: Contemporary Sacred Narratives*, Bristol: Intellect, pp. 35–60.

Sumner, G. and Haines, S. (2010), *Cranial Intelligence: A Practical Guide to Biodynamic Craniosacral Therapy*, London: Singing Dragon.

Sutherland, W. (1990), *Teachings in the Science of Osteopathy*, London: Cranial Teaching Foundation.

Todres, T. (2007), *Embodied Enquiry: Phenomenological Touchstones for Research, Psychotherapy and Spirituality*, London: Springer Publications.

Tolle, E. (1997), *The Power of Now: A Guide to Spiritual Enlightenment*, London: Hodder & Stroughton.

Tuhovsky, I. (2017), *Zen: Happy, Focused and Peaceful Lifestyle Forever*, UK: Amazon.

Upledger, J. (1997a), *Your Inner Physician and You*, Berkeley: North Atlantic Book.

Upledger, J. (1997b), *Your Inner Physician: CranioSacral Therapy and SomatoEmotional Release*, Berkeley: North Atlantic Books.

Upledger, J. (2001), *CranioSacral Therapy: Touchstone for Natural Healing*, Berkeley: North Atlantic Books.

Upledger, J. (2008), *CranioSacral Therapy: What It Is: How It Works*, Berkeley: North Atlantic Book.

Warren, S. (2019), *The Pain Relief Secret: How to Retain Your Nervous System: Heal Your Body, and Overcome Chronic* Pain, n.p.: TCK Publishing.

Webster, S. and Wreede, R. (2016), *Embryology at a Glance: Second Edition*, Chichester: John Wiley & Sons.

Whatley, S., Garrett Brown, N. and Alexander, K. (2015), *Attending to Movement: Somatic Perspectives on Living in This World*, Axmister: Triachary Press.

Whitehouse, M. (1999a), 'Physical movement and personality', in P. Pallaro (eds), *Authentic Movement: Essays by Mary Starks Whitehouse, Janet Adler and Joan Chodorow*, London: Jessica Kingsley, pp. 51–57.

Whitehouse, M. (1999b), 'Reflections on a metamorphosis', in P. Pallaro (eds), *Authentic Movement: Essays by Mary Starks Whitehouse, Janet Adler and Joan Chodorow*, London: Jessica Kingsley, pp. 58–62.

Whitehouse, M. (1999c), 'The transference and dance therapy', in P. Pallaro (eds), *Authentic Movement: Essays by Mary Starks Whitehouse, Janet Adler and Joan Chodorow*, London: Jessica Kingsley, pp. 63–72.

Whitehouse, M. (1999d), 'C.G. Jung and dance therapy', in P. Pallaro (eds), *Authentic Movement: Essays by Mary Starks Whitehouse, Janet Adler and Joan Chodorow*, London: Jessica Kingsley, pp. 73–101.

Wilber, K. (2000), *Integrated Psychology: Consciousness, Psychology, Therapy*, Boulder: Shambhala Press.

Williamson, A. (2009), 'Formative support and connection: Somatic movement dance education in community and client practice', *Journal of Dance & Somatic Practices*, 1:1, pp. 29–45.

Williamson, A. (2010), 'Reflections and theoretical approaches to the study of spiritualities within the field of somatic movement dance education', *Journal of Dance & Somatic Practices*, 2:1, pp. 35–61.

Williamson, A. (2014), 'Professorial reflections: Carla Walter interviewed by Amanda Williamson', *Dance, Movement & Spiritualities*, 1:3, pp. 451–49.

Williamson, A. (2015a), 'Somatically inspired movement and prepatriarchal religious symbolism', *Dance, Movement & Spiritualities*, 2:3, pp. 323–55.

Williamson, A. (2015b), 'Editorial and some personal weaves on existential limitations and articular freedoms', *Dance, Movement & Spiritualities*, 2:2, pp. 93–117.

Williamson, A. (2015c), 'On dance and phenomenology: An essay interview with Professor Sondra Fraleigh', *Dance, Movement & Spiritualities*, 2:2, pp. 199–217.

Williamson, A. (2015d), 'Interview with Harrison Blum', *Dance, Movement & Spiritualities*, 2:1, pp. 73–79.

Williamson, A. (2016a), 'A few weaves on suffering and existential phenomenology', *Journal of Dance, Movement and Spiritualities'*, 4:2, pp. 345–90.

Williamson, A. (2016b), 'Reflections on applied existential phenomenology to spirituality in somatics movement education and therapy', *Journal of Dance and Somatic Practices*, 8.4, pp. 589–638.

Williamson, A. (2016c), 'Reflections on existential phenomenology, spirituality, dance and movement-based Somatics', *Journal of Dance & Somatic Practices*, 8:2, pp. 273–99.

Williamson, A. (2018), 'Falling in love with language', in S. Fraleigh (ed.), *Back to the Dance Itself: Phenomenologies of the Body in Performance*, Illinois: University of Illinois Press, pp. 301–47.

Williamson, Amanda (2020a), 'Bio-somatic dance movement naturotherapy: The occiput, scapulae and sacrum – Fulcrums of support and reorganization', *Dance, Movement & Spiritualities*, 6:1&2, pp. 49–85.

Williamson, Amanda (2020b), 'Post-Newtonian anatomy and physiology: The gravitational and parasympathetic experience in bio-somatic dance movement naturotherapy', *Dance, Movement & Spiritualities*, 6:1&2, pp. 171–98.

Williamson, Amanda (2020c), 'Sympathetic holding and parasympathetic release: Vagal tone and beta, alpha and theta in bio-somatic dance movement naturotherapy', *Dance, Movement & Spiritualities*, 6:1&2, pp. 199–229.

Williamson, Amanda (2020d), 'Sensing her: Matrifocal symbolism in the field of somatic movement dance education and therapy', in A. Williamson and B. Sellers-Young (eds), *Spiritual Herstories: Call of the Soul in Dance Research*, Bristol: Intellect, pp. 132–79.

Williamson, Amanda (2020e), 'Your feet and my hands – Fulcrums of support and reorganization: Bio-somatic dance movement naturotherapy', *Dance, Movement & Spiritualities*, 7:1&2, pp. 139–63.

Williamson, A. and Eddy, M. (2014), 'Reflections on the spiritual dimensions of somatic movement education', *Journal of Dance & Somatic Practices*, 2.1, pp. 35–61.

Williamson, A. and Hayes, J. (2012a), 'Dance, movement and spiritualities', *Journal of Dance and Somatic Practices*, 4:1, pp. 10–31.

Williamson, A. and Hayes, J. (2012b), 'Editorial: Dance, movement and spiritualities', *Journal of Dance & Somatic Practices*, 4:1, pp. 3–9.

Williamson, A. and Hayes, J. (2014), 'Dancing the sacred in secular higher education contexts', *Dance, Movement & Spiritualities*, 1:1, pp. 11–20.

Williamson, A. and Sellers-Young, B. (2020d), *Spiritual Herstories: Call of the Soul in Dance Research*, Bristol: Intellect.

Williamson, A., Batson, G., Whatley, S. and Weber, R. (2014a), *Dance, Somatics and Spiritualities: Contemporary Sacred Narratives*, Bristol: Intellect.

Williamson, A., Batson, G., Whatley, S. and Weber, R. (2014b), 'Introduction', in A. Williamson, G. Batson, S. Whatley and R. Weber (eds), *Dance, Somatics and Spiritualities: Contemporary Sacred Narratives*, Bristol: Intellect, pp. xxvi–xxxiii.

Williamson, A., Batson, G., Whatley, S. and Weber, R. (2014c), 'Part 1', in A. Williamson, G. Batson, S. Whatley and R. Weber (eds), *Dance, Somatics and Spiritualities: Contemporary Sacred Narratives*, Bristol: Intellect, pp. 1–9.

www.ingramcontent.com/pod-product-compliance
Ingram Content Group UK Ltd.
Pitfield, Milton Keynes, MK11 3LW, UK
UKHW051043120926
8556IPUK00031B/862

9 781789 386905